OPTIONS
THE ALTERNATIVE CANCER THERAPY BOOK

Richard Walters

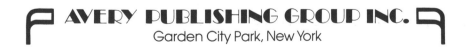

AVERY PUBLISHING GROUP INC.
Garden City Park, New York

The author and publisher do not advocate the use of any particular form of health care but believe that the information presented in this book should be available to the public. This book is not intended to replace the advice and treatment of a physician. Any use of the information set forth herein is entirely at the reader's discretion.

Because there is always some risk involved, the author and publisher are not responsible for any adverse effects or consequences resulting from the use of any of the preparations or procedures described in this book. Please do not use this book if you are unwilling to assume the risk. Each person and situation are unique, and a physician or other qualified health professional should be consulted when there is any question regarding the presence or treatment of any abnormal health condition. It is a sign of wisdom, not cowardice, to seek a second or third opinion.

In-House Editor: Elaine Will Sparber
Typesetters: Bonnie Freid and Antoinette Mason

The material on pages 368–376 is used with the permission of Patrick McGrady, Jr., © 1992 by Patrick McGrady, Jr.

The material on pages 377–379 is used with the permission of Catherine J. Frompovich. It is from the brochure "Proposed Amendment XXVII to U.S. Constitution, the Healthcare Rights Amendment," © 1990 by Catherine Frompovich.

Library of Congress Cataloging-in-Publication Data
Walters, Richard, 1947–
    Options : the alternative cancer therapy book / Richard Walters.
        p.   cm.
    Includes bibliographical references and index.
    ISBN 0-89529-510-5
    1. Cancer—Alternative treatment.   I. Title.
    [DNLM: 1. Alternative Medicine. 2. Neoplasms—therapy.   QZ266 W235a]
    RC271.A62W35   1992
    616.99'406—dc20
    DLC
    for Library of Congress   92-49901
                                                                CIP

Printed in the United States of America by Paragon Press, Honesdale, PA.

10   9   8   7

CONTENTS

ACKNOWLEDGMENTS

Many people read portions of the text or the complete manuscript and offered valuable comments and suggestions. Any remaining errors, of course, are solely my responsibility. I would especially like to thank the following individuals: Elaine Alexander; Steve Austin, N.D.; Robert O. Becker, M.D.; Abram Ber, M.D.; Christopher Bird; Gerard Bodecker, Ed.D.; Lawrence Burton, Ph.D.; Stanislaw Burzynski, M.D.; Brian Clement; Marcus A. Cohen; Michael Culbert, D.Sc.; Erik Enby, M.D.; Charles Farr, M.D.; Richard D. Fischer, D.D.S., F.A.G.D.; David Frawley, O.M.D.; Gary Glum, D.C.; Joseph Gold, M.D.; Nicholas Gonzalez, M.D.; Alex Jack; Roger Jahnke, O.M.D.; David Kingsley; Jim Lake; Ed McCabe; Gaston Naessens; Ingrid Naiman; Hans Nieper, M.D.; William Philpott, M.D.; Paul W. Scharff, M.D.; Hari Sharma, M.D.; David A. Steenblock, D.O.; G. G. Strating-IJben; Gerard Sunnen, M.D.; Le Trombetta; Dana Ullman; Vivian Virginia Vetrano, D.C., M.D.; Julie Anne Wagner; Morton Walker, D.P.M.; Patricia Spain Ward; Tim Wead; Ann Wigmore; Julian Winston; and Ralph S. Wolfstein, M.D. Special thanks also to Rudy Shur and Elaine Will Sparber of Avery Publishing Group for their invaluable assistance and suggestions.

PREFACE

This book serves a twofold purpose. First, it is a practical guide for cancer patients who are interested in exploring alternative therapies that may be used instead of, or as a complement to, conventional treatment. Second, for the general reader curious about why there has been so little progress in the "war on cancer," it examines the political forces that have worked to actively block or suppress so many promising nontoxic, noninvasive cancer therapies. If the book helps to save lives, and also generates momentum for drastic, long-overdue reforms in cancer treatment and research, it will have accomplished its purpose.

Many cancer patients who recovered using alternative therapies share their inspirational stories in these pages. Most of these people had been written off as "hopeless" or "terminal" by their orthodox doctors, but they sought out alternative treatment, followed it, and got well. Their moving stories, while not intended as endorsements for any particular therapies, do illustrate how specific therapies work and may give hope and strength to readers.

There is currently no book available that takes a comprehensive, unbiased look at the full range of alternative cancer therapies. *Options* is intended to fill that gap. For each therapy, it explains in clear language the underlying rationale, proposed mechanism of action, supportive evidence, and what patients can expect in the course of treatment. An effort has been made to evaluate the strengths and weaknesses of the therapies whenever possible. Some new findings and statistics are presented that may upset both supporters and detractors of alternative cancer therapies. Only those therapies that have shown some degree of efficacy and that have reputable physicians or researchers behind them have been included.

The plan of the book is as follows. Chapter 1 attempts to dispel the most common myths and stereotypes surrounding alternative cancer therapies. Chapters 2 through 29 are devoted to specific therapies: biologic, nontoxic pharmacologic, immune, herbal, nutritional, metabolic, and adjunctive treatments; energy medicine; and mind-body approaches. There is some overlap between these categories; most therapies do not fit into neat, tight compartments. Each therapy chapter includes a Resources section at the end. Two methods that have received some sanction from official medicine—hyperthermia and hydrazine sulfate—are included because they are not well-known. Chapters also cover homeopathy, Indian Ayurvedic medicine, and Chinese medicine, systems that are followed by a large segment of humanity and deserve to be better known. The Conclusion focuses on the politics of cancer and discusses pressing issues of patient empowerment. The appendices list further information resources and present documents that could be instrumental in securing rights for the cancer patient, and for all patients.

Cancer is this century's Black Plague. At least one in three Americans will develop cancer; of those, roughly two-thirds will die within five years. The number of Americans with cancer will *double* in the 1990s, and by the year 2000, cancer will surpass heart disease as the nation's leading cause of death, according to *MediTrends 1991–1992,* a report by the American Hospital Association. (The report can be ordered by calling 800-AHA-2626.) To end this epidemic, scientists and researchers should be making every effort to impartially explore innovative treatment approaches, even those that fall outside of orthodox medicine. Unfortunately, this is not happening. On the contrary, promising alternative therapies have been thwarted or destroyed by a medical establishment that seems more interested in preserving its vested interests.

This book is not intended to replace the advice or treatment of a physician. It offers a critical examination of orthodox, alternative, and potential cancer therapies. The author is not a physician, though nearly every chapter has been read by one or more physicians for accuracy. No statement included in this book should be taken as medical advice. The author and publisher assume no responsibility for any decision made by the reader regarding treatment.

Note: This book cites a number of clinical (human) and animal studies that were done in support of alternative cancer therapies. The animal experiments are part of the scientific record. However, the author in no way endorses laboratory animal experiments or condones arrogance, lack of compassion, or torture of fellow creatures by researchers. Animal experiments waste time and lives and have been shown to be of dubious or negative benefit to science. Carefully controlled clinical, epidemiological, and other human-based studies are the best means of investigating the treatment and prevention of human illness. There are many sophisticated nonanimal research methods that can be used in the development of treatments for cancer patients. Former American Cancer Society President Dr. Marvin Pollard, interviewed on the television science show *Walter Cronkite's Universe* on August 24, 1982, acknowledged the problems with animal studies: "My own belief is that we have relied too heavily upon animal testing, and we believed it too strongly. Now, I think we're commencing to realize that what goes on in an animal may not necessarily be applicable to humans." Persons interested in more information on this important issue should contact People for the Ethical Treatment of Animals (PETA) at P.O. Box 42516, Washington, DC 20015, 301-770-PETA, for a detailed information packet.

GUIDELINES FOR CHOOSING A THERAPY

A bewildering variety of options confronts the person trying to choose a therapy as an alternative or complement to conventional cancer treatment. A patient may despair of understanding the array of choices. You may feel like simply entrusting your life to the doctor, which seems the easiest way. But if you want to take an active part in your recovery, you should take the time to learn about all treatment possibilities, conventional and alternative, in order to make an informed personal choice.

A good place to begin is by evaluating the conventional treatments. One or more of them may offer high rates of remission and long-term survival for the kind of cancer you have. Even if you are oriented toward the alternative therapies, you owe it to yourself to learn what the conventional therapies have to offer. Find out as much as you can about your type of cancer. Don't be intimidated by your doctor. Ask tough questions.

Approach *all* therapies—conventional and alternative—with healthy skepticism and suspicion. You should regard all cure and remission rates with caution. The cancer cure rates promoted by the American Cancer Society and the National Cancer Institute are suspect for a number of reasons. For one thing, these rates represent people who are alive five years after diagnosis. But about half of all cancer patients die between their fifth and tenth year after diagnosis. Also, the official cancer statistics come mainly from a small handful of cancer hospitals where patients receive the best technological care available. At some poorer hospitals, cancer death rates are twice as high. Orthodox medicine uses a number of other devices to sugar-coat or inflate cancer statistics. And there are many alternative practitioners who fabricate their statistics.

Find out exactly what the doctor—any doctor—means by "response." Conventional as well as unorthodox practitioners frequently mislead patients by referring to, say, an "80 percent response rate." Pin down whether this is supposed to mean short-term improvement, long-term survival, reduced pain, enhanced well-being, or something else.

Get a second or third opinion. While it is rare for an oncologist to call cells cancerous when they are not, a misdiagnosis in which one type of cancer is mistaken for another is more common than one might assume. Getting more than one opinion not only enables you to verify the type and stage of cancer, it may also bring to light different treatment paths. Even within orthodox medicine, there is an enormous range of approaches to treating the same form of cancer. A second opinion often generates a second, completely different treatment strategy, with each doctor arguing eloquently for his or her proposed course of action. The ultimate decision, of course, rests with you.

Don't be pushed. Too often, patients are rushed into treatment immediately after diagnosis. They are led to believe that any delay will have dire consequences. Patients are rarely informed of the value of a second opinion and are seldom encouraged to explore complementary, let alone alternative, therapies. In a state of shock from a diagnosis of cancer, many patients go along with whatever the doctor tells them without making a genuinely informed personal choice. True, in rare instances, there may be a need for immediate action—for example, a lung mass is hampering breathing, a tumor is obstructing the bowel or causing significant bleeding, the blood count of a patient with acute leukemia is rising every few hours. But for most people, there is time to get a second opinion and weigh all the options.

If conventional treatment does not offer the methods or long-term survival results you want, then consider alternative treatment. Your regular doctor may not be very helpful in this regard. Most, but not all, oncologists still dismiss alternative therapies as "worthless quackery." If you broach the subject with them, they may treat you with derisive contempt and anger, as if you have lost your senses. Even the idea of complementing your orthodox treatment with nutrition and immune-enhancing supplements may be mocked by close-minded physicians. Not all doctors will react this way, however. In one study, published in the July 1984 issue of *Annals of Internal Medicine,* 30 percent of cancer patients' conventional doctors *supported* the use of alternative treatments.

The chances are that your oncologist will not be very knowledgeable about nonorthodox therapies. Fortunately, there are educational organizations and patient referral services for people who wish to explore these therapeutic options (see page xv). This book, too, is a good starting point. Talking with survivors who had the same type of cancer as you may instill confidence and inspiration. It will also help you to learn more about the doctors whose services you are considering. The names and phone numbers of patients who recovered through alternative therapies are available from a number of the organizations listed in the following pages and also from some clinics. These people will gladly share their experiences with you.

Just because an alternative therapy is nontoxic and noninvasive doesn't mean it will work. You'll want to ask a lot of focused questions when you screen alternative practitioners and clinics. What is the doctor's success in treating your specific type of cancer? How many cancers of your type does he or she see every year? A therapy that is effective against one type of cancer may not get good results with another cancer. Try to pinpoint your type of cancer and the stage of the disease. If a particular therapy involves treatment at a clinic or hospital, what is the required length of stay? What are the side effects of the treatment? What self-care procedures will you have to do once you leave?

Some alternative practitioners exaggerate their results, inflating the rates of cure and remission. There are also scrupulously honest alternative practitioners who lack the resources to compile thorough statistics and do proper follow-up. Reliable, accurate figures in the alternative cancer-treatment field are extremely hard to come by. You can ask to see supportive studies, documented cases, and patients' testimonials. Some doctors and clinics have lists of recovered and recovering patients whom you can call or write. Another thing of which to be aware is that some alternative therapists tend to tout their own system as the only road to health and deride other approaches even if they are sadly unfamiliar with them. There seems to be as much ego, territoriality, exclusiveness, and passion in the alternative field as there is in mainstream science and medicine. Don't base your choice on therapists' persuasive tactics or glossy brochures. You have to sort through the conflicting claims, theories, and approaches to find the treatment, or combination of treatments, that works best for you.

Does a therapy fit in with your lifestyle, personality, tolerances, and belief system? Some nutritional therapies, for example, demand a degree of commitment that many people simply do not want to make. Or a therapy may involve frequent, regular injections that will cause extreme stress in some people. Some therapies require travel. For others, you may need hands-on assistance from a relative or friend to make self-care feasible. There could be special medical procedures to perform or foods to buy and prepare a certain way, tasks that you may not be able to easily accomplish on your own.

The choice of a therapy is a deeply personal one. Try to get an intuitive feeling about the therapy and whether you could work with it productively. Does the therapy promote healing along lines that make sense to you?

It may be helpful to augment some therapies with parts of others. However, this might be inappropriate and the practitioner may advise against it. If he does, ask yourself whether this advice is medically well-founded or reflects the practitioner's lack of openness toward other systems. If you are following a nutritional or metabolic program, you may be able to enhance it with herbs or immune stimulation. Again, seek medical advice. Whatever therapy you choose, you can work toward good health on the physical, nutritional, emotional, psychological, and spiritual levels all at once. Maintaining a positive, determined outlook is important. Mind-body techniques such as guided imagery, relaxation, psychotherapy, prayer, and spiritual exercises can assist you on the road to recovery.

Give the therapy you finally choose a fair chance. Some herbal regimens, for example, may work gradually and may not yield decisive results for three to six months, perhaps longer. Is the tumor shrinking, slowly but steadily? Follow through on whatever approach you choose and be alert to any progress. But if the therapy is clearly not working, you need to go back to square one, formulate a different strategy, and choose another treatment. There are people who did not respond to one alternative therapy, chose a different therapy, and then recovered. There are people who attained complete remission using just one therapy. There are also patients who combined therapies. There are those who used a number of different therapies successively before recovering. The whole field is unsystematized, and you will need to stay open to all possibilities.

Treatment costs are a factor for most people, and they vary widely. But a program's costs shouldn't necessarily be the deciding factor in your choice of a therapy if you feel strongly that a program is right for you. On the other hand, you may not need the added financial and emotional stress that comes from a therapy you can't afford. An excellent source of information on alternative cancer-care programs, doctors, clinics, and hospitals is *Third Opinion,* by John Fink (see Appendix A). This comprehensive, unique directory lists therapists and treatment centers in the United States and abroad, with concise information on each practitioner's approach, treatment offered, types of illness treated, length of treatment or stay, and costs. In addition, the directory provides basic information on scores of support groups, educational centers, and information services for cancer patients considering alternative or complementary treatment.

For guidelines to choosing an alternative or conventional therapy, ask the People's Medical Society to send you its eight-page bulletin *Cancer Care: Today's Treatment Options.* Another useful bulletin the group publishes is *How to Choose a Doctor.* Contact the People's Medical Society at 462 Walnut Street, Allentown, PA 18102; 215-770-1670.

What follows is an alphabetical listing of some of the principal organizations for cancer patients seeking information or referrals for alternative or complementary treatment.

Arlin J. Brown Information Center
P.O. Box 251
Fort Belvoir, VA 22060
Phone: 703-451-8638

This clearinghouse for information on nontoxic cancer therapies publishes a newsletter, *Health Victory Bulletin,* and sells books and pamphlets, including *March of Truth on Cancer,* a typed manual containing concise descriptions of seventy-nine different cancer treatments. Arlin Brown, a retired physicist with the United States Army, is a long-time crusader for medical freedom of choice, and his center, which he founded in 1963, was the first organization of its kind in the United States. He emphasizes dietary, herbal, and metabolic approaches aimed at detoxifying the system, eliminating the malignancy, and regenerating the body.

Cancer Control Society
2043 North Berendo Street
Los Angeles, CA 90027
Phone: 213-663-7801

An educational and informational nonprofit organization, the Cancer Control Society (CCS) provides listings—with names, addresses, and phone numbers—of alternative practitioners as well as patients treated with nontoxic cancer therapies. It publishes the bi-monthly *Cancer Control Journal*, geared to patients, and offers a large selection of mail-order books. Its annual cancer convention, held during the Fourth of July weekend in Los Angeles, features well-known alternative practitioners. Cassette tapes of talks given at conventions are available from Tapeco, Inc. (800-643-8645). Founded in 1973, CCS sponsors a bus tour of Tijuana clinics about four times a year.

CANHELP
3111 Paradise Bay Road
Port Ludlow, WA 98365-9771
Phone: 206-437-2291

CANHELP prepares individualized reports for persons seeking information about alternative, complementary, experimental, or conventional cancer therapies. Drawing on medical data banks, professional literature, and feedback from a network of doctors around the world, it provides a computer print-out telling which cancer specialists or centers get the best results treating patients with the cancer you're interested in. You also receive a typewritten interpretation of these data for you and your physician, copies of reports from CANHELP's files when applicable, and a synopsis of the conversations held on your behalf with CANHELP's network of medical advisors. Patrick McGrady, Jr., who launched CANHELP after his father's death from cancer in 1980, is not a doctor and does not prescribe therapies. He is a medical writer who translates medical jargon into plain English, a former *Newsweek* Moscow bureau chief, and the coauthor of *The Pritikin Program for Diet and Exercise*, by Nathan Pritikin.

Center for Advancement in Cancer Education
300 East Lancaster Avenue
Suite 100
Wynnewood, PA 19096
Phone: 215-642-4810

The Center for Advancement in Cancer Education is a nonprofit information, counseling, and referral agency that helps cancer patients evaluate conventional and alternative therapies and find appropriate treatment programs. Its emphasis is on nutritional, metabolic, and biologic approaches as nontoxic alternatives or adjuncts to conventional therapy. The center offers counseling for patients and their families in person or by telephone; there is no fee for this service. It also functions as a clearinghouse for information on immunotherapy, cellular therapy, herbal medicine, psycho-emotional issues, and so forth. Its library is open to the public by appointment. The center conducts a support group for the family and friends of cancer patients, dispenses books and information packets, and offers food-preparation classes. "We believe in an integrative, total-person approach to cancer," says Susan Silberstein, executive director. "If attention is not given to the entire organism's functioning, the cancer is likely to recur no matter what therapy is used." Silberstein founded the center (formerly called the Delaware Valley Foundation for Advancement in Cancer Therapy) in 1977 after her husband died of terminal cancer.

> Foundation for Advancement in Cancer Therapy
> P.O. Box 1242
> Old Chelsea Station
> New York, NY 10113
> Phone: 212-741-2790

An information clearinghouse and referral agency, the Foundation for Advancement in Cancer Therapy, also known as FACT, emphasizes biologic, nutritional, and metabolic approaches that can be used either as adjuncts or alternatives to orthodox cancer treatment. Its brochure states: "We believe that if given the support that nature intended it to have, the body's own immune system can prevent or control cancer in the majority of cases. . . . Our interest focuses on several factors which work together to optimize the body's ability to repair itself. Among these are: Early noninvasive diagnosis; Nutrition; Detoxification; Structural balance; Mind-body connection. Nontoxic programs may include: Fever therapy; Immunotherapy; Cellular therapy; Botanicals." Founder-director Ruth Sackman, in her seventies and with over twenty years of experience, offers counseling to patients and their families in person, by phone, or by mail. There's no fee involved. FACT publishes *Cancer Forum* magazine and sells books and tapes.

> The Health Resource
> 209 Katherine Drive
> Conway, AR 72032
> Phone: 501-329-5272

Janice Guthrie, a former cancer patient, founded The Health Resource in 1984 after her medical research skills led her to treatment that facilitated her recovery from a rare form of ovarian cancer. The service provides an individualized, in-depth report on your specific medical problem, with information from medical texts and journals; lay-oriented newsletters, books, and magazines; and computer databases. The reports range in length from 110 to 150 pages and include the latest information, pro and con, on both orthodox and alternative therapies. They address your individual situation (for example, "Should I take chemotherapy for node-negative breast cancer?") and are designed to help you survey your treatment options and locate conventional and holistic practitioners who may be helpful. A shorter report format is also available.

> International Association of Cancer Victors and Friends
> 7740 West Manchester Avenue
> Suite 110
> Playa del Rey, CA 90293
> Phone: 213-822-5032

With a worldwide membership and chapters throughout the United States, Canada, and Australia, the International Association of Cancer Victors and Friends (IACVF) emphasizes nontoxic therapies for persons seeking an alternative to conventional cancer treatment. This nonprofit organization provides a contact list of recovered patients and their specific type of cancer as well as a compilation of alternative practitioners and clinics. Founded in 1963 by a recovered cancer patient who conquered her own disease using nontoxic therapies, IACVF disseminates new information about alternative treatments, publishes *Cancer Victors Journal,* and operates a cancer hotline offering information on promising therapies for specific tumors and conditions. It also acts as a consumer advocate on behalf of cancer patients and physicians.

> World Research Foundation
> 15300 Ventura Boulevard
> Suite 405
> Sherman Oaks, CA 91403
> Phone: 818-907-5483

Health tools and therapies available worldwide but overlooked or in limited use in the United States are the focus of the World Research Foundation (WRF). For a nominal fee, the staff of this nonprofit information network will perform a library search on alternative therapies or a computer search, using its worldwide databases, on conventional, allopathic therapies. The library, open to the public at no charge, contains information on such topics as homeopathy, acupuncture, color and light therapy, electromagnetic therapies, nutrition, visualization, relaxation, and herbal medicine. Cancer, diabetes, arthritis, multiple sclerosis, and immune deficiencies are the diseases for which WRF receives the greatest number of queries. WRF publishes *World Research Journal* and sells books and videocassettes.

Chapter 1

ALTERNATIVE CANCER THERAPIES

This year, one million Americans will learn they have cancer. Roughly two out of three cancer patients will die of the illness (or related therapy) within five years of diagnosis. While the news media periodically announce major cancer breakthroughs, the cures are occurring mainly in the press releases. The "war on cancer" has been a colossal failure despite hundreds of billions of dollars spent on research and treatment.

The three "proven" methods of treating cancer—chemotherapy, radiation, and surgery—may actually shorten your life in many instances. Each of these treatments is invasive, has devastating side effects, and treats only symptoms. Each can cause the spread or recurrence of cancer. While these immunity-damaging approaches may at times be necessary, their successes have mostly been limited to relatively rare forms of cancer or the early stages of the disease. For most adult cancers, the orthodox therapies are virtually noncurative, though they may buy some time. For many patients, the standard therapies shorten the life span: "Most cancer patients in this country die of chemotherapy," observes Dr. Alan Levin of the University of California Medical School. "Chemotherapy does not eliminate breast, colon, or lung cancers. The fact has been documented for over a decade. . . . Women with breast cancer are likely to die faster with chemotherapy than without it."[1]

Only 2 to 3 percent of the nearly one-half million Americans diagnosed of cancer every year are being saved by chemotherapy, according to Dr. John Cairns of the Harvard University School of Public Health.[2] Yet over half of all cancer patients routinely receive chemotherapy drugs, which can cripple a person's chance of survival. All chemotherapy drugs are toxic and many are carcinogenic—they can cause cancer. The overuse of chemotherapy—a $750 million-a-year racket in drug sales alone—is a national scandal.

Disillusioned with standard cancer treatments—which often have devastating side effects and typically cost $30,000 or more—thousands of patients are turning to alternative or nontoxic therapies. Often called complementary, unorthodox, or nonconventional, these therapies include nutritional, herbal, metabolic, immune-enhancing, biologic, nontoxic pharmacologic, and psychological-behavioral approaches. While the alternative therapies exhibit great variation, all of them are rooted in the idea that a truly healthy body will not develop cancer. Alternative practitioners believe the cause of cancer is often found in a disorder of the immune system or a bodily imbalance that allows the tumor to develop.

Alternative therapies share certain common features. They are relatively nontoxic, unlike chemotherapy and radiation, which destroy normal cells. They aim to cleanse the body, to stimulate its natural defenses and tumor-destroying capacity. They have relatively high safety levels compared to the orthodox treatments. Many or most alternative therapies combine special diets; supplementation with vitamins, minerals, and enzymes; detoxification; oxygenation measures; immune stimulation; and psychological or spiritual regimens to promote gentle healing.

To mainstream doctors, cancer is a *localized* disease, to be treated in a localized manner. By cutting out the tumor, irradiating it, or flooding the body with toxic (and often carcinogenic) drugs, the orthodox physician hopes to destroy the tumor and thus save the patient. But all too often, the cancer is still present and has metastasized (spread elsewhere). The allopathic, conventional approach, for all its high-tech trappings, is based on a primitive medical philosophy: aggressively attacking an "enemy" disease. Often, the patient is devastated in the process, while the cancer and its underlying causes remain.

In contrast, the alternative healer regards cancer as a *systemic* disease, one that involves the whole body. In this view, the tumor is merely a symptom and the therapy aims to correct the root causes. Instead of aggressively attacking the tumor, many alternative therapies focus on rebuilding the body's natural immunity and strengthening its inherent ability to destroy cancer cells. A number of alternative therapies also include natural measures to directly attack and destroy the tumor, whether by herbs, enzymes, or other means.

Many cancer patients who were pronounced "terminal" or "hopeless" by their orthodox doctors went on to use alternative therapies, recovered fully, and are alive and well five, ten, twenty, or more years after their fatal diagnoses. Other patients who follow alternative protocols experience prolonged survival times and relief from pain and suffering. Not everyone does well on alternative cancer therapies; many die. There are no "magic bullets," no guarantees. Unfortunately, there are no reliable statistics on the results of alternative treatment. Some of the therapies work some of the time for some people.

The medical establishment ignores the existence of these cancer survivors or contemptuously dismisses them as "anecdotal evidence." Another establishment trick is to claim that people who got well through alternative therapies somehow magically recovered due to prior treatment—even if the toxic chemotherapy or immunity-destroying radiation that had been administered months or years earlier was of absolutely no benefit in slowing a rapidly advancing or metastasized malignancy.

Another favorite establishment ploy is to say that cancer patients who were cured through alternative therapies simply underwent "spontaneous remissions." This is medical lingo for "unexplained recovery," a fig leaf to cloak doctors' ignorance of what happened. Actually, there is no such process as spontaneous remission, as many doctors acknowledge. There must always be a cause or mechanism for the seemingly spontaneous tumor regression.[3] The most comprehensive study ever undertaken on the spontaneous remission of advanced cancers turned up a paltry total of 176 such cases in the world medical literature from 1900 to 1965. This means the odds of a doctor meeting with several spontaneous remissions in one lifetime are virtually zero.[4] Yet there are alternative doctors who have hundreds of so-called spontaneous remissions of advanced cancer to their credit.

Reviewing 200 cases of so-called spontaneous regression of cancer, Canadian professor Harold Foster, Ph.D., found in 1988 that *the great majority of these people (88 percent) had made major dietary changes*—usually switching to a strictly vegetarian diet and avoiding white flour, sugar, and canned or frozen foods—before their dramatic tumor regression or complete remission occurred.[5] Most of these patients also used vitamin, mineral, and herbal supplements as well as detoxification measures. These are all prominent features of several of the alternative cancer therapies discussed in this book.

Cancer is a biologic puzzle. There is no unanimous agreement on what makes cells grow abnormally, in endless, uncontrolled multiplication. There could be many different valid ways to treat cancer. According to Michael Evers, executive director of Project CURE, "There are serious, scientifically based approaches to cancer which do not happen to fit the mainstream model. We're not talking about quackery or snake-oil medicine here." A patient advocacy group, Project CURE supports "a pluralistic medical system" that would make nontoxic cancer therapies available to patients as part of standard medical practice. Most Americans, it seems, endorse this goal. An Associated Press–Media General national poll in September 1985 revealed that half of all Americans believe alternative cancer clinics should be allowed to operate in the United States—even if the treatments they offer are opposed by the orthodox medical establishment. Over half of the respondents said they would seek such treatment themselves if they were diagnosed with cancer.

Despite the public's support and growing interest in nontoxic, noninvasive alternative approaches, the medical establishment has waged a fierce campaign against such therapies, labeling them quackery. Treatment centers have been padlocked. Doctors who prescribe nutrition or herbs have been thrown in jail. Responsible, caring physicians who verbally support or practice alternative therapies have been fired, demoted, or ostracized or have had their medical licenses revoked. While official medicine suppresses or thwarts promising alternatives, it pours billions of dollars into narrow research supporting chemotherapy, radiation, and surgery as the major weapons in the "war on cancer." That war has been a total failure in slowing the death rate. The overall age-adjusted cancer death rate has *risen* by 5 percent since the war against cancer began.

"Everyone should know that the 'war on cancer' is largely a fraud," wrote Dr. Linus Pauling, two-time Nobel Prize winner. Another Nobel winner, Dr. James Watson, codiscoverer of the DNA double helix, put the matter more bluntly. Watson served for two years on the National Cancer Advisory Board. Asked in 1975 what he thought of the National Cancer Program, he promptly replied, "It's a bunch of shit."[6] Death rates for the most common cancers—cancers of the lung, colon, breast, prostate, pancreas, and ovary—have either stayed the same or increased during the past fifty years. As noted in the September 22, 1986, issue of *Business Week*, "Surgery, radiation, and highly toxic drugs all tend to fail for a stunningly simple reason: a tumor the size of your thumb has one billion malignant cells in it. Even if a treatment gets 99.9% of them, a million remain to take root all over again."

You may live longer by having no conventional treatment at all. That was the conclusion of the late Dr. Hardin Jones, professor of medical physics at the University of California at Berkeley. After carefully analyzing the cancer survival statistics for twenty-five years,

Jones told an American Cancer Society meeting in 1969 that *untreated patients do not die sooner than patients receiving orthodox treatment–and in many cases they live longer.*[7] Three studies by other researchers support this negative assessment, which has never been refuted.

MYTHS SURROUNDING ALTERNATIVE CANCER THERAPIES

Many myths and misconceptions surround alternative cancer therapies. What follows is an attempt to clarify the most common.

Myth #1: All alternative cancer therapies are worthless.

This is the official position of the $80 billion-a-year "cancer industry," which has a vested stake in the orthodox therapies. But the facts tell a very different story. Patients with advanced, metastasized cancers, given up as medically incurable by their conventional doctors, have reversed their illnesses using alternative therapies and are today completely cancer-free. Many more patients on nontoxic therapies have at least been able to keep their cancers under control and lead active, productive lives. Some alternative physicians have amassed clinical evidence, including studies and carefully documented case histories, to demonstrate the safety and effectiveness of their methods. This evidence is routinely rejected by the medical orthodoxy on the grounds that it does not meet certain criteria, such as double-blind controlled trials (in which half the patients do not receive the treatment in question).

These cures do not mean that all of the nonconventional methods work. Some may by ineffective or fraudulent. "Most alternative therapies are almost totally useless—just like the conventional therapies," says Patrick McGrady, Jr., founder of CANHELP.

Estimates of success rates with alternative therapies vary widely. What works for one patient or type of cancer may fail with another patient having the same or a different malignancy. Holistic health advocate Gary Null, who spent years investigating alternative clinics and interviewing patients, claims that success rates have ranged "from 2 to 20 percent" in cases of terminal cancer. Some alternative practitioners exaggerate their results, claiming five-year remission rates of 60 percent or more. Patrick McGrady is skeptical of all such claims. "It would be good, if it were true."

"My subjective impression," says Ralph Moss, publisher of *The Cancer Chronicles* newsletter, "is a baseline 4 to 5 percent five-year remission rate in all of the alternative clinics. Then the figure goes up with less severe cases. If I found a 20 percent rate of five-year remission, that would be really exciting." But Moss feels that this posited success rate is highly significant. "After all, these therapies are not supposed to cure anybody, according to orthodox medicine." He points out that the chance for recovery in many patients has been undercut by prior radiation and chemotherapy, both of which can severely damage the body's immune response and normal functioning.

Myth #2: Alternative cancer therapists are quacks–unscrupulous, unlicensed, untrained in medicine, out for a fast buck.

This stereotype may apply to some practitioners. Too often, though, it's used to paint with one brush all doctors and therapists who work beyond the limits of conventional medicine. The reality turns out to be just the opposite.

In a 1984 study in *Annals of Internal Medicine,* Barrie Cassileth, Ph.D., and fellow researchers found that 60 percent of the 138 alternative cancer practitioners they investigated were medical doctors (M.D.'s). Of the remaining 40 percent, many held doctorates in biology, chemistry, or other related sciences and had extensive research backgrounds.[8]

The American Cancer Society (ACS) maintains a compendium of "Unproven Methods of Cancer Management," which serves as the cancer establishment's chief tool to label alternative therapies as pseudoscience. To the ACS, *unproven* means *disproven.* Yet the ACS judges' pronouncement that "there is no acceptable evidence" for a particular therapy usually amounts to a blatant disregard of all the supporting data.[9] The inclusion of a doctor's name and therapy on this ugly official blacklist leads to loss of funding, a sudden inability to get articles published, the rejection of testing applications, and Food and Drug Administration (FDA) harassment, if not jail. The ACS blacklist "resembles the list of 'subversive' organizations once maintained by the House Un-American Activities Committee," notes Ralph Moss in his hard-hitting exposé *The Cancer Industry* (see Appendix A). "Merely including a scientist's name on the list has the effect of damning that researcher's work and putting the tag of quackery on him and his efforts."[10]

Moss's analysis of the unorthodox therapists whose names appear on the ACS Unproven Methods list reveals that 65 percent of them were M.D.'s, many from prestigious medical schools; an additional 13 percent held Ph.D.'s in medical or scientific disciplines.

"A number of the scientists on the ACS Unproven Methods list were undoubtedly persons of genius," observes science writer Robert Houston.[11] Among the examples he cites is Max Gerson, M.D., whose dietary treatment of cancer anticipated many current research trends. Gerson was hailed by Nobel laureate Dr. Albert Schweitzer, who wrote, "I see in him one of the most eminent medical geniuses in the history of medicine."

These practitioners hardly fit the image of snake-oil salesmen.

Myth #3: Patients who seek alternative therapies are driven by desperation. They're ignorant, gullible, or both.

Contrary to the stereotype, recent studies have shown that alternative cancer therapies are more popular among affluent, well-educated patients—and that some conventional physicians are surprisingly supportive of them. "The stereotype of the less-educated, poor person succumbing to the sideshow lures of the quack has been exploded," Dr. LaMar McGinnis told a San Francisco conference organized by the American Cancer Society in 1990. McGinnis, ex-chairman of the ACS Committee on Unproven Methods and no friend of alternative treatment, based his remarks on an unpublished ACS study of 5,047 patients.

"Many patients receiving alternate care do not conform to the traditional stereotype of poorly educated, terminally ill patients who have exhausted conventional treatment," wrote Barrie Cassileth in her landmark 1984 study (see Myth #2). She found that cancer patients on alternative therapies were significantly better educated than were patients on conventional treatment only. Many were attracted to therapeutic alternatives emphasizing personal responsibility and nutrition and moving away from what the patients viewed as deficiencies of orthodox medical care. Most of the patients paid less than $1,000 for the first year of alternative treatment. Even taking into account inflation and sharp variations in fees, these costs are modest compared to the expenses of *$2,500 per day* that the medical establishment demands for its invasive procedures. Cassileth also found that alternative therapy was actually approved by patients' primary physicians 30 percent of the time.

Myth #4: Alternative cancer therapies are "unproven," therefore untested and unscientific.

The American Cancer Society has seventy-two alternative cancer therapies on its Unproven Methods list. In his revealing analysis of the ACS blacklist, Ralph Moss notes that for 44 percent of these condemned therapies, *no investigation at all had been carried out by the ACS or any other agency.* For another 11 percent, the investigations had actually yielded *positive* results. Inconclusive findings were reported for 16 percent. And for the remaining 29 percent, the ACS judges had determined the methods in question to be ineffective, yet, as Moss points out, "Virtually all of the ACS judges are orthodox physicians with a vested interest in the system. In making their assessments, they rely on second- or third-hand reports like magazine articles and foreign medical associations."

Hyperthermia, or heat therapy—once branded as a "worthless remedy" and "quackery" by the ACS—was removed years later from the Unproven Methods list. Today, hyperthermia is in trial use at major medical centers; it has been hailed by some oncologists as the fifth modality in cancer treatment after surgery, radiation, drugs, and immunotherapy. This is the same method that the ACS banished into limbo in 1967.

Four other unorthodox cancer treatments once stigmatized by their inclusion on the ACS blacklist were later removed from it: hydrazine sulfate, the Coley therapy, the Lincoln therapy, and Hendricks Natural Immunity therapy. Their Stalinist-like "rehabilitation" came about through pressure from prestigious researchers and institutions with a keen interest in exploring these methods.

These examples demonstrate the bias built into the ACS's unscientific system, which is largely designed to protect the monetary interests of chemotherapy, radiation, and surgery. One should keep an open mind about all the available options.

THE MYTH OF "PROVEN" THERAPIES

Most of the everyday practices of modern medicine are unproven if we go by the government's own standards. In 1978, the Office of Technology Assessment (OTA), an arm of the United States Congress, issued a major research report that concluded "only 10 to 20 percent of all procedures currently used in medical practices have been shown to be efficacious by controlled trial." In other words, 80 to 90 percent of what doctors do to you is scientifically unproven guesswork. By this government-supported definition, most of modern medicine is quackery.[12]

Chemotherapy and radiation, two of the three principal "proven" methods of treating cancer, seem to fall within the OTA definition of unproven, potentially dangerous quackery, at least in much of their current usage in the United States. Chemotherapy, radiation, and surgery are all harmful to the body as well as to the tumor and all cause physical suffering and emotional trauma that frequently make them an excruciating ordeal. Each of these methods deserves a closer look.

Chemotherapy

Chemotherapy has scored dramatic successes in treating cancers of the lymph and blood cells: the leukemias, the lymphomas, and Hodgkin's disease (a type of lymph cancer). These cancers are treated by combination chemotherapy, which uses "cocktails" of several different toxic drugs at once. Chemo cocktails, when preceded by surgery and radiotherapy, have achieved significant cure rates, mostly with rare types of solid tumors such as choriocarcinoma.

The Janker Klinik in Bonn, Germany, is famous for its short-term, high-dosage chemotherapy, usually administered over a one- or two-week period. Published (but nonscientific) reports credit the Klinik with an incredible 70 percent remission rate and cures in patients who had widely metastasized cancers. This figure seems questionable because most patients go there as a last resort, their systems already devastated by conventional treatment. Skeptical American doctors say that the remissions are very short-lived and that when the cancer returns, it is quickly fatal.[13]

Virtually all of the anticancer drugs approved by the FDA are *toxic* at the applied dosages and markedly *immunosuppressive*, destroying a patient's natural resistance to many diseases, including cancer. Most of these FDA-approved chemo drugs are also *carcinogenic*, that is, highly cancer-causing in lab animals and capable of causing cancer in human beings.

All these drugs are poisonous not as a *side effect* but as a *primary effect*. Because these poisons cannot distinguish between cancerous and normal cells, they disrupt or kill normal, healthy cells throughout the body besides attacking the tumor. They attack the bone marrow, thereby destroying the white blood cells, which fight infection; the red blood cells, which carry life-sustaining oxygen to the body's organs; and the platelets, which help the blood to clot. Unfortunately, these immune-system cells are a major part of the body's built-in defense against cancer.

Patients undergoing chemotherapy—with their immune systems completely destroyed or compromised—frequently die of pneumonia or common infections. Death from toxicity is also quite common. In one study, 10 percent of 133 patients using the chemo drug 5-FU (5-fluorouracil) died as a direct result of the drug's toxicity.[14] Doctors jokingly refer to this popular chemotherapy drug as "Five Feet Under." Chemotherapy patients come down with the whole range of blood diseases, such as aplastic anemia, in which the bone marrow can no longer make blood cells; leukopenia, an abnormal decrease in the amount of white blood cells; and thrombocytopenia, an abnormal reduction in platelets. The long-term effects of chemotherapy can include heart damage weeks, months, or years after treatment; loss of fertility; and an increased risk of recurrence of cancer.

Most chemo drugs cause secondary cancers, especially of the gastrointestinal tract, ovaries, and lungs. These are among the most difficult cancers to treat. They can appear five, ten, fifteen years after the "successful" chemotherapy. In one study, 18 percent of the survivors developed unrelated cancer up to fifteen years later. Reports like the following are fairly typical: "Secondary cancers are known complications of chemotherapy and irradiation used to treat Hodgkin's and non-Hodgkin's lymphomas and other primary cancers" (*New England Journal of Medicine*, September 21, 1989). "Chemotherapy drugs that were long ago used to treat ovarian cancer may have done as much harm as good by sharply increasing the risk of leukemia. . . . Among women treated from 1960 through 1985, the risk of leukemia was 12 times higher in those who received chemotherapy than in those who only underwent surgery" (Associated Press, January 5, 1990). Between 5 and 10 percent of all patients who survive chemotherapy die of leukemia in the first ten years after treatment, according to Harvard microbiologist Dr. John Cairns. When chemotherapy and radiation are given together, secondary tumors occur *about 25 times more than the expected rate*. This depressing assessment was made by Dr. John Laszlo, the American Cancer Society's senior vice president for research.[15]

Chemotherapy can be one of the most physically and emotionally devastating of all treatments. Most of the forty FDA-approved chemo drugs on the market cause baldness; hair may take years to return to normal. Other common side effects include extreme nausea and vomiting, bleeding gums, sores around the mouth, bleeding and ulceration of the gastrointestinal tract, and candida (thrush). Numerous patients say they find the side effects worse than the disease itself. A number of autopsy studies have shown that many patients die from the standard treatment they receive before the tumor has a chance to kill them.[16]

The cancers from which most people die—the big killers like breast, colon, and lung cancer—generally do not respond to chemotherapy. Chemotherapy has only a limited effectiveness against any tumor that is large or has spread; its successes are generally with small, very early tumors. Several studies indicate that chemotherapy has no survival value in breast cancer. "Survival may even have been shortened in some [breast cancer] patients given chemotherapy," according to six British cancer specialists writing in the prestigious British medical journal *The Lancet.*[17]

"Practicing physicians are intimidated into using regimes which *they know do not work.* One of the most glaring examples is chemotherapy, which does not work for the majority of cancers," Alan Levin, M.D., told a national conference on abuses in medicine held in 1985. A distinguished professor of immunology at the University of California at San Francisco Medical School, Levin added, "Despite the fact that most physicians *agree* that chemotherapy is largely ineffective, they are *coerced* into using it by special interest groups which have vested interest in the profits of the drug industry."[18] Prescribing chemotherapy when it has little or no chance of working "is at best stupid and at worst criminal," notes Dr. Robert Atkins, well-known practitioner of complementary medicine.[19] Yet mainstream cancer doctors do this on a daily basis.

Radiation

Radiation therapy, or radiotherapy, used on about half of American cancer patients, employs high-intensity X-rays to cripple cancer cells' ability to reproduce. Radioactivity emanating from artificial implants—such as cobalt-60 or radium "seeds" inserted directly into the cancer—is also used. The problem with radiation is that like chemotherapy, it damages normal, healthy cells in the process of killing cancer cells. Radiation severely depresses immunity and can cause serious chromosomal damage at both diagnostic- and therapeutic-dose levels. Radiotherapy is a powerful carcinogen; it causes secondary cancers in many patients exposed to it. In one study, as many as 17 percent of the patients treated with radiotherapy developed secondary cancers within twenty years in the sites exposed to the radiation.

Radiation can achieve five-year remission in 80 percent of very early Hodgkin's disease patients and is effective in treating lymphosarcoma, inoperable local prostate cancer, and localized tumors of the head, neck, and cervix. It is probably preferable to surgery for some cancers, such as cancer of the larynx or prostate. In treating breast cancer, lumpectomy combined with radiotherapy appears to decrease the chances of recurrence in the affected breast, although this is disputed since later cancers can occur ten years after exposure.

Other than these successes, radiation appears to be of limited value in the treatment of cancer and often does more harm than good.

Several studies have shown that people who undergo radiation therapy are *more* likely to have their cancer metastasize to other sites in their bodies. This was noted by oncologist Dr. Lucien Israel, consultant to the National Cancer Institute, in his book *Conquering Cancer*.[20] The radioactivity used to kill cancer cells can also trigger the process of mutation that creates new cancer cells of other types.

Radiation therapy causes damage and dysfunction in body organs and tissues. Various studies have shown that it offers no survival advantage for most cancers. "The majority of cancers," writes John Cairns in the November 1985 issue of *Scientific American,* "cannot be cured by radiation because the dose of X rays required to kill all the cancer cells would also kill the patient." Cairns is a professor at the Harvard University School of Public Health.

Radiotherapy following breast surgery *increases* death rates, according to several clinical trials and a study published in *The Lancet.*[21] Yet 50 percent of radiologists still radiate women following surgery for breast cancer. "Complications following high-dose radiotherapy for breast cancer are: fibrous, shrunken breasts, rib fractures, pleural and/or lung scarring, nerve damage, scarring around the heart . . . suppression of all blood cells, immune suppression," according to Robert F. Jones, M.D., writing in the *Seattle Times* on July 27, 1980. "Many radiation complications do not occur for several years after treatment, giving the therapist and the patient a false sense of security for a year or two following therapy. . . . The bone marrow, in which blood cells are made, is largely obliterated in the field of irradiation. . . . This is an irreversible effect."

There is very little agreement in the medical fraternity about the proper role of chemotherapy combined with radiation therapy in the treatment of malignant tumors. Opinions among oncologists range from enthusiastic approval to strong condemnation. As noted earlier, people who undergo both chemotherapy and radiation experience later cancers twenty-five times more often than the general population.

The side effects of radiation therapy include severe, prolonged immune deficiency and chromosomal damage resulting in later cancer. "Even very moderate amounts of radiation of the testicles and ovaries may cause sterilization or induce genetic mutations," notes Dr. Israel.[22] Radiotherapy can permanently stunt growth in children. Its other side effects include:

- Nausea, vomiting, and excessive weakness and fatigue, sometimes rendering patients bedridden.

- "Sores or ulcers . . . in the mouth, throat, intestines, genital areas and other parts of the body. . . ." (American Cancer Society, *Cancer Book*, 1986.) Mouth sores can make it difficult to eat.

- Bone death in the mouth following irradiation of the tongue, mouth, or gums.

- Temporary or permanent hair loss, depending on the dosage.

- Welts and extensive burns of the skin and mucous membranes.

- Permanent dilation of the small capillaries and arteries under the skin in patients who have a wide area irradiated, as with breast cancer.

- Amenorrhea in women close to menopause who are exposed to as little as 400 rads of radiation. (*Rad* stands for "radiation absorbed dose," which is the basic unit of ionizing radiation.)

- "Rectal ulcers, fistulas, bladder ulcers, diarrhea, and colitis" in "women undergoing radiation of the pelvic cavity." (ACS, *Cancer Book*, 1986.)

- The swelling of tumors after a single large dose of radiation. This is especially dangerous for brain tumors. Patients may receive corticosteroids in an attempt to prevent this effect.

Many doctors believe that radiotherapy is relatively harmless, so they continue to recommend this highly lucrative treatment to patients as a palliative. But even "safe" levels of radiation are suspect. Early studies at Memorial Sloan-Kettering Cancer Center in New York showed that radiotherapy was deadly and that patients who received *no* radiation lived longer than those who were irradiated. These and similar findings were presented to Congress in 1953 in the famous Fitzgerald Report, which charged that the medical establishment was actively conspiring to suppress promising alternative cancer therapies.[23] But these important studies were ignored, and the radiotherapy industry got its way. "For 30 years radiologists in this country have been engaged in massive malpractice," charged Dr. Irwin Bross in 1979.[24] Bross, former director of biostatistics at Roswell Park Memorial Institute, was unable to get adequate funding to research the thirty-year cover-up of what he calls doctor-caused cancer from radiation therapy.

Surgery

Surgery is sometimes a necessary, lifesaving procedure in treating cancer. It is effective as a cure for early, small tumors that have not spread to other parts of the body. For example, surgery achieves roughly 70 percent five-year survival in uterine cancers, 85 percent in skin cancers, 60 percent in breast cancers, and 40 percent in colon cancers. But once a tumor has grown beyond a certain size or has spread to other sites, it is frequently inoperable. There is no reliable way to tell whether a tumor is localized or has metastasized. In early-stage breast cancer, 30 percent or more of women given a favorable prognosis after surgery experience recurrences of their cancer, according to the latest figures from the National Cancer Institute.[25]

Surgeons routinely tell cancer patients, "I got it all," but many studies have shown that some cancer cells are left behind in 25 to 60 percent of patients, allowing malignant growths to recur. Surgery itself is often responsible for the spread of the cancer, according to many physicians. A microscopic miscue or careless manipulation of tumor tissue by the surgeon can "spill" literally millions of cancer cells into the bloodstream. Surgical biopsy, a procedure used to detect early-stage cancer, can also contribute to the spread of cancer. "Often while making a biopsy the malignant tumor is cut across, which tends to spread or accelerate the growth. Needle biopsies can accomplish the same tragic results," observed Dr. William Kelley.[26]

Surgery weakens immunity, places great systemic stress on the patient, and can cause sudden death. Many cancer patients have died on the operating table, or shortly after leaving it, from complications of surgery. Some surgical operations are performed needlessly. "Even though it's been proven conclusively that lymph node excision after radiation does not prevent the spread of cervical cancer, you will still see lymphadenectomies performed all over the country routinely. This despite the fact that lymphadenectomies make women feel so bad they wish they were dead—and are a proven useless procedure."[27]

Pain, disfigurement, and restriction of function often accompany surgery. Many cancer patients are left debilitated, crippled, traumatized, or humiliated after the operation. A surprising number of "cured" cancer patients have had their lives ruined by the "successful" surgery. For all these reasons, cutting up the body is not the final answer to cancer.

Part One

BIOLOGIC AND PHARMACOLOGIC THERAPIES

Cancer has been described as approximately 150 different diseases with many causes and patterns. All of these diseases share two basic characteristics: the uncontrolled growth of cells and the ability of these cells to invade and damage normal tissues. Why cells start dividing uncontrollably in mindless multiplication is not definitely known. The explanation most frequently advanced today is that damage to the DNA or chemical damage to cell membranes leads to cell mutation.

All of the therapies discussed in Part One of *Options* were developed by highly qualified, distinguished physicians or scientists. All of them employ one or more biologic substances or nontoxic pharmacologic agents. Each of the innovators has gathered medical evidence that his therapy is based on scientific principles and shows effectiveness in treating cancer patients. Yet each of the therapies, in its own way, goes against some current dogma, or entrenched belief, about cancer.

An example of a dogma is the belief that cancer is not caused by a microbe. Mainstream researchers in this country once widely believed that cancer was caused by a germ or microorganism. Today, a minority of doctors and scientists keep this theory alive, even though it goes against the prevalent outlook. Another dogma of today's medical orthodoxy is the widespread assumption that chemotherapy must be toxic in order to work. Two of the approaches discussed in Part One are nontoxic chemotherapies.

Besides challenging the dominant assumptions, the therapies discussed here also pose an economic threat to establishment medicine. As well-known nutritional expert Robert Atkins, M.D., has noted, "The entire concept of a biologic, nontoxic cancer therapy would signal the beginning of the end of the highly profitable chemotherapy industry." Dr. Atkins, who practices complementary medicine synthesizing conventional and alternative approaches, points out that medical conferences in Europe are devoted to high-quality research into successful nontoxic, biologic cancer treatments, yet in the United States, official medicine displays a "calculated ignorance" of these promising discoveries.[1]

One example of a promising biologic therapy neglected by the medical establishment is the treatment pioneered by German bacteriologist Guenther Enderlein (1872–1968). Examining live blood under the microscope for several decades, Enderlein came to believe in *pleomorphism,* the theory that certain bacteria living within the human body can change in size and shape, transforming from harmless agents into disease-causing bacteria or fungi. Enderlein developed medicines designed to halt the pleomorphic microbes' attack on body cells and tissues. These remedies are said to foster self-healing by changing the disease-causing forms of the pleomorphic microbes back into harmless forms.[2]

Abram Ber, who is both a medical doctor and a practicing homeopath in Phoenix, Arizona, has successfully used the Enderlein remedies, some of which are potentized through homeopathic dilution. Out of thirty-eight cancer patients treated during a recent twelve-month period, Dr. Ber reports that only one—a very advanced case of cancer of the pharynx—was lost. All the rest are either in remission or doing well. Two other physicians who have reported good results with the Enderlein remedies in treating cancer patients are Harvey Bigelsen, M.D., of Scottsdale, Arizona, and Erik Enby, M.D., of Gothenberg, Sweden.

Pleomorphic (form-changing) microorganisms are also central to the therapies of Gaston Naessens (Chapter 3), Virginia Livingston (Chapter 7), and Royal Rife (Chapter 25).

Chapter 2

ANTINEOPLASTON THERAPY

"The body itself has a treatment for cancer," says Dr. Stanislaw Burzynski. The Polish-born physician-biochemist, based in Houston, Texas, discovered that a group of *peptides* (short chains of amino acids) and amino-acid derivatives occurring naturally throughout our bodies inhibit the growth of cancer cells. In his view, these substances are part of a *biochemical defense system* completely different from our immune system. Unlike the immune system, which protects us by destroying invading agents or defective cells, the biochemical defense system reprograms, or corrects, defective cells. It carries "good" information to abnormal cells, instructing them to develop normally.

Dr. Burzynski named these peptides *antineoplastons* because of their ability to inhibit neoplastic, or cancerous, cell growth. He discovered that cancer patients have a drastic shortage of these compounds in their bodies—blood samples of advanced cancer patients reveal only 2 to 3 percent of the amount typically found in healthy individuals. By simply reintroducing the peptides into the patient's bloodstream, either orally or intravenously, he brings about tumor shrinkage or complete remission. In many cases, just weeks after the start of treatment, tumors have shrunk in size or disappeared. Most types of cancer reportedly respond to the therapy, which is safe and nontoxic. The natural substances used are well tolerated by the body, even in high doses, without any of the disastrous side effects routinely associated with toxic chemotherapy and radiation.

Since the Burzynski Research Institute (BRI) opened in 1977, Dr. Burzynski has treated some 2,000 cancer patients, most of them in advanced stages. He has saved or prolonged hundreds of lives with his innovative approach. A significant number of persons treated have been in complete remission for five years or more, even though they were pronounced "terminal" or "incurable" by their conventional doctors. However, Dr. Burzynski advises that antineoplaston treatments are not effective against all types of cancer nor for all patients.

A front-page article in the July–August 1990 issue of *Oncology News* was devoted to antineoplastons, "a completely new type of antitumor agent that is nontoxic and seems to make malignant cancer cells revert to normal." Dvorit Samid, Ph.D., a Bethesda, Maryland, researcher, was quoted as saying, "Such a dramatic phenomenon is seldom seen. . . . I am very excited about these findings." This report on the Ninth International Symposium on Future Trends in Chemotherapy, held in Geneva, Switzerland, presented favorable preclinical and clinical results achieved with antineoplaston therapy by researchers from Japan, Poland, China, and the United States.

A complete remission in a Japanese patient with inoperable metastatic ovarian cancer and complete remissions in American patients with advanced prostate cancer were among the results presented. These types of cancer are very rarely cured by conventional forms of treatment.

Some of the most exciting results obtained with antineoplastons have been with the tumors that usually do not respond to chemotherapy, radiation, or immunotherapy. These include malignant brain tumors (astrocytoma, stages III and IV, and glioblastoma), advanced cancer of the prostate, certain forms of lung cancer, bladder cancer, and even cancer of the pancreas. For example, in a Phase II trial involving astrocytoma, a highly malignant form of brain cancer, twenty patients—nearly all of them in advanced stages of the disease— were treated with antineoplastons. All but one had received and failed prior standard therapies.

Four patients achieved complete remission, and two others, partial remission. Ten other patients showed objective stabilization (less than 50 percent decrease of tumor size). Since the end of this study, in May 1990, some of the ten patients classified as stabilized have achieved complete or partial remission.[1]

Clinical studies are also underway with patients in Poland. Researchers in Japan, Great Britain, Italy, the United States, and China have reproduced and are expanding Dr. Burzynski's preclinical work. In September 1990, the Burzynski Research Institute entered into a letter of intent with Ferment, a major Soviet pharmaceutical firm, to conduct clinical trials with antineoplastons on cancer patients in the Soviet Union.

While Burzynski's breakthroughs are being eagerly pursued abroad, here in the United States, where he lives and sees patients, the doctor has been the target of an ill-informed, multipronged attack aimed at discrediting him and closing down his clinic. Despite the fact that he has published 150 scientific papers and holds twenty patents for antineoplaston treatment covering sixteen countries, his work has been dismissed as quackery by such interlocking government agencies and private-sector vested-interest groups as the Food and Drug Administration and the American Cancer Society. Close-minded oncologists, when asked by their patients about Dr. Burzynski, have said that he has published nothing. Some insurance companies have sent pleasantly worded form letters denying all payment for his services.

The American Cancer Society in 1983 put Burzynski's antineoplaston therapy on its Unproven Methods blacklist, where it remains to this day. Yet, as Ralph Moss notes in *The Cancer Industry*, the ACS's condemnatory report on the therapy "included data which undercut its own conclusions," such as the fact that 86 percent of far-advanced cancer patients treated with antineoplastons showed clinical improvement in one 1977 study! Four patients (19 percent) had complete remission, and another four had partial remission. Yet the ACS twisted the facts and said it "does not have evidence that treatment with antineoplaston results in objective benefit."[2]

The FDA filed suit against Dr. Burzynski in March 1983 in an attempt to drive him out of business. It ordered Burzynski and his institute to stop all further research, development, manufacture, and use of antineoplastons. A federal judge allowed the doctor to continue his research and treatment within the state of Texas but ruled that he could not ship the drugs across state lines.

In July 1985, FDA agents and federal marshals, armed with an illegal search warrant to look for vague "violations," raided the Burzynski Research Institute and seized over 200,000 confidential documents, including private medical records. They went through Dr. Burzynski's personal correspondence and rifled his briefcase. The federal officers loaded eleven of his filing cabinets onto their truck in an outrageous violation of his (and patients') constitutional and civil liberties. Dr. Burzynski sued the FDA for the return of his records, but all the documents remain in the FDA's hands to this day.

The Texas State Board of Medical Examiners tried to revoke Burzynski's medical license in 1988 on hairsplitting technical charges that had no connection whatsoever with the quality of care he provides. Hundreds of letters of support were sent to the board by

Burzynski's patients and their families and friends. The following letter from a Midwestern teenager was typical:

> I am 13 years old and I have a 7 year old brother. We love our father very much. Thanks to Dr. Burzynski's treatment, my father's tumor has stopped growing. All of the doctors in my home state of Missouri said there was no cure for my father's disease. Dr. Burzynski gave him a chance for life again. Please don't take that away from us.

The board's investigation has been slowed but not stopped.

For five years, the Justice Department has unsuccessfully sought an indictment against Dr. Burzynski on trumped-up charges of mail fraud. This investigation has been centered not on the treatment's efficacy but on how insurance is billed by the clinic. The charges are not based on any patient's complaint nor on harm caused to any patient. BRI and Aetna Life Insurance Company have sued each other; the outcome is pending.

To the American medical monopoly, Dr. Burzynski and his therapy are a threat in at least three ways. First, if his theory about a biochemical defense system separate from the immune system is correct, the biology textbooks will have to be rewritten. His theory is revolutionary in its implications. Second, although he is an alternative healer, Burzynski plays by the rules, publishing his findings openly and widely in the peer-reviewed medical literature, which makes it much harder to smear him as a quack. Third, and most important, his safe, nontoxic cancer treatment, with its tremendous promise, is perceived as a threat by the mega-billion-dollar cancer business with its vested monetary interests in toxic chemotherapy, radiation, and surgery. Orthodox doctors and the huge drug companies would not welcome a safe, relatively inexpensive cancer cure— such as naturally occurring peptides, an herbal brew, or something similar—that can't be marketed to reap superprofits.

At present, antineoplaston therapy is not cheap. The monthly minimum cost of outpatient treatment is between $3,000 and $5,000, excluding the expense of room and board in Houston, transportation, and so forth. The minimum length of treatment time is averaging from four months to one year. The costs are spelled out in detail in the Burzynski Clinic's patient brochure. A number of insurance companies accept antineoplaston treatment for full or partial reimbursement.

The treatment costs reflect the enormous expenses involved in developing and manufacturing the drugs, which are produced by BRI without the advantages enjoyed by the big pharmaceutical companies. However, if antineoplastons ever gain wide acceptance and are mass-produced by a big pharmaceutical company, the cost to the patient would drop drastically.

Ten-year-old Ryan Werthwein was diagnosed by doctors in August 1989 with advanced (Stage IV) thalamic glioblastoma, a brain tumor with the highest grade of malignancy. Under conventional care, persons with this type of cancer usually don't live longer than six to nine months after diagnosis. This cancer is considered incurable.

Orthodox doctors told Ryan's parents that the boy, an identical twin from Marlboro, New Jersey, had six months to a year to live. If Ryan took a highly toxic experimental drug, the doctors said, he might survive a year, just possibly a year and a half, but in a progressively debilitated condition. Ryan underwent radiation therapy for five weeks starting in early October, but it proved ineffective. The tumor remained the same size, as indicated by a Magnetic Resonance Imaging (MRI) scan of the brain in January 1990. "The radiation burnt out most of Ryan's pituitary gland, stunted his growth, and hurt his mental functioning," according to Sharon Werthwein, the boy's mother. "We were never told about radiation's possible long-term effects."

After reading up extensively on alternative therapies, Ryan's parents decided to forego chemotherapy and take their son to Houston for treatment by Dr. Burzynski. "The doctors really beat us up over not doing chemo. We were discouraged at every turn from pursuing a safe, nontoxic alternative. They also told us Burzynski was a quack," recalls Sharon. "The American Cancer Society said they have an arrangement with the Hilton to keep rooms available for cancer patients' families, but when we mentioned Dr. Burzynski's name, they said to 'forget it.' The Corporate Angel Network, which boasts in TV ads how it flies young cancer patients around the country for free, refused to fly our son because the National Cancer Institute won't let them fly Burzynski's patients. The system is a disgrace."

Ryan's treatment with antineoplastons began in mid-April 1990. One month after the intravenous infusions were started, there was a major breakdown of the tumor mass, and from then on, it steadily shrank as the therapy continued. "It felt as if a miracle had occurred," says Sharon. An MRI scan of the brain on May 15—after four weeks of treatment—showed only barely visible tumor remnants. On November 1, 1990, Ryan displayed complete remission. Subsequent MRI scans have shown him to be cancer-free.

"When I called the radiologist to tell him the good news, he said, 'I thought you were calling to tell me your son had passed away,'" says Sharon. "In utter disbelief, he begged me to come in the next day with my son's brain scan. After inspecting it, he admitted that he had never seen anything like this before but refused to discuss his earlier negative evaluation of Dr. Burzynski."

Ryan continues to receive antineoplaston treatment, but the dosage is gradually being reduced. He wears a miniature infusion pump, carried in a waist pack, that injects antineoplastons through a catheter in his chest twenty-four hours a day. There is no pain or discomfort. The ambulatory pump, similar to the one used by diabetics, is reloaded with medicine every two to three days. A patient can inconspicuously carry it in a moderately sized shoulder bag or waist pack. Patients can function and walk about with minimum inconvenience.

Ryan's physical growth and metabolism have slowed. At the age of thirteen, he is over three inches shorter than his identical twin brother, which the Werthweins attribute to the radiation therapy. "The thing that attracted us to Dr. Burzynski's approach," explains Sharon, "is that it is safe and nontoxic, without the horrendous damage and pain that chemotherapy and radiation cause. We figured, 'Our boy is dying. What have we got to lose by trying this method?' It is criminal that the American medical system would attempt to suppress Dr. Burzynski's therapy, which has saved our son's life. It is wrong that we can only get this treatment for our son in Texas, rather than right here where we live."

Dr. Burzynski reports that he continues to see very encouraging results in the majority of his patients with advanced, high-grade malignant brain tumors.

Some of Dr. Burzynski's patients receive the antineoplastons orally, through capsules. For others, the treatment is administered intravenously, through a catheter. The insertion of a catheter is a simple procedure, performed by a qualified medical doctor outside the clinic.

Another of Dr. Burzynski's patients was a thirty-six-year-old female diagnosed by the University of California Medical Center with advanced (Stage IV) astrocytoma of the brain stem. The patient was initially treated with radiation therapy but showed clear, debilitating progression of the disease before starting on an antineoplaston protocol. She was given oral doses of Antineoplaston A10 (one of the specific peptide compounds) as well as intravenous injections of Antineoplaston AS2-1. She did not show objective response to the treatment, however, and was switched to Antineoplaston A10 and AS2-1 infusions. After six months on this regimen, she was documented to be in complete remission, and she continues to be cancer-free three years later.[3]

There's a telling irony in the saga of a scientist fleeing Poland for the United States in search of freedom to do his work, only to encounter harassment and repression by the government and medical establishment. At age twenty-five, Stanislaw Burzynski graduated from the prestigious Lublin Medical Academy in Poland, ranked first in his class of 250. The next year, in 1968, he received a Ph.D. in biochemistry, becoming one of the youngest people in Europe ever to receive both advanced degrees. It was in 1967, at age twenty-four, that Burzynski discovered the cancer-growth-inhibiting properties of peptides.

When Burzynski refused to join the communist party in Poland, his position became precarious. He emigrated to the United States in 1970, becoming an assistant professor at Baylor College of Medicine in Houston. A research grant from the National Cancer Institute allowed him to continue his investigation of peptides part-time.

Over the next few years, Burzynski isolated 119 peptides and classified them according to activity. He elaborated on his original finding that "messenger" peptides bond to potential cancer cells, feeding them the complex information they need to revert to normal and perform their intended function. Without this corrective biochemical defense system, asserts Burzynski, we would soon succumb to the cancer-causing forces that continually trigger abnormal cell development, such as carcinogenic chemicals, radiation, and viruses.

Burzynski's work on peptides convinced him that cancer is "a disease of information processing." Some peptides spur cellular growth, others inhibit it, but they all accomplish their mission by sending messages the body can obey. The peptides in the bloodstream, which he named antineoplastons, are said to correct the DNA's chemical program inside the cell and force the cell toward normal development.

Dr. Burzynski discovered that antineoplastons exhibit three distinct modes of action. In the first mode, the antineoplastons inhibit the incorporation of glutamine (an amino acid) into the protein of cancerous cells. In the second mode of action, the antineoplastons intercalate (insert) themselves into the double-helix strand of DNA.

Since carcinogens also do this, the antineoplastons are believed to work because they pre-emptively take up the carcinogen's "parking spot" on the DNA strand. This mechanism is not new; some conventional anticancer drugs act in precisely this manner, but they also bind with normal cells and are highly toxic. In the third mode of action, the antineoplastons inhibit methylation (introduction of a methyl group) in the DNA and RNA of cancer cells, thus inducing malignant cells to differentiate and enter a normal cell cycle.[4]

At first, Burzynski derived the antineoplaston compounds from blood serum. Then he discovered that the body eliminates these peptides in the urine. Today, most antineoplastons are synthesized from off-the-shelf chemicals, but some of them are still derived from purified human urine. Critics have twisted these facts to paint Burzynski's therapy as bizarre. In reality, the investigation of urinary peptides and amino acids in human urine has been pursued by researchers for over half a century. As Dr. Burzynski observed, "Urine is not really waste material, but probably the most complex chemical mixture in the human body, and therefore it can deliver us virtually any information about the body. So from the cybernetic point of view it is just a treasure of information. Blood is not such a complex mixture. It contains fewer chemicals."[5] Far from being bizarre, Burzynski's method of isolating antineoplastons falls squarely within mainstream science.

Antineoplastons, being species-specific, are not generally effective in experiments on laboratory animals. Because of this, Dr. Burzynski received permission to do clinical trials on cancer patients at Houston's Twelve Oaks Hospital. The results were extremely impressive, with the antineoplastons having a pronounced effect on cancers unresponsive to chemotherapy and radiation. But, just as the doctor was proving the efficacy of antineoplastons on human patients, the hospital withdrew its permission for him to do further tests, the National Cancer Institute got cold feet and cancelled his funding, and the American Cancer Society refused him research money.

So, with entrepreneurial spirit, an undaunted Dr. Burzynski quit his job at Baylor University in 1977 and struck out on his own, establishing his own laboratory so that he could manufacture antineoplastons and treat patients himself. His only savings was $5,000, and he was forced to turn to bank loans to keep the operation alive. Today, the Burzynski Research Institute has three facilities in Houston, including a large pharmaceutical plant, and employs a staff of doctors, engineers, and lab technicians.

In 1983, Burzynski submitted an Investigational New Drug (IND)

Application, which took the foot-dragging FDA six years to approve. As a result of the approval, the doctor is currently seeking funding to do a Phase II trial on the effects of Antineoplaston A10 on patients with advanced breast cancer, to be conducted at an institute independent of his clinic.

Perhaps the most important preclinical study on antineoplastons, according to Dr. Burzynski, was done by the pathology department of the United States Department of Defense in Bethesda, Maryland, in 1989. Researchers there demonstrated that using Antineoplaston AS2-1 in tissue culture changes cancer cells into normal cells after approximately two to three days. These "corrected" cells behave completely like normal cells until they die, unless the medicine is removed from the culture medium too soon.[6]

"This means that when we are treating a patient who has cancer . . . we have to maintain a certain consistent concentration of antineoplastons in their body, in their blood," comments Dr. Burzynski. "If we slow down too soon, then we have to start from scratch, because the cell will begin to multiply again and simply go toward the cancerous way of life."

Antineoplastons appear to be remarkably effective in the early diagnosis and prevention of cancer. Researchers at the Medical College of Georgia in Augusta demonstrated that Antineoplaston A10 significantly delayed the appearance of inborn tumors in mice.[7] Low doses of synthetic Antineoplaston A10 administered orally can prevent lung, breast, and liver cancer in animals, according to research carried out at the University of Kurume Medical School in Japan and the Burzynski Research Institute. Antineoplastons show great promise as part of a preventive program against cancer in humans. Seemingly healthy individuals who have low levels of antineoplastons, such as smokers, would be prime candidates for that type of program. The possibilities of Burzynski's "new medicine" appear endless since, in addition to cancer, errors in cell programming can lead to such diverse disorders as benign tumors, certain skin diseases, AIDS (acquired immune deficiency syndrome), genital warts, and Parkinson's disease.

All patients at the Burzynski Clinic are treated on an outpatient basis. The initial patient response to treatment can be evaluated by standard medical tests, usually within the first three to six weeks of care. While patients receive treatment, clinical evaluations are made, including tumor measurements, radiologic studies, and a total laboratory profile. Most patients show virtually no side effects; a small percentage experience just minor adverse reactions such as skin rashes, slightly changed blood pressure, chills, or fever. In contrast to toxic chemotherapy and radiotherapy, antineoplaston therapy can actually create beneficial side effects, including increases in white- and red-blood-cell counts and decreases in blood cholesterol.

According to the clinic, the treatment does not interfere with surgery, radiation, nor various forms of conventional chemotherapy or immunotherapy. In fact, for some types of cancer, antineoplastons are used together with a small dose of chemotherapy. Such combination treatments are usually free of chemo's adverse reactions because the dose of chemotherapy given is very small. In addition, the depression of bone marrow that occurs under chemotherapy is offset by the antineoplastons, which actually stimulate bone-marrow function.

In addition to the successes against brain tumors, the clinic reports its most favorable results are obtained against lymphomas, such as non-Hodgkin's lymphoma; prostate cancer; certain forms of breast cancer; and bladder cancer. The clinic claims an objective response in treating advanced cancer of the pancreas, with two patients in remission for three years. Certain types of cancer do not respond well to antineoplaston therapy. For instance, the clinic does not accept patients with childhood leukemia or testicular cancer.

A small number of AIDS patients have been treated at the Burzynski Clinic. Most of them reportedly had marked improvement in their white-blood-cell counts, with their *T4 cells* (the white blood cells particularly affected by AIDS) increasing after the first four weeks of treatment. Most AIDS patients take Antineoplaston AS2-1 orally, in capsule form. According to Dr. Burzynski, "Antineoplaston AS2-1 will block the 'AIDS program' which is in the DNA of the cell. The cell will undergo specialization and function normally. The virus will not be able to multiply in a cell which is not dividing, and when the cell dies, the virus will die also. Hopefully, this will be the main benefit for the patient."

While scientists in countries such as Japan, Poland, and the Commonwealth of Independent States (formerly the Soviet Union) actively pursue antineoplaston research, the American medical establishment has been dragging its heels. At the time of this writing, the National Cancer Institute finally agreed to conduct four independent Phase II trials of antineoplaston therapy on patients with brain tumors.

Dr. Burzynski maintains a calm, single-minded perseverance in the face of opposition. With philosophical detachment, he once said, "Most medical breakthroughs have happened because there was some lack of suppression by the supervisors of people doing some innovative work. For instance, the introduction of insulin happened after experiments were performed by Dr. Banting in the absence of the head of his laboratory. He went for a vacation to Europe, and this allowed Dr. Banting to have some freedom to do the experiments. . . .

"That they leave you alone—this is the best you can hope for, yes. Louis Pasteur's discovery was suppressed for about 22 years, and the reason why it was finally accepted was because Louis Pasteur was allowed to do a final experiment to indicate the effectiveness of his vaccinations. The experiment was constructed in a way that his adversaries thought would never succeed, and they set it up this way to prove that the discovery was not working. But they made an error. They allowed a certain degree of freedom. They allowed him to do the experiment, hoping that it would fail—but it succeeded."[8]

Resources

Burzynski Clinic
6221 Corporate Drive
Houston, TX 77036
Phone: 713-777-8233

For further information on antineoplaston therapy and details on treatment.

Reading Material

Gary Null's Complete Guide to Healing Your Body Naturally, by Gary Null (see Appendix A for description).

The Cancer Industry: Unravelling the Politics, by Ralph W. Moss (see Appendix A for description).

Burzynski Clinic, written and published by the Burzynski Clinic (see above for address and phone number). Patient brochure.

Chapter 3

GASTON NAESSENS

A French biologist now living in Canada, Gaston Naessens developed a nontoxic treatment for cancer and other degenerative diseases. Called 714-X, the compound is an aqueous solution of nitrogen-enriched camphor molecules. Camphor is a natural substance derived chiefly from the camphor tree of eastern Asia. The camphor-nitrogen compound is injected into the body's lymphatic system, usually via the lymphatic area in the groin. Circulating in the body, it is said to strengthen the patient's debilitated immune system, which then rids the body of disease.

Based on forty years of microscopic and biologic research, Naessens' treatment has restored to health hundreds of cancer patients, many of them diagnosed by orthodox doctors as terminal. It seems to have also helped stabilize several dozen cases of AIDS. Many patients experience dramatic benefits, including relief of pain, improved appetite and weight gain, increased strength, cessation of vomiting, and feelings of well-being.

A course of treatment consists of daily injections for at least three 21-day periods, with a 3-day rest between each period. For advanced or metastatic cancer, an average of seven to twelve periods is recommended. Patients can be taught to self-administer the treatment.

Despite his therapeutic successes and important scientific discoveries, Naessens has been relentlessly persecuted by Canada's medical establishment. His theories and methods compete with vested interests and challenge conventional dogma. The Canadian media have imposed a virtual blackout on his work. In Canada, where Quebec's medical-drug complex has dismissed Naessens' treatment as worthless, 714-X is available through the emergency drug branch of the federal government for patients suffering from degenerative diseases. Treatment is also currently available through the Centre d'Orthobiologie Somatidienne de l'Estrie (C.O.S.E.), located in Rock Forest, Quebec. For patients outside of Canada, the Naessens remedies can be obtained with a special export permit by doctor's prescription. They are also readily available in Western Europe, where they are distributed by a Swiss pharmaceutical firm. A number of doctors in the United States are currently using 714-X. In Mexico, 714-X treatment can be obtained at certain clinics, including Genesis West–Provida in Tijuana.

One physician who has had positive results with 714-X is Warren Harrison, who practices in Washington, D.C. Dr. Harrison has treated six cancer patients with 714-X since April 1991. "All results have been favorable thus far," he reports. One patient, whose breast cancer had been surgically removed three years earlier, came to Dr. Harrison with a malignant node under her arm "at least as large as a walnut." Through treatment with the 714-X compound, the node has been reduced to one-fifth of its previous size and the woman's constant fatigue has disappeared.

Another of Harrison's patients had an ovarian cyst so large that it made her appear four or five months pregnant. The cancer had also metastasized. By the end of four months of treatment with the Naessens compound, the mass had grown dramatically smaller. The woman had regained her appetite, and her strength had greatly improved. "With all six patients," says Dr. Harrison, "a feeling of calm and well-being was observed within two to three days of commencing treatment, followed by reduction in the size of the tumor and relief from discomfort." Though he only began treating cancer patients with 714-X recently and thus cannot make a definitive judgment, he finds the results highly encouraging.[1]

Two doctors from Hanover, Massachusetts, Richard Cohen, M.D., and David Ganong, D.D.S., are overseeing cases in which patients are using 714-X on themselves. They attended a June 1991 symposium on Naessens in Quebec with Dr. Ganong's father, who had lung cancer. The elder Ganong's blood picture, shown on-screen during the live demonstrations, looked "the worst of all," said the younger Ganong. After two weeks of 714-X treatment, the blood picture cleared up remarkably and Mr. Ganong began to look better. Less than two months after the symposium, "his cancer doctor decided they could go in and get the tumor, which had been changed into an apparently nonthreatening jellylike mass he'd never seen the likes of before," Dr. Ganong told science reporter Peter Tocci.[2]

In 1990, Naessens put together a thick file of medical dossiers documenting cancer victims brought into remission or substantially helped by his therapy. This was in response to a request from Canada's Health Ministry. One of the cases involved a fifty-two-year-old man diagnosed in 1977 with a prostate cancer affecting the lymphatic ganglia and surrounding tissue. After exploratory surgery, the hospital's cancer committee recommended cutting out the prostate and all cancerous tissue. The patient refused and also turned down all other forms of aggressive conventional treatment. Instead, he undertook a complete course of 714-X treatment and was brought into remission. Follow-up hospital tests in 1989 revealed that he was cancer-free. Many other dramatic cases are presented in Christopher Bird's book *The Persecution and Trial of Gaston Naessens: The True Story of the Efforts to Suppress an Alternative Treatment for Cancer, AIDS, and Other Immunologically Based Diseases* (see Resources).[3]

While in France in the 1950s, Naessens invented a high-powered microscope capable of viewing living organisms far smaller than can be seen with the best light microscopes today. Using ultraviolet and incandescent light, with a magnification of 30,000, Naessens' microscope represents a major advance over the electron microscope, which requires specimens to be in a vacuum, thus killing them. With Naessens' Somatoscope, as his microscope is called, the tiniest known *live* microorganisms can be seen swimming, metabolizing, and reproducing with unparalleled clarity. In a letter dated September 6, 1989, Rolf Wieland, senior microscopy expert for the world's foremost optics firm, Carl Zeiss, described the Naessens microscope in these words: "What I have seen is a remarkable advancement in light microscopy. . . . It seems to be an avenue that should be pursued for the betterment of science."[4]

Using this remarkable microscope, Naessens discovered a previously unknown, infinitesimal living and reproducing microorganism in the blood, which he named a *somatid* ("tiny body"). Somatids circulate by the millions in the bloodstream and are also present in animals and in plant sap. Naessens believes they are a precursor of DNA, something leading to DNA's creation. He succeeded in culturing (growing under glass) these ultramicroscopic specks of life and discovered that they are pleomorphic, or form-changing. They normally go through a three-stage developmental cycle: somatid, spore, double spore. Naessens postulated that this three-stage cycle allows normal cell division to occur in the body through the somatids' production of a special growth hormone.

Through years of painstaking observation, Naessens learned that when the immune system of a human or animal is weakened by pollution, radiation, stress, shock, or some other trauma, the somatid goes through thirteen additional stages, for a total of sixteen separate forms, with each evolving into the next. By following the somatid cycle in the blood of people suffering from various degenerative diseases, he has correlated the somatid forms in the sixteen-stage disease cycle with specific disorders such as cancer, rheumatoid arthritis, multiple sclerosis, and lupus. He maintains that through an analysis of somatid conditions in the blood, all of these illnesses can be diagnosed up to eighteen months *before* the onset of clinical symptoms.

Naessens says the sixteen-stage somatid cycle is an indicator or herald of disease, rather than the cause of disease. His work appears to offer an important new way of evaluating the status of immune defense systems and assessing disease states or their absence. In June 1991, he unveiled a new light-gathering condenser—adaptable to most light microscopes—which he says enables anyone to see the phenomena he has been observing for nearly forty years.

Naessens has photographed and filmed the dance of the somatids. A fifty-five-minute videocassette that he recently released shows somatids in all the growth stages in full microscopic view. Other scientists and physicians have attested to the validity of Naessens' discoveries. Raymond Keith Brown, M.D., hired by the Sloan-Kettering Institute for Cancer Research to investigate alternative treatment methods, dispatched the following memo on Naessens in 1974 to the director of New York's Memorial Sloan-Kettering Cancer Center:

> What I have seen is a microscope that reveals with spectacular clarity the motion and multiplicity of pleomorphic organisms in the blood which are intimately associated with disease states.
>
> The implications of what this microscope has revealed are staggering. . . . It is imperative that what its inventor, a dedicated biological scientist, is doing, and can do, be totally reviewed. I am convinced that he is an authentic genius and that his achievements cut across and illumine some of the most pertinent areas of medical science.
>
> If the review of his work is confirmatory, this man should be brought to New York and given unlimited support and facilities to continue his research.
>
> To quote from anesthesia annals: *"Gentlemen, this is no hoax!"*[5]

Brown published sharp color photographs of somatids in his 1986 book *AIDS, Cancer and the Medical Establishment.*[6] Dr. Jan Merta de Velehrad, a Czech-born Canadian, successfully replicated most of Naessens' observations using the Somatoscope; he also produced the 714-X compound and other Naessens remedies in a Scottish laboratory. Boston biochemist Boguslaw Lipinski, Ph.D., D.Sc., reviewed firsthand the ongoing investigations in Naessens' Canadian lab and wrote: "I believe that Monsieur Naessens' work should be given proper attention in order to fully explore the potential value of his research for the benefit of humanity. It might turn out that the cure for cancer is already available."[7]

Some researchers who accept pleomorphism nevertheless remain unconvinced of the existence of the somatid and its cycle. Among them are Beverly Rubik, Ph.D., director of Temple University's Center for Frontier Sciences in Philadelphia, and Neil Riordan of Wichita's Center for the Improvement of Human Functioning. "I've looked through the Somatoscope, and unless there's something I haven't been shown, I see no more there than I do through my modified dark field unit," says Riordan. Neither he nor Rubik believes that Naessens has provided a repeatable procedure for isolating and culturing the alleged somatid particle.[8]

Naessens views cancer as a disease of the whole organism, reflecting impaired immunity. In a healthy person, he says, the somatid cycle is limited to just three stages because inhibitors found in the blood control the pleomorphism. But when stress or biologic disturbances lower the concentration of the blood inhibitors, the somatid cycle goes wild, that is, it continues its natural evolution into thirteen more forms—bacterial, mycobacterial, yeastlike, filamentous, and so forth. This creates an abnormal build-up of trephones (growth hormones), which in turn have a disastrous effect on cellular metabolism.

Cells revert to a more primitive form. They start to get their energy by fermenting glucose (sugar) in oxygenless reactions instead of through normal oxidation, or respiration. (Otto Warburg, the German biochemist, won a Nobel Prize for his work demonstrating that deficient oxygenation of fermenting cells contributes to cancer.) The primitive cell loses the individualized functions that attach it to a particular organ: the cell "remembers" its earliest properties, especially the ability to multiply rapidly. Cancer is the ultimate result.

If the immune system is strong, it swings into action and fights to eliminate the precancerous agglomerations of cells that are constantly forming in the body. But if the immune system is weak, according to Naessens, the primitive cells attain a "critical mass" and form a tumor, which needs enormous amounts of nitrogen for subsistence. Naessens discovered that cancerous cells emit a substance, dubbed *CKF* (*Cocancerogenic K Factor*), that enables the tumor to rob the body of nitrogen derivatives. At the same time, CKF paralyzes the immune system's germ-destroying and tumor-fighting cells, leaving the body defenseless against the abnormal cell growth.

Naessens designed a therapy to reverse this situation. He found one answer to cancer in nitrogen-enriched camphor. The compound 714-X carries to the tumor cells all the nitrogen they need, thereby shutting down the tumor's production of CKF. This helps the immune system "come to its senses" and consider the tumor cells as a foreign body to be rejected or destroyed. The *leukocytes* (white blood cells that fight invaders) resume their activity, as do the other *phagocytes* that ingest and destroy foreign cells and microorganisms in the body.[9]

Some people associate camphor, a white, strong-smelling, crystalline substance, with mothballs. Camphor, originally from the wood of a tree, has been used in medicine for centuries as a stimulant and inhalant. Naessens' immune-boosting camphor derivative, 714-X, is not an *antimitotic* (a substance that retards cell growth). Its effectiveness against cancer stems from its ability to give nitrogen-hungry tumor cells all the nitrogen they require; this suppresses the secretion of immune-destroying CKF. And this is all done without side effects. (The high-tech-sounding name "714-X" has a simple origin: the "7" and "14" refer to the seventh and fourteenth letters of the alphabet— "G" and "N," Naessens' initials. "X" is the twenty-fourth letter of the alphabet, echoing the year of Naessens' birth, 1924.)

A criminal trial was brought against Naessens in late 1989 at the instigation of the Quebec Corporation of Physicians (a provincial equivalent of the American Medical Association). He was accused of causing the death of an already terminally ill woman who had come to him for treatment in an advanced condition after she had refused all other medical treatment. Naessens was fully acquitted on all five counts by a jury of his peers in a trial held in Sherbrooke, Quebec, just thirty miles north of Vermont. The jury refused to believe the allegation that Naessens had contributed in any way to the woman's death. Had he been found guilty of the most serious charge, he could have been sentenced to life in prison, which is exactly what Canada's medical establishment had hoped would happen.

Christopher Bird, who has closely followed Naessens' work for over fifteen years, attended the trial each day as the only foreign journalist-observer present. In his book *The Persecution and Trial of Gaston*

Naessens, Bird tells how ten witnesses, including one doctor—all of them recovered from serious forms of cancer—came from France to testify under oath to the success of Naessens' therapy. Because of their testimony, along with that of many other cancer survivors, the jury became convinced that the soft-spoken, distinguished biologist was a true scientist who had discovered something of potentially vast importance to humanity and not a charlatan, as the Quebec medical corporation's president had branded him.

One witness, a Canadian translator, Belgian-born Arnault de Kerckhove Varent, had been diagnosed in the late 1970s with a melanoma of the eye, one of the most lethal and fast-growing cancers. Cancer surgeons had strongly recommended enucleation (removing the eyeball from its socket). They told Varent he could expect to live nine to twelve months if he did not have the operation. Asked what Varent's survival time might be if he did have the procedure, the surgeons only said, "Then you begin to *pray!*" Refusing to take the orthodox medical advice, Varent sought out what he called a systemic treatment, one that would affect his whole body, not just the site of the tumor. He opted for 714-X, regained his health, and has outlived the death sentence handed down by the conventional physicians.[10]

Dr. Raymond Brown of New York City, a former Sloan-Kettering cancer researcher, told a pretrial press conference how he had treated one of his own patients with 714-X for a pancreatic cancer that had proven resistant to all other forms of treatment. Naessens' therapy had prolonged the patient's life well over expectancy and kept him free of side effects, he said. Dr. Brown declared that while 714-X was not a panacea, it deserved a place in the arsenal of weapons available to official medicine. Also, Belgian physician Florianne Piers reported that over a four-month period, she had treated seven cancer patients with 714-X. "The product prolonged the lives, and eased the deaths, of two terminally afflicted patients," she said, "and has allowed the other five, who came to me with seriously advanced cancerous states, to see every one of their symptoms disappear and to take up their lives as if they had never incurred the disease."[11]

Ironically, Naessens had fled to Canada hoping to find the freedom to pursue his work without the legal harassment he had endured in France. He had begun his scientific studies at the University of Lille just before France was occupied by the Nazis during World War II. Evacuated to southern France, he received the equivalent of a university education under the tutelage of displaced professors. He was awarded a diploma from the Union Nationale Scientifique Française, but because he neglected to seek an "equivalence" from the new republican government, he has often been falsely accused of never having received any academic certification.

Naessens developed innovative anticancer products in France as well as remedies for a variety of degenerative diseases. When word of his successful treatments spread, the French medical authorities hauled him into court for the illegal practice of medicine. In the early 1960s, to escape harassment, he opened a small research laboratory on the Mediterranean French island of Corsica. Having developed a treatment for leukemia, he was besieged by desperate patients from all over the world. This incurred the wrath of France's medical orthodoxy, which took him to trial for the unlicensed practice of medicine. A top-ranking member of the French police bureaucracy—whose terminally ill wife, Suzanne Montjoint, Naessens had restored to health—confided in the biologist that he faced many years in prison. Naessens abruptly left his native country and, with the same official's help, settled in Quebec.

Not a physician, Naessens does not practice medicine, under the constant threat of legal persecution. Instead, he consults with doctors and advises them about how to use his remedies.

Naessens' scientific discoveries are potentially revolutionary in their implications for medicine, biology, and our understanding of life itself. Through careful, repeated experiments, Naessens has found that the somatids are virtually indestructible. They are totally unaffected by the strongest acids. They survive exposure to 50,000 rems of nuclear radiation, far more than the dosage needed to kill any living organism. They shrug off carbonization temperatures of 392°F (200°C) and higher. They cannot be cut with a diamond knife. Somatids seem imperishable! Surviving the death of their hosts, such as humans, they may return to the earth and live for millions of years. Exactly how or why or from what somatids take shape is not known.

"My belief," Naessens told a medical symposium in June 1991, "is that the somatid constitutes a transitional link between matter and cosmic energy. It may well be the first cosmic manifestation of life."[12]

If all this sounds like science fiction, it nevertheless has a scientific foundation. Antoine Béchamp (1816–1908), the great French bacteriologist, a contemporary and adversary of Louis Pasteur (1822–1895), discovered that all animal and plant cells contain tiny "grains," or granules, that under certain conditions evolve into bacteria and continue to live after the host organism dies. Béchamp called these living, indestructible granules of life *microzymas* ("small ferments") because the bacteria into which they evolve have fermentative proper-

ties. Clearly, Béchamp's microzymas are cousins of Naessens' somatids—or perhaps, they are one and the same thing.

Béchamp insisted that microzymas are not the cause of disease.
Rather, he said, they become destructive only when a host's internal
environment, or bodily "terrain," has deteriorated. Béchamp was a
distinguished medical doctor and professor who also had a doctorate
in chemistry. Through precise observation and experimentation, he
discovered that some microorganisms are pleomorphic. His theory
of disease was opposed to that of Pasteur, who posited eternally
nonchangeable microbes as the primary cause of illness. Pasteur, a
master of self-promotion, wove much of Béchamp's work into his own
without acknowledging Béchamp's priority. Pasteur plagiarized
Béchamp's discovery of the cause of wine fermentation, and he
allegedly plagiarized Béchamp's major discovery of antisepsis, the
technique of preventing infection. Pasteur ultimately acknowledged
the existence of microzymas in the blood, yet he continued to dispute
Béchamp's theory even after other researchers had observed the
same form-changing microorganisms.

Today, a large body of research on pleomorphic microbes is aggressively opposed by mainstream biologists, who stubbornly refuse to even
examine the evidence. Yet a number of alternative cancer therapies
besides Naessens' are based on firsthand, detailed observation of pleomorphic organisms. These include the immune therapy of Virginia
Livingston, M.D. (Chapter 7) and the electromagnetic frequency generator developed by American microscope inventor Royal Raymond Rife
(Chapter 25).

Naessens' work also ties in with the work of another unorthodox
genius, Wilhelm Reich, M.D., the Austrian-born psychoanalyst-
turned-biophysicist. Reich witnessed strange blue forms, living
particles that he called *bions*. Under the microscope, the bions
changed form when cancer developed, and Reich claimed to see
them spontaneously proliferate from specially treated grass, sand,
or coal. In cancer patients, he observed bions being transformed
into what he called T-bacilli ("T" for *tod*, which is German for
"death"). When injected into mice, the bions caused cancer.

Naessens was recently asked whether his somatids might be the
same as Reich's bions. He replied, "*Peut-être* [maybe]," as he simply
did not know.[13]

While Naessens is hailed by eminent doctors as one of the greatest
scientists of this—or any—century, the medical mainstream remains
blissfully ignorant of his discoveries and treatment methods. His

therapy, condemned without any investigation by the American Cancer Society, remains on the ACS Unproven Methods blacklist, that fertile repository of innovative and lifesaving treatments that threaten the profits of the medical monopoly.

Resources

C.O.S.E., Inc.
5270, Fontaine
Rock Forest, Quebec J1N 3B6
Canada
Phone: 819-564-7883

For further information on 714-X as well as a list of doctors in the United States who can provide information on it.

Genesis West–Provida
P.O. Box 3460
Chula Vista, CA 91902-0004
Phone: 619-424-9552

For further information on 714-X and details on treatment.

Reading Material

The Persecution and Trial of Gaston Naessens: The True Story of the Efforts to Suppress an Alternative Treatment for Cancer, AIDS, and Other Immunologically Based Diseases, by Christopher Bird, H. J. Kramer (P.O. Box 1082, Tiburon, CA 94920; 415-435-5367), 1991.

"Gaston Naessens vs. $cientific Medicine," by Christopher Bird, *Townsend Letter for Doctors*, vol. 94, May 1991.

Other Material

Video: *The Somatidian Orthobiology of Gaston Naessens*, 1991. Fifty-five minutes. Shows the complete cycle of the somatid in photomicrographs and animated diagrams. Also has sequences showing how 714-X treatment is administered and how the new condenser is adapted to popular models of light microscopes such as Zeiss, Nikon, Olympus, and Leitz. Available from C.O.S.E. (see above for address and phone number).

Chapter 4

REVICI THERAPY

Dr. Emanuel Revici has developed an original approach to the treatment of cancer. His nontoxic chemotherapy uses *lipids,* lipid-based substances, and essential elements to correct an underlying imbalance in the patient's chemistry. *Lipids*—organic compounds such as fatty acids and sterols—are important constituents of all living cells. They are a separate, critical system in the body's defenses against illness, according to research conducted by Dr. Revici early in his career.

The Romanian-born physician, who practices in New York City, has applied his wide-ranging discoveries for over sixty years to the treatment of cancer as well as many other disorders, including AIDS, arthritis, Alzheimer's disease, chronic pain, drug addiction, schizophrenia, allergies, shock, and burns. The great majority of his cancer patients are in advanced stages of the illness. Five, ten, sometimes twenty years after receiving treatment, some of these patients are in remission with no signs of active disease.

Revici, in his mid-nineties, is fiercely dedicated, still makes occasional house calls, and has patients call him at home. To critics, his approach is far too complex, too theoretical, and inconsistent in its results. Even friendly critics within the alternative health field say he cures very few cancer patients. But to admirers, he is a man who has saved the lives of cancer patients pronounced hopeless by orthodox doctors, a scientific genius who has opened up whole new vistas and whose theories and discoveries may serve as a principal basis for future medicine.

Commenting on Revici's 1961 book, *Research in Physiopathology as a Basis of Guided Chemotherapy With Special Applications to Cancer,* Dr. Gerhard Schrauzer, a leading authority on selenium, wrote, "I came to the conclusion that Dr. Revici is an innovative medical genius, outstanding chemist and a highly creative thinker. I also realized that few of his medical colleagues would be able to follow his train of thought and thus would be all too willing to dismiss his work."[1]

Dr. Revici views health as a dynamic balance between two opposing kinds of activity that occur in all living systems. One process, the *anabolic*, or constructive, fosters the growth and build-up of natural patterns. The other process is *catabolic*, or destructive, involving the breakdown of structure, the liberation of energy, and the utilization of stored resources. According to Dr. Revici, a long-term predominance of either activity leads to abnormality and disease.

In his "guided lipid" therapy with cancer patients, Revici has found two basic patterns of lipid imbalance—one, the result of an excess of sterols, and the other, the result of an excess of fatty acids. Sterols are solid unsaturated alcohols such as cholesterol. In treating cancer, Revici first determines whether the anabolic or catabolic phase of activity is currently progressing unchecked. Then he administers lipid-based compounds to renormalize the balance between the body's opposing forces.

Revici describes the body's overall defense system as consisting of four successive phases. When an antigen, or foreign substance, such as a virus or microbe, enters an organism, it activates the defense system. In the first phase, the antigen is broken down by *enzymes*. This is followed by the *lipidic* phase, followed in turn by the *coagulant antibody* phase, and succeeded finally by a phase mediated by *globulinic antibodies* able to fully neutralize the antigen.

The key point about this defense system is that a new phase does not start until the previous phase has been successfully completed. At any point where the agents available are qualitatively insufficient to defend against the noxious influence, the sequence breaks down. Then the body overcompensates by manufacturing excessive amounts of the defense agents from the breakdown point, and it does not progress to the next phase. Revici found that most chronic diseases, including cancer, are characterized by such abnormal conditions. When the body's defense is arrested in the lipidic phase, either fatty acids or sterols are produced in abnormally large quantities, leading to a variety of disorders, including cancer.

Patients diagnosed with an excess of sterols are treated with fatty acids to correct the imbalance. Conversely, patients found to have a predominance of fatty acids are treated with sterols and other agents.

This "biologically guided chemotherapy," as Dr. Revici calls it, is highly individualized to suit each person's specific metabolic character and condition. "There are simply no two cancers which are alike, just as no two individuals are alike," he has said.[2] The substances and dosages used are unique for each patient and can be changed if analytical tests reveal a change in the body's balance. Through regular tests, such as the urine pH, specific gravity, surface tension, and chloride index, Dr. Revici can detect systemic changes in the body produced by lipid imbalances.

Revici's research has demonstrated that lipids have an affinity for tumors and other abnormal tissues. Because of this, the lipids or lipid-like synthetic compounds administered to the patient, either by mouth or injection, travel directly to the tumor or lesion. Cancerous tissue is abnormally rich in free lipids, and the lipidic agents introduced into the bloodstream are readily taken up by the tumor.

Revici's nontoxic cancer therapy has been denied both fair testing and funding in the United States, though it has been studied and put into practice in France, Italy, and Austria. A distinguished physician and research scientist who graduated first in his class at the University of Bucharest, Dr. Revici has been stereotypically portrayed by the American media as a quack who should have been put out of business a long time ago. The American Cancer Society put Revici's therapy on its Unproven Methods blacklist in 1961, and in 1984, the State of New York tried to revoke his medical license permanently on grounds of deviation from standard medicine, negligence, incompetence, fraud, the use of unapproved experimental drugs, and similar charges. After four years of struggle, Revici triumphed in July 1988 with a decision that placed him on probation but allows him to continue treating cancer patients.

To save his license, Revici's patients and several medical civil-liberties groups undertook intensive lobbying at the state capitol. At the federal level, New York Congressman Guy Molinari held an all-day hearing in March 1988 to address the Revici matter and the whole field of alternative cancer therapies. Dr. Seymour Brenner, a respected radiation oncologist in private practice in New York, testified on Revici's behalf. He had investigated a number of patients in very advanced stages of cancer, incurable by orthodox means, whom Revici had put into long remissions. Dr. Brenner had an independent panel of pathologists confirm the diagnosis and stage of illness prior to each patient's initial visit to Revici. He testified that his personal findings strongly suggest Revici has a cancer treatment deserving further study, and he proposed that such an evaluation be conducted by the FDA.

In a letter to Congressman Molinari, Brenner outlined a protocol in which a panel of doctors would monitor cancer patients placed on alternative therapies after their conditions had been deemed unamenable to the standard forms of treatment. The letter contained the detailed case histories of ten advanced cancer patients whom Revici had healed.

One patient, a forty-three-year-old man, was diagnosed with an invasive, high-grade cancer of the bladder at Memorial Sloan-Kettering Cancer Center in September 1980. "They said, 'The only way you can be treated is if we take your bladder out and give you a colostomy on the side.' He said no."[3] The patient visited Dr. Revici in October and went on the therapy. He has had no other treatment. In 1987, he returned to Sloan-Kettering for a cystoscopy, which revealed him to be cancer-free.

Another patient, a twenty-nine-year-old woman, was operated on at Memorial Sloan-Kettering in October 1983 for a chordoma, a brain tumor. The tumor was incompletely resected, and the patient was given a course of radiation therapy. The young woman's condition progressively worsened during the twelve months following surgery. She was seen by Dr. Revici in May 1984, at which time she was confined to a wheelchair, with limited function. Since she started the Revici program, she has had two babies and functions well. Her only problem is that she walks with a cane.

Marianne Dimetres achieved remission from preterminal uterine cancer through a combination of Revici's nontoxic medications, wheatgrass therapy, diet, and psychological support. See her story on page 157.

Revici, who holds patents for his numerous chemical compounds, claims to have devised a novel technique to open double bonds in molecules of unsaturated fatty acids in order to incorporate different metallic elements at precise points in the molecules. The result is an entirely new series of therapeutic compounds, exceedingly low in toxicity and incorporating selenium, copper, sulfur, zinc, calcium, nickel, beryllium, mercury, lead, and other elements. In general, these compounds reportedly have a toxicity less than one-thousandth of that of the elements in the forms normally available. The technique converts toxic substances into safe anticancer agents. "Through this method, Revici has opened up an entirely new field for the therapeutic use of these elements," according to Dr. Dwight McKee, one of Revici's medical associates.[4]

Revici's use of selenium in the treatment of cancer predates mainstream interest in this mineral by more than twenty years. Selenium is one of the major trace elements always found deficient in cancer-prone populations. Research has shown that it is of value not only in preventing cancer but also in treating it. Revici uses a special molecular form of selenium (bivalent-negative selenium) incorporated in a molecule of fatty acid. In this form, he can administer up to 1 gram of selenium per day, which corresponds to 1 million micrograms per day, reportedly with no toxic side effects. In contrast, too much selenite (hexavalent-positive selenium) has toxic effects on animals, so human intake of commercial selenite is limited to a dosage of only 100 to 150 micrograms by mouth. Dr. Revici often administers his nontoxic form of selenium by injection, usually considered to be four times more powerful than the form given orally.

Extra selenium in the diet drastically reduces the spontaneous occurrence of cancer in mice. In human populations, high selenium intake correlates with low cancer rates. In a 140-patient study of cancer victims treated with selenium, Dr. R. Donaldson of the St. Louis Veterans' Administration Hospital reported in 1983 that some patients deemed terminal with only weeks to live were completely free of all signs of cancer after four years; all the patients showed a reduction in tumor size and in pain.[5]

Dr. Revici uses the Periodic Table of Elements as one of several guides when choosing the best course of treatment for a patient. This ties in with his view that cancer is part of a hierarchical organization found throughout Nature, from the precellular level to the entire organism. All the known elements, in his view, can be classified as supporting either anabolic or catabolic activity, and each element's biological activity correlates with its position in the Periodic Table. Revici maintains that the vertical rows in the table all share either anabolic or catabolic activity, whereas the horizontal rows indicate at which level of biological organization a particular element acts—whether at the level of a subnuclear particle (nucleoprotein), nucleus, cell, tissue, organ, or whole body. By this means, Dr. Revici determines the body level (or levels) most affected by the illness and therefore most in need of therapeutic intervention. This information is correlated with diagnostic tests indicating which imbalance is present at which level.

Harassed for decades by the American medical monopoly, Revici, ironically, had originally come to the United States seeking freedom to do his work. A scientific prodigy, he had written his first research manuscript at the age of twelve and entered the University of Bucharest at seventeen. In 1936, after serving as an assistant professor on the Faculty of Medicine, he moved with his family to Paris, where he spent three years investigating the biochemistry of cancer. When World War II erupted, the Revicis fled to Nice, where the doctor joined the French Resistance and gave medical aid to wounded Resistance fighters sought by the Nazis. His anti-fascist activities so endangered him and his wife and daughter that the leaders of the French

Underground had to arrange for the family's passage out of Europe.[6] The Revicis settled in Mexico, where Dr. Revici founded the first Institute of Applied Biology, in Mexico City.

Eager to advance his research in the United States, Dr. Revici was granted three special visas through the intercession of Sumner Welles, a special aide to President Franklin D. Roosevelt.[7] Revici moved to Chicago, then to New York, establishing the institute anew in Brooklyn in 1947. Today, his office is located in a two-story building in Manhattan, where he treats patients aided by a small support staff.

By 1948, Revici had begun exploring the use of selenium in treating cancer and as a means for rendering radiation less harmful. His promising findings on radiation came to the attention of United States Navy scientists testing A-bombs in the Pacific. Twice, the scientists invited him to join them in studying radiation's harmful effects.

In 1954, Revici's fund-raising organization financed the purchase of Beth David Hospital in Manhattan. Renamed Trafalgar Hospital, this general-care facility employing over 200 resident and visiting physicians enabled Revici, as the chief of oncology, to provide round-the-clock care for critically ill patients. Its animal research laboratories were staffed by 35 scientists and technicians, all involved in projects related to Revici's theories and therapeutic approach. Revici served as chief of Trafalgar's oncology department for over twenty years. The hospital closed in 1978 due to financial difficulties.

Revici's treatment agents were used in Belgium with favorable results by Professor Joseph Maisin, president of the International Union Against Cancer and director of the Cancer Institute of the University of Louvain. Between 1965 and his death from a car accident in 1971, Maisin corresponded with Revici to describe how he treated patients with advanced metastatic cancer who had failed conventional therapies. Maisin used several Revici preparations, at times coupled with low-dose radiation. He reported that in nine of the twelve terminal-cancer patients on the Revici medicines, significant improvements occurred, including regression of tumors, disappearance of metastases, and cessation of hemorrhage. Incredibly, paralyzed patients were able to walk again.

Dr. Revici developed successful treatments for heroin and alcohol addiction. His detoxification agent for heroin addicts, called Perse, was almost chosen over methadone as the nation's treatment of choice. Perse, which incorporated selenium in a lipid base, physically detoxified addicts within five to eight days. At the request of Congress, Revici presented over 2,000 case histories of successful uses of this nontoxic and nonaddictive agent. The idea for Perse had arisen from Revici's cancer practice after he observed that patients previously on addictive narcotic analgesics exhibited no withdrawal symptoms when placed on his lipid analgesics.

At a 1971 congressional subcommittee hearing that took testimony about Perse for a full day, Congressman Charles Rangel of New York said, "The results and what we witnessed with patients was so unbelievable that the doctor from Municipal Hospital has now gone back on a daily basis in order to continue with this chance to see the miraculous results that have taken place."

Barron's ran a full-page feature on Revici's treatments for narcotic and alcohol addiction in 1972. Both Congress and the FDA promised Dr. Revici full support for large-scale clinical testing, signaling that Perse could be the most important breakthrough in drug treatment. Because selenium is normally toxic in high doses, Revici reformulated the medication to eliminate it. The new substance, called Bionar, worked just as well—in the same amount of time, with no withdrawal symptoms. (The selenium incorporated in Perse was a bivalent-negative form, very active and virtually nontoxic.)

The stage seemed set for a major advance in the war on drugs. But less than one month after the congressional hearing, the FDA reversed its position and recommended methadone, an addictive and toxic drug, as the treatment of choice. Why?

One possible answer is provided by Marcus Cohen, who helped coordinate the campaign to save Revici's license. He suggests, "Hospitalization was required for treatment with Perse, and because many of the patients were poor, Medicaid was asked to pick up the tab. As in the case of most drug addicts, they presented with other conditions besides addiction which needed medical attention. . . . Methadone, addicting in itself, nevertheless was favored by State and City officials as a means of controlling the mostly black and Hispanic drug population. . . . The drug companies and health care professionals that profited from exclusive use of methadone did not welcome competition, least of all from a treatment which did not cause a lifelong dependency."[8]

Dr. Revici's nontoxic treatment for AIDS applies his findings on the antiviral and immune-enhancing properties of certain lipids. He views AIDS as a "quadruple pathological condition," consisting of:

1. a primary viral infection, inducing
2. a deficiency in the body's natural lipidic defense, followed by
3. secondary opportunistic infections or specific neoplasms (cancers) due to the lack of certain lipids, resulting in
4. an exaggerated imbalance, usually catabolic.

Each of the four conditions is addressed with a specific therapeutic approach. Antiviral agents are given to inactivate, or kill, the human immunodeficiency virus (HIV). To counteract the patient's nonspecific loss of defense against opportunistic infections, Dr. Revici administers, via injection, a group of phospholipids that he calls refractoriness lipids. These compounds appear to induce a generalized resistance (refractoriness) toward many different antigens. The doctor claims impressive results with these preparations in the clinical manifestations of AIDS and AIDS Related Complex (ARC). Antibiotics are also given to combat the secondary opportunistic infections. To redress bodily imbalances, the appropriate anticatabolic or antianabolic agents are used.

Two of Revici's therapeutic compounds for cancer, amyl selenide and tri-thioformaldehyde (TT), tested positive in trials conducted in the late 1970s by the National Cancer Institute and Roswell Park Memorial Institute.[9] Another selenium compound that Revici developed showed activity against four tumor systems in tests conducted in England. However, the dose at which antitumor activity was found was "fairly close to the toxic dose," and further studies of the compound were recommended.

An unpublished study of the 1,047 cancer patients treated with the Revici regimen between 1946 and 1955 was made by Robert Ravich, M.D., who worked closely with Revici. Most of the patients were far advanced or terminal, and most had prior conventional treatment. Of the 1,047 cases, Ravich found that 100 had favorable response (objective and subjective); 11 had objective response only; 95 had subjective response only; 296 showed no response; and 545 had equivocal or undetermined response (380 of this last group were treated for less than three months).[10]

The only published clinical study of Revici's treatment for cancer appeared in the *Journal of the American Medical Association* (*JAMA*) in 1965. It was written by a panel of nine New York physicians after Revici himself requested that a scientific panel review his cancer-management program. After two years of observation, the panel concluded that the Revici therapy was "without value." The authors reported that 22 of the 33 patients in the study died of cancer or its complications while on the Revici treatment and 4 more died after discontinuing the regimen. None of the 33 showed signs of objective tumor regression, according to the authors.

Dr. Revici wrote a detailed rebuttal in which he stated that the panel had ignored evidence indicating several tumor remissions, multiple reductions in tumor size, and relief of pain in many advanced patients. He noted that of the nine physicians on the panel, only two had actually seen the patients during the entire two-year study. He further commented that he had requested the study in the "hope that the demonstration of positive results in even a few of these advanced cases would excite sufficient interest to lead to a large-scale study of our approach. . . . To conclude from a limited study, such as this, that the method should be discontinued, *in all cancers*, is to say that since surgery and radiation have failed in these same terminal patients, these 'recognized' methods should also be discontinued, not only in these types of cancer but in all cancers in general." Although Dr. Revici submitted substantiating pathological data in his lengthy rebuttal, *JAMA* refused to publish it.

It is now more than forty years since Revici developed his nontoxic chemotherapy. An open-minded, unbiased evaluation of it is long overdue.

Resources

Emanuel Revici, M.D.
26 East 36th Street
New York, NY 10016
Phone: 212-685-0111

For further information on Revici therapy and details on treatment.

Reading Material

Cancer and Consciousness, by Barry Bryant, Sigo Press (P.O. Box 8748, 25 New Chardon Street, Boston, MA 02114; 508-281-4722), 1990. Contains an interview with Emanuel Revici.

"Research and Theoretical Background for Treatment of the Acquired Immunodeficiency Syndrome (AIDS)," by Emanuel Revici, M.D., *Townsend Letter for Doctors*, vol. 45, February–March 1987. Contains an in-depth discussion of aspects of Revici's treatment for cancer and AIDS.

Emanuel Revici, M.D.: A Review of His Scientific Work, by Dwight L. McKee, M.D., Institute of Applied Biology (see above for address and phone number), March 1985. A fairly technical nineteen-page booklet.

"On Emanuel Revici, M.D.," by Marcus A. Cohen, Institute of Applied Biology (see above for address and phone number), 1988. Typescript. A valuable source of information on Dr. Revici's life and work.

Chapter 5

HYDRAZINE SULFATE

Hydrazine sulfate, a simple, off-the-shelf chemical, dramatically reverses cachexia (ka-KEK-si-a), the wasting-away process that kills two-thirds of all cancer patients. This inexpensive drug, with little or no side effects, also has a clinically documented antitumor action. It causes malignant tumors to stop growing, to reduce in size, and, in some cases, to disappear. A growing number of cancer patients diagnosed as terminal have experienced tumor stabilization and remission through hydrazine sulfate therapy.

About half of all patients who take hydrazine sulfate experience weight gain, restored appetite, extended survival time, and a significant reduction in pain and suffering. Many patients report an increase in vigor and strength and the disappearance of symptoms of the disease, along with feelings of well-being and optimism.

While hydrazine sulfate may not be a sure-fire cancer cure, large-scale clinical trials suggest that it affects every type of tumor at every stage. It can be administered either alone or in combination with cytotoxic chemotherapy or radiation to make the cancer more vulnerable to these standard forms of treatment.

Hydrazine sulfate is now undergoing Phase III trials sponsored by the National Cancer Institute. It is available to patients as a "compassionate IND [Investigational New Drug]," a designation conferred by the Food and Drug Administration on a case-by-case basis, so it is no longer, strictly speaking, an "unconventional therapy." Yet even though hundreds of patients across the country are using the drug, it is not widely discussed or disseminated among practicing physicians and its promise remains largely untapped twenty-four years after it was first proposed as an anticancer treatment by Dr. Joseph Gold. Meanwhile, hydrazine sulfate is widely available in the Commonwealth of Independent States (formerly the Soviet Union), where researchers have followed up on Gold's pioneering work with over ten years of investigation supporting the drug's effectiveness.

"We've gone from a red light to a yellow light, and hopefully will go to a green light," says Dr. Gold, director of the Syracuse Cancer Research Institute in Syracuse, New York, which he founded in 1966. Since his discovery in 1968 that hydrazine sulfate can prevent the wasting-away process in cancer patients and inhibit tumor growth, Gold has waged a courageous uphill battle to win acceptance for his nontoxic chemotherapy by the medical establishment.

The American Cancer Society put hydrazine sulfate on its Unproven Methods blacklist in 1976. It condemned and stigmatized the drug following a clinical trial on twenty-nine patients at Memorial Sloan-Kettering Cancer Center in New York. But it is now widely acknowledged that the Sloan-Kettering tests were botched.

When Dr. Gold made an unannounced visit to the hospital in 1974, he discovered, to his horror, that "many patients in the study were either being underdosed or overdosed. Some people who were beginning to show anticachexia response were suddenly being given 90 to 100 milligrams at one time. All this was in clear violation of the drug protocols and of our joint agreements," said Gold.[1] The study's protocol called for patients to receive 60 milligrams once a day for the first three days, twice a day for the next three days, and three times a day for the following six weeks. Therefore, some patients were getting a 67 percent overdose.

In a letter of protest to Sloan-Kettering,[2] Gold pointed out that some patients were receiving a massive, single dose of approximately 120 to 190 milligrams a day (instead of the usual two or three 60-milligram doses), "which quickly wiped out whatever good response they were beginning to show." The study was so poorly executed that it could never be published today, he maintains.

Nevertheless, the damage was done. The ACS's blacklisting of hydrazine sulfate caused Gold's funding to dry up and scared away other researchers from following up on his early papers.

But Gold refused to give up. In 1975, he did a study of the drug's effects on eighty-four advanced cancer patients. A total of 70 percent of them experienced weight gain (or the cessation of weight loss) and reduced pain. Only 17 percent showed tumor improvements. Meanwhile, Russian scientists at Leningrad's Petrov Research Institute were getting impressive results. In one study of forty-eight terminal cancer patients treated with hydrazine sulfate, 35 percent had tumor stabilization or regression and 59 percent showed "subjective response" (ability to function normally, complete disappearance or marked reduction of pain, and so forth).

As a result of these and other favorable studies, the American Cancer Society announced in 1979 that it was removing hydrazine sulfate from its official blacklist. Only four other "unproven methods" that were once stigmatized on the ACS list as "quackery" have been removed from it. However, the ACS included hydrazine sulfate in the 1979 edition of the Unproven Methods list, and that edition continued to be circulated until 1982. Hydrazine sulfate was finally removed from the list the next time the list was revised, in July 1982.[3]

Tim Hansen, now in his early twenties, of Minneapolis, Kansas, is one person grateful for the existence of hydrazine sulfate therapy. In August 1984, when he was eleven years old, Tim was diagnosed with three inoperable malignant tumors that were growing quickly in his brain. He was placed on radiation therapy, but his health steadily deteriorated until, by early 1985, his weight had dropped to fifty-five pounds. "The radiation harmed his mental functioning, and in January 1985 the surgeon told me that Tim had one week to live," says Gloria Hansen, Tim's mother.

In February, after reading a short item about hydrazine sulfate in *McCall's*, Gloria and her husband, Ray, got in touch with Dr. Gold, and Tim was put on hydrazine sulfate therapy by his physicians in Kansas. By August, his weight was up to seventy-five pounds. By early 1987, two of Tim's tumors had completely vanished. In January 1991, a computerized axial tomograph (CAT scan) revealed further shrinkage of the remaining tumor, located in the base of the brain. Dr. Gold plans to keep Tim on the hydrazine sulfate protocol until the tumor is completely gone. Tim graduated from high school in 1990 and is now studying electronics at a trade school, getting A's and B's.

Dr. Gold first stumbled upon hydrazine sulfate's anticancer properties during his methodical quest for a specific type of therapy. Cancer has two principal devastating effects on the body. One is the invasion of the tumor into the vital organs, with the destruction of the organs' functions—the most common cause of cancer death in the public's mind. In reality, however, this accounts for only about 23 percent of the country's half-million annual cancer deaths.

The other devastating effect of cancer is cachexia, the terrible wasting away of the body, with its attendant weight loss and debilitation. In cancer, as in AIDS, patients succumb to the accompanying illnesses, which they would otherwise survive if not for the wasting syndrome.

"In a sense, nobody ever dies of cancer," notes Dr. Harold Dvorak, chief of pathology at Beth Israel Hospital in Boston. "They die of something else—pneumonia, failure of one or another organs. Cachexia accelerates that process of infection and the building-up of metabolic poisons. It causes death a lot faster than the tumor would, were it not for the cachexia."[4]

Halting the wasting syndrome instead of directly attacking the cancer cells with poison was Dr. Gold's plan of attack. As he explains, "Each of these processes [the tumor invasion of vital organs and cachexia] has its own metabolic machinery, each is amenable to its own therapy, and each is to some degree functionally interdependent on the other. In the interest of treating the totality of malignant disease, each of these processes warrants intervention. Such an approach, dealing with *both* major underpinnings of the cancerous process—mitogenic and metabolic—affords the greatest promise for eliciting long-term, symptom-free survival and the potential for disease eradication."[5]

But what causes cachexia? Cancer cells gobble up sugar ten to fifteen times more than normal cells do. The sugar consumed by the cancer cells is generated mainly from the liver, which converts lactic acid into glucose. (Normal cells are far more efficient users of glucose, which they derive from the food we eat, not from lactic acid.) When cancer cells use sugar (glucose) as fuel, they only partially metabolize it. Lactic acid—the waste product of this incomplete combustion—spills into the blood and is taken up by the liver. The liver then recycles the lactic acid (and other breakdown products) back into glucose, and the sugar is consumed in ever-increasing amounts by voracious cancer cells. The result is a vicious cycle, what Dr. Gold calls a "sick relationship" between the liver and the cancer. The patient's healthy cells starve while the cancer cells grow vigorously. Some healthy cells even *dissolve* to feed the growing tumor.

To break this sick relationship, Gold reasoned, all he needed was to find a safe, nontoxic drug that inhibits *gluconeogenesis* (the liver's recycling of lactic acid back into glucose). In 1968, he outlined his theory in an article published in *Oncology*. "The silence was deafening," he recalls.

A year later, by a remarkable coincidence, Gold heard biochemist Paul Ray deliver a paper explaining that hydrazine sulfate could shut down the enzyme necessary for the production of glucose from lactic acid. Gold had chanced upon an eminently logical way of starving cancer. He immediately tested hydrazine sulfate on mice and found that in accord with his theory, the drug inhibited both gluconeogenesis *and* tumor growth.

Over the years, many dramatic remissions in patients on hydrazine sulfate therapy have been reported. In one case, a sixty-two-year-old woman with widely disseminated cancer of the cervix, in a very debilitated condition, was put on the drug. After one week, a secondary tumor the size of an orange had completely disappeared, much to the amazement of the woman's doctors, and neck nodes had become markedly smaller. After three weeks on the therapy, the patient had gained weight and was active and in good spirits. The woman was discharged from the hospital a short time later.[6]

In 1987, Erna Kamen, a sixty-three-year-old lung cancer patient, was administered hydrazine sulfate after her discharge from a Sarasota, Florida, hospital. "Basically, my mother was sent home to die," says Jeff Kamen, an Emmy-winning television reporter. "She'd lost a significant amount of weight by then, and she had no appetite and virtually no will to do anything."

A doctor had told Jeff's father, Ira Kamen, that hydrazine sulfate offered at least "a shot in the dark." So one Monday in August 1987, a home nurse gave Mrs. Kamen one hydrazine sulfate pill shortly before serving lunch. "On Tuesday morning," recalls Jeff, "there was a commotion in the house. My mother had risen from her bed like the phoenix rising from the ashes. She was demanding that the nurse bring her downstairs so that she could have breakfast with me. . . . When people you love get into this kind of facedown with death, you're just incredibly grateful for each moment."[7]

As Jeff describes his mother's recovery, "her searing pain was gone; her appetite returned at a gallop." Within three weeks, her racking cough had vanished and she could walk unaided. "In the months before her death, she went on television with me to tell the nation about hydrazine sulfate. The National Cancer Institute stopped trashing hydrazine sulfate and began referring inquiries to the UCLA Medical School team whose work had validated the effectiveness of the drug long before Erna Kamen began taking it."[8] Jeff attributes his mother's death months later to her being "mistakenly taken off hydrazine sulfate and subjected to an unproven experimental substance."

With cancer patients, hydrazine sulfate is usually administered orally in 60-milligram capsules or tablets, approximately one to two hours before meals. It is given at first once a day for several days, then twice a day, then three or four times daily, depending on the patient's response and the physician's judgment. On such a regimen, many terminal and semiterminal patients have derived considerable benefit, although patients in the early stages of the disease derive the most benefit from the treatment.

Approximately half of the patients to whom the drug is properly administered in the early stages of the disease show an almost immediate weight gain and reversal of symptoms; in some instances, the tumor eventually disappears. The common types of cancer most frequently reported to benefit from hydrazine sulfate therapy are recto-colon cancer, ovarian cancer, prostatic cancer, lung (bronchogenic) cancer, Hodgkin's disease and other lymphomas, thyroid cancer, melanoma, and breast cancer. Some less common types of cancer also benefit.

"Whether hydrazine sulfate should be used in conjunction with other agents seems to be dependent on whether these agents are doing the patient any demonstrable good," according to Dr. Gold. "In the instances in which these agents have been doing good, hydrazine sulfate should be used in conjunction with them. However—and especially with those cases on toxic drugs—in instances in which the drugs have been doing no evident good, it is probably best to withdraw such drugs and use hydrazine sulfate alone." Many alternative therapists disagree. They see hydrazine sulfate as mainly an adjunctive treatment, albeit a potentially powerful one.

Critics have made much of the fact that hydrazine sulfate, a common industrial chemical, is found in such products as rocket fuel, insecticides, and rust-prevention agents. For medical purposes, however, the salt is refined, purified, and used in reagent-equivalent grades. Given to patients in minuscule amounts, it occasionally produces mild, transient side effects such as nausea, dizziness, itching of the skin, drowsiness, and euphoria, but such side effects are minimal, especially when compared with the devastating effects of standard chemotherapy.

A very small percentage of patients undergoing long-term, high-dosage hydrazine sulfate therapy experience pain or temporary numbness in their extremities, but this condition is quickly controlled by reducing the dosage and administering vitamin B_6. In no known cases has hydrazine sulfate depressed or destroyed white blood cells or bone marrow, as conventional chemotherapy often does. In general, toxicity has been exceedingly low or nil.

The most recent study of this drug, however, concluded that hydrazine sulfate appears not to be beneficial and may even have neurological side effects. This study involved a nationwide, twenty-month trial with 291 advanced non-small-cell lung cancer patients, all of whom received chemotherapy. In the double-blind phase, half were given hydrazine sulfate, while the other half received a placebo. Patients receiving hydrazine sulfate had a median survival of 7.62 months, while the comparable figure for those on placebo was 7.5 months. Hydrazine sulfate had no effect on cancer cachexia, according to Michael Kosty, M.D., an oncologist with Scripps Clinic and Research Foundation in La Jolla, California, who was the study's principal investigator, nor were differences noted between the two groups in anorexia or weight gain. Furthermore, the placebo group rated their quality of life higher than did those patients taking hydrazine sulfate, and some hydrazine sulfate patients experienced loss of sensation and motor function. "Therefore, the best we can say about this drug is that it has no effect and may even be deleterious," Dr. Kosty was quoted as saying in a summer 1992 issue of *ASCO Highlights*, a publication of the American Society of Clinical Oncology.

Dr. Rowan Chlebowski, director of a UCLA research project on hydrazine sulfate, conservatively estimates that the drug could benefit about half a million cancer patients each year in the United States alone.[9] His team has conducted many clinical studies of hydrazine over two decades. Dr. Chlebowski says that the drug's indirect mode of action against tumors is problematic to more cautious investigators. "We found that hydrazine sulfate was an anticachexia agent that indirectly induced antitumor responses without much toxicity. Its action is not directed at cancer cells yet it may profoundly affect them."[10]

Dr. Chlebowski and his colleagues at the Harbor-UCLA Medical Center in Torrance, California, recently found evidence that hydrazine sulfate added to conventional chemotherapy improves the nutritional status and prolongs the life of patients with non-small-cell lung cancer, especially deadly forms of the disease. In the January 1990 issue of the prestigious *Journal of Clinical Oncology*, he reports that earlier-stage patients have a median survival time of at least 328 days, compared to 209 days for the placebo group. There is no curative therapy for this type of lung cancer, so the results, if confirmed, seem promising.

The wasting syndrome seen in cancer patients is also a prime risk factor for AIDS patients with Kaposi's sarcoma. There is evidence that hydrazine sulfate's capacity to stop cachexia may save many AIDS patients. Currently, Dr. Chlebowski is planning a study to test hydrazine sulfate as an anticachexia agent in patients who are infected with HIV and have lost weight.

Even though hydrazine sulfate is now undergoing extensive Phase III trials sponsored by the National Cancer Institute, resistance to this inexpensive, nontoxic chemotherapy in orthodox medical circles persists. Dr. Vincent DeVita, former director of the NCI, told a

Washington Post reporter in 1988 that he thought hydrazine was a "ho-hum idea." Dr. Gold, until recently, has been frozen out of the "war on cancer." Two articles on cachexia published in July 1990 in the prestigious *Cancer Research* journal fail to reference any of Gold's path-breaking work, and one even denies there is any effective treatment for the wasting-away syndrome.

Dr. Gold, who does not treat patients, says that the cost of hydrazine, at most, should be nominal—comparable to the daily cost of insulin and other supplies for diabetics. "Until a pharmaceutical company sponsors the drug through the FDA, it will not be widely in use," he predicts, adding, "However, with the new studies, drug companies have suddenly begun to take notice of this most exemplary drug."

Resources

Syracuse Cancer Research Institute
Presidential Plaza
600 East Genesee Street
Syracuse, NY 13202
Phone: 315-472-6616

For further information on hydrazine sulfate and details on treatment.

Reading Material

The Cancer Industry: Unravelling the Politics, by Ralph W. Moss (see Appendix A for description).

Part Two

IMMUNE THERAPIES

The immune system is your body's major line of defense in the battle against cancer and infection. Specialized cells in your immune system can recognize cancer cells as foreign and destroy them. The aim of immune therapies is to bolster those parts of the immune system that combat and eliminate cancer cells. Most other alternative therapies, though not strictly immuno-therapies, also stimulate the body's natural defenses.

Several forms of orthodox immunotherapy are currently being explored in clinics and cancer centers. They are still used almost totally as adjuncts to chemotherapy, radiation, and surgery. While these orthodox immune therapies are said to hold great promise, they remain largely experimental. In contrast, the three alternative immune therapies discussed in Part Two of *Options* are used by many patients as full-fledged programs, though these treatments have been condemned, persecuted, or shunned by the medical establishment without an in-depth investigation into their possible merit. Most conventional physicians, trained to be aggressive in their approach to fighting disease, are cool toward the idea of strengthening the body's gentle self-healing powers and its natural resistance to cancer.

Cancer cells are believed to form every day in the healthy person, but a strong immune system can easily detect and destroy them before they have an opportunity to divide and proliferate. Unfortunately, for various reasons—poor nutrition, the massive pollution in our environment, stress, aging—the immune system sometimes fails to recognize the cancer cells as an enemy, and the cancer begins its slow, insidious growth over a number of years while you continue to be unaware of it.

Your immune system is normally on constant alert, scanning your body for "foreigners" such as bacteria, viruses, and abnormal cells. As soon as a foreign body is recognized, your whole system springs into action. Highly mobile *natural killer cells,* specialized to destroy foreigners, are your body's first line of defense. If the cancer cells evade the natural killer cells, they proliferate and manufacture *antigens,* which are telltale substances detected by the *T-cells,* your immune system's second line of defense against tumor growth. Specialized T-cells (or *T-lymphocytes*) destroy cancerous and virus-infected cells. (The "T" in *T-cell* stands for "thymus-derived" because these white blood cells, created in the bone marrow, are carried to the thymus gland, which transforms them into T-cells.) Other white blood cells, *macrophages* (Greek for "big eaters"), ingest the cancer cells. A wide range of other cells and substances that make up the immune system help to orchestrate a coordinated attack against almost any invader.

Altogether, there are five major types of orthodox immunotherapy. The first is *BCG,* a tuberculin vaccine used in the treatment of cancer that stimulates macrophages to kill cancer cells. Consisting of a weakened strain of the tuberculosis bacillus, BCG (which stands for *bacillus Calmette-Guérin*) apparently works best when combined with chemotherapy; yet as a solo treatment, it has brought about some complete remissions and many cases of temporary or prolonged remission. Used by conventional as well as alternative doctors, BCG has been particularly successful in treating malignant melanoma. It appears to work well when injected directly into tumors visible on the skin, though it has also been used to treat lung cancer and other forms of the disease. One of the researchers who discovered BCG's anticancer potential was Dr. Lloyd Old, who later became director of the Sloan-Kettering Institute for Cancer Research.

Interferon is a family of proteins produced by the white blood cells in response to viral infection. It stimulates the production of macrophages and *lymphocytes* (white cells), blocks the growth of tumor cells, and transforms some lymphocytes into natural killer cells. Hyped as a wonder therapy and miracle cure when it was first synthesized in 1980, synthetic interferon turned out to be very expensive and have toxic side effects. It produces fever, chills, and muscle contractions so severe that they may require morphine.[1] Today, interferon is approved for use in the treatment of two rare forms of cancer, hairy-cell leukemia and juvenile laryngeal papillomatosis. It may have limited value in a number of other rare conditions. The FDA approved its use for AIDS patients in 1988, but it has largely been a failure in ARC-AIDS trials. Infected people who received it had flu-like symptoms, fatigue, swelling, headaches, and even hallucinations.

Interleukin-2, a protein produced by the T-cells, was also hyped by the cancer industry and the major news media as a cancer breakthrough. The results to date, however, have been disappointing. IL-2, as it is called, has reportedly been effective in some patients with melanoma and renal cancer, but its drawbacks are major and became evident early on. Charles Moertel, M.D., of the Mayo Clinic, charged that IL-2 is highly toxic, hugely expensive, and not particularly effective.[2] Its side effects include fever, chills, malaise, swelling of the spleen, anemia requiring multiple transfusions, severe bleeding, shock, and confusion. Treatment with IL-2, according to Dr. Moertel, may require weeks of hospitalization in an intensive care unit "to survive the devastating toxic reactions."[3] After a few patients died because of interleukin-2, the National Cancer Institute, which had eagerly presented it to the public as a miracle drug, withdrew such claims.[4]

Tumor necrosis factor (TNF), produced in the body in minute quantities, seems to kill cancer cells by destroying their cell membranes, although why this happens is not clear. Side effects occur regularly; most patients develop fever and chills as well as some nausea and vomiting.[5] Injected into cancerous mice, TNF causes their tumors to melt away. It is currently being tested to determine its potential efficacy in treating human cancer patients. Some observers believe that TNF, upon which the cancer establishment has spent millions, is simply *tumor antibody,* one of the four blood fractions used by Lawrence Burton, pioneer of a nontoxic immune therapy used in the diagnosis and treatment of cancer (see Chapter 6).

Monoclonal antibodies are synthetic antibodies created through gene-splicing, fusing a cancer patient's white blood cells with his or her cancer cells. When these bizarre *hybridomas* are reintroduced into the patient's body, they manufacture specific antibodies said to attack only the cancer cells. Attached to anticancer drugs or natural toxins, monoclonals serve as "guided missiles" by directing the antibodies they manufacture toward their malignant prey. Still in the investigative stage, monoclonals—like interferon, interleukin-2, and TNF—promise to be tremendously expensive, a boon to the pharmaceutical-medical monopoly if they are ever used in cancer treatment. They are frequently touted by the media as the next cancer breakthrough.

The American Cancer Society freely admits that it will take "many years to find the proper role of these [orthodox immunotherapy] agents in cancer treatment."[6] Observers say this means twenty years or more. Meanwhile, the ACS continues to use its enormous power and influence to restrict or suppress safe, nontoxic cancer therapies that have produced remarkable clinical results in human beings, such as the immune therapies of Lawrence Burton, Ph.D. (Chapter 6) and Virginia Livingston, M.D. (Chapter 7), or the biologically based therapy of Stanislaw Burzynski, M.D. (Chapter 2).

Ironically, *Coley's mixed bacterial vaccine,* which has perhaps shown a greater cure rate than any other cancer treatment, is totally unavailable. Dr. William Coley (1862–1936), an eminent New York City surgeon and Sloan-Kettering researcher, in the 1890s developed a vaccine made of bacterial toxins that activated immune-resistance mechanisms in cancer patients and cured hundreds. His daughter, Helen Coley Nauts, D.Sc., has preserved and carried forward his important work. Yet, despite the successful use of bacterial vaccines amply reported in the medical literature since the turn of the century, today's big drug companies have no interest in what they view as merely an unprofitable item.

Staphage Lysate, a nonspecific bacterial vaccine made from *staphylo-cocci,* is legally sold today as a specific therapy for acute and chronic staphylococcal infections. Unofficially, it has been widely used by pragmatic doctors who have had encouraging results in treating multiple sclerosis, cancer, herpes, allergies, arthritis, asthma, and many other conditions.[7] Relatively inexpensive and almost totally nontoxic, Staphage Lysate can be inhaled, injected, or taken orally. It is known to increase the production of T-lymphocytes and to induce the natural formation of interferon and *inter-leukin-1,* the predecessor of interleukin-2.

Immune therapies, whether orthodox or alternative, are generally used as a treatment of last resort after patients have received toxic chemotherapy or radiation. Many doctors believe that the prior use of immune-destroying, often carcinogenic conventional treatments lowers a patient's chances for recovery through immune therapy. Chemotherapy often accomplishes the destruction of the immune system, and radiation can cause severe, pro-longed immune deficiency. At any one time, there are thousands of cancer patients in the United States undergoing aggressive chemotherapy who would benefit from any immune-enhancing measures whatsoever, even supportive nutrition or vitamin supplementation.

Chapter 6

BURTON'S IMMUNO-AUGMENTATIVE THERAPY

Dr. Lawrence Burton uses four blood proteins—substances occurring naturally in the body—to treat cancer. His Immuno-Augmentative Therapy (IAT), developed while he was a senior oncologist at St. Vincent's Hospital in New York City in the 1960s, does not "attack" the cancer. Instead, it aims to restore normal immune functioning so that the patient's own immune system will destroy the cancer cells.

Burton discovered that these components, or *blood fractions*, which he isolated, are deficient in the cancer patient. When present in the correct balance, they work synergistically to control cancer-cell growth and kill tumors. His therapy involves replenishing the deficient blood fractions by injecting patients with them in amounts based on daily or twice-daily blood analyses. Patients continue to self-administer the injections of serum for the length of time deemed necessary, much as a diabetic takes insulin. IAT is nontoxic and has minimal or no side effects, unlike orthodox immunological treatments, toxic chemotherapy, and radiation.

Dr. Burton does not claim that Immuno-Augmentative Therapy is a cure, describing it instead as a means to control and combat cancer. Yet, according to clinical records, 50 to 60 percent of patients experience tumor reduction, many undergo long-term regression, and some, even those with terminal cancer, have achieved complete remission. Many cases of metastatic cancer of the colon and abdomen, treated with Burton's serum-injection therapy, are now well beyond five years of recovery—a remarkable achievement since the National Cancer Institute says that these types of cancer have a *zero* five-year survival rate. Positive results have also been achieved in brain cancer, advanced pancreatic cancer, melanomas, cancers of the bladder and prostate, and malignant lymphoma, among many other types.

A follow-up study of 277 IAT patients—most of them with "hopeless," terminal cancer—who were treated at Burton's clinic in 1977 revealed that at least 18 percent of the patients were in good health five years later. (The normal one-year survival rate in terminal cancer patients is less than 1 percent.) The results overall are especially impressive, given that most patients undergoing IAT have been pronounced terminal by orthodox medicine, their immune systems severely weakened by extensive chemotherapy, radiation, or both.

Burton's innovative concepts were almost accepted as mainstream in immunotherapy by the mid-1980s. His great heresy, from the standpoint of orthodox medicine, was to effectively *treat* cancer patients with the techniques he pioneered, many years before his ideas became popular. Because his nontoxic, noninvasive therapy was perceived as a competitive threat by the medical monopoly, he was virtually driven from American soil and forced to relocate in order to continue treating patients, many grateful to him for saving their lives. Today, the Immuno-Augmentative Therapy Center, an outpatient facility directed by Dr. Burton, operates on Grand Bahama Island. The clinic has treated over 4,000 patients in Freeport, The Bahamas, since it opened its doors in 1977. Satellite clinics also provide IAT in Dusseldorf and Regensburg, Germany. New satellite clinics will soon open in Italy and Switzerland.

Meanwhile, Memorial Sloan-Kettering Cancer Center is pursuing research into tumor necrosis factor, a blood substance that reportedly causes the rapid shrinkage or destruction of tumors. Sloan-Kettering claims that TNF was discovered by accident in 1971 when its scientists injected serum into mice. But Burton believes that TNF developed directly out of the original research conducted by his team at St. Vincent's between 1953 and 1963. Dr. Robert Kassel, who worked on the Burton research team that shrank mouse tumors using cancer-growth-inhibiting blood fractions, later went to Sloan-Kettering. Burton maintains that TNF is identical to tumor antibody, one of the four substances he uses to treat cancer patients.

Another tumor-shrinking blood substance, called *humoral recognition factor* (*HRF*), has been studied extensively by investigators at Tulane and McGill universities. Its composition is very similar to two of Burton's other blood fractions. Thus, TNF and HRF represent a stunning confirmation at major medical centers of the validity of Burton's approach.

Born in the Bronx, New York, in 1926, Lawrence Burton earned a Ph.D. in experimental zoology from New York University. He was an oncologist for fifteen years at St. Vincent's Hospital in New York City, where he and a team of cancer researchers discovered a tumor-inhibiting factor that reduces or inhibits cancer in leukemic mice.

In 1966, Dr. Burton astonished the medical world. At an American Cancer Society science writers' seminar in Phoenix, Arizona, he and an associate, Dr. Frank Friedman, injected their serum into a group of mice with large, rock-hard tumors. An hour and a half later, the tumors were almost gone. Within a few hours, the tumors had totally disappeared. This unprecedented demonstration was carried out in the presence of 70 scientists and 200 science writers. The next day, the experiment got front-page newspaper coverage around the world. The *Los Angeles Herald Examiner*'s headline provocatively posed the question: "Fifteen Minute Cancer Cure for Mice: Humans Next?"

In September of the same year, the two doctors (both experimental zoologists by training) repeated their demonstration before an audience of oncologists at the New York Academy of Medicine. This time, skeptical members of the audience selected which of the sixteen mice were to be treated. Once again, the tumors rapidly dissolved an hour or so after the mice were injected with the newly isolated tumor-inhibiting factors.

Incredibly, even these two scientific demonstrations—one conducted under American Cancer Society auspices—did not stop the ACS from putting Burton's therapy on its Unproven Methods blacklist, first in a condemnatory informal summary in 1977, then as a full-fledged unproven method in 1984. To the ACS, the NCI, and their friends, Burton's dramatic discoveries about the immunological treatment of cancer were seen as a threat that could eventually render obsolete the deadly triad of chemotherapy, radiation, and surgery, the economic support and mainstay of the cancer industry.

Shortly after Burton's two sensational public experiments, the cancer establishment attempted to buy out Burton for a song and co-opt his discoveries. The American Cancer Society dispatched its senior vice president of research to make a proposal to the St. Vincent's oncology team. The emissary offered Burton and his co-workers a one-year, $15,000 grant; in exchange, the Burton researchers would reveal their tumor-dissolving techniques to the NCI, the ACS, and Sloan-Kettering. Dr. Burton and his team had hoped for substantial, long-term support and a lifetime fellowship, which are often given by the ACS to promote research. Naturally, they rejected the offer.

Early in 1967, the National Cancer Institute tried again. It dispatched another official to visit the St. Vincent's researchers to find out about their methods and data. After spending two weeks at St. Vincent's, the NCI official encouraged Burton to apply to the government for a $500,000 grant, with the proviso that in return, Burton would reveal his extraction methods and data. In July 1967, Burton was informed that the grant proposal had been approved and was told to turn over the information sought by the NCI. But, through a clerical mix-up, the NCI's hand was revealed: an NCI letter *rejecting* the proposal had been prematurely mailed and was received by one of Burton's team members just as Burton was being ordered to turn over his data. Naturally, Burton refused to do so.

Within a few months, all of Dr. Burton's major research funding was cut, including a grant from the United States Public Health Service. From that time onward, medical and scientific journals refused to publish papers submitted by Burton or his team members, even though the researchers had previously published their findings in prestigious, peer-reviewed journals. A coauthor, Dr. John Harris, senior scientist at Sloan-Kettering, was fired from the cancer center for publishing with Burton and his team. Out of discouragement, Burton subsequently gave up trying to publish. Lecture forums that had once welcomed Burton no longer sent invitations. In short, he and his colleagues were frozen out of the "war on cancer."

In 1974, Drs. Burton and Friedman left St. Vincent and founded a clinic in Great Neck, New York. With affiliated physicians, they treated close to 200 mostly terminal cancer patients over the next three years. A total of 30 of these patients reportedly had complete remission, and 80 others experienced tumor regression.

John Beaty, M.D., of Greenwich Hospital, Greenwich, Connecticut, sent 20 advanced patients to Burton. Tumors regressed in 50 percent of them. "All ten," Dr. Beaty said, "owe their very survival to Dr. Burton's treatment. . . . They also show tumor shrinkage, appetite improvement, weight gain, and loss of pain. I believe this is a breakthrough in the treatment of cancer—the single best frontier in cancer therapy today."[1]

In July 1974, *New York* magazine published a front-cover feature story about Burton and Friedman entitled, "The Politics of Cancer—Why Won't the Medical Establishment Pay Attention to These Two Men?" The article greatly interested Howard Metzenbaum, United States Senator from Ohio, whose wife had died of cancer. Senator Metzenbaum tried to arouse the National Cancer Institute to investigate Burton's therapy. In reply, the NCI contemptuously dismissed the article.

Around this time, the American Cancer Society approached Burton with a research proposal that included a stipulation calling for experiments on a human control group. In other words, half of the terminally ill cancer patients in the study would *not* receive Burton's treatment. To Dr. Burton, the ACS's twisted priority of putting statistics above the welfare of patients was unethical. He refused the ACS proposal.

After Burton and Friedman were awarded three patents in 1975, the FDA refused to permit clinical trials. It sent pages and pages of irrelevant questions, some of which required Burton to undertake ten-year studies on tangential matters before being answered. The FDA had employed its endless-questions technique many times in the past to block other alternative therapies.

Faced with obstacles and harassment, and interested in treating real cancer patients, Dr. Burton closed his Great Neck clinic and opened the treatment center in the Bahamas in 1977 despite the NCI's strenuous arm-twisting of Bahamian government officials to block the new clinic. Over the years, the National Cancer Institute has repeatedly attempted to induce Bahamian authorities to shut down the clinic but without success.

Then, in July 1985, Burton was ordered by the Bahamian health ministry to padlock the clinic and discontinue treatment until further notice. The charges: contaminating patients with AIDS and hepatitis and spreading AIDS-contaminated serum to patients returning to the United States. The trumped-up charges were false, a scare concocted by health officials of the National Cancer Institute and the United States Centers for Disease Control (CDC). In fact, there were *no* reported cases of HIV antibodies in IAT patients; there were *no* reported cases of AIDS in IAT patients; and the test results for the clinic's blood sera were *negative* for HIV antibodies. The CDC reported just two cases of hepatitis B among Burton's thousands of patients over eleven years. This is a remarkable record of safety, considering that the hepatitis B virus, an epidemic infection, has contaminated much of the American blood supply.

The Bahamian clinic was reopened eight months later but only after lawsuits were filed against NCI and CDC. Weeks after the clinic was closed, Burton's patients marched on Washington, D.C., lobbied Congress, and demanded help. This led New York Congressman Guy Molinari to hold a hearing at which impressive medical testimony of Burton's immune therapy was presented.

Among those testifying was distinguished cancer surgeon Dr. Philip Kunderman, former chief of thoracic surgery at Roosevelt Hospital in New York. Dr. Kunderman told how his own metastasized cancer of the prostate was successfully controlled on Burton's Immuno-Augmentative Therapy. As a lung surgeon, he was also amazed at the results Burton obtained in treating mesothelioma, a deadly type of lung cancer for which there is no effective orthodox treatment.

Dr. Kunderman has observed extraordinary remissions in other IAT patients labeled "incurable" by their orthodox doctors, including patients with metastatic carcinoma of the pancreas, brain lesions, malignant melanoma of the skin, cancer of the pharynx, and cancer of the colon with liver metastases. "I have seen patients arrive in wheelchairs and stretchers who appeared to be terminal, respond to Immune Augmentation Therapy and regain their weight and strength to the point where they were walking about, free of pain. This is a remarkable feat in this series of cases, none of which have been controlled or cured by conventional therapies."

Mesothelioma, a usually incurable form of cancer caused by exposure to asbestos, typically attacks the lungs and sometimes the stomach or heart. There is no known treatment for it—only pain management—according to a National Cancer Institute treatise on the subject. The survival rate in conventional medicine is zero, with a prognosis of four to eleven months survival time. Eleven IAT-treated patients with advanced mesothelioma, according to a 1988 report by Dr. Robert John Clement, medical director of the Bahamian clinic, achieved survival rates two to three times greater than those of the traditional therapies, with a number of unusual remissions and cases of prolonged survival.[2] Five patients were alive at the time the study was concluded, with survival ranging from twenty-two to eighty months; the mean (average) survival for those living was forty-three months. The total group had a mean survival of thirty-five months.

A 1987 study conducted at the University of Pennsylvania showed that IAT patients live nearly twice as long after diagnosis as patients undergoing conventional treatment and are expected to go on living much longer. Dr. Barrie Cassileth and her colleagues surveyed seventy-nine long-term IAT patients and reported that the average survival time was more than five years from diagnosis, with 63 percent of the patients still alive at the time of analysis. Three-fourths of the group had come to the Burton clinic with advanced cancer unresponsive to conventional treatment, and most had metastatic or inoperable cancer.

Dr. Cassileth, who is no friend of alternative methods, refused to publish her study after circulating prepublication copies. In fact, she downplayed the implications of her findings, alleging methodological flaws and calling for "an appropriately designed study of IAT." In an analysis of Cassileth's refusal to publish, medical writer Robert Houston observed that "the Cassileth team appears to be genuinely embarrassed by the positive results of their survey."[3]

Dick Jacobs, a Michigan candidate for the United States Senate in 1988 and a former candidate for the governorship of his state, had exploratory surgery in the summer of 1987 that revealed a malignant tumor, seven inches long by two inches wide, wrapped around his aorta. After surgery, he was told that he needed to undergo first chemotherapy, then radiation, providing the chemo succeeded in reducing the size of the tumor. An oncologist advised him that the standard procedure for treating his type of cancer was chemotherapy involving three different drugs, one of which was experimental. The drugs' side effects could cause heart problems, destroy his white blood cells, prevent his blood from clotting properly, and damage his kidneys. "There was also the problem of hair loss, skin discoloration, plus the possibility of getting a new type of cancer from the drugs themselves," recalls Jacobs.[4]

After reading about Burton's Immuno-Augmentative Therapy, Jacobs decided to go to the Bahamas and take the treatment. When he told his oncologist of his plan and explained that he had decided against the use of any chemotherapy or radiation, "my doctor, supposedly a professional person, became so upset with me that he threw my medical records on his desk, jumped up, and told me that if I was going to be treated by a quack he didn't want anything to do with me. He then stormed out of his office, leaving my wife and I sitting there in utter dismay."

In mid-September, Dick Jacobs flew to the Bahamas, and though his first week was rough, he found the clinic "an upbeat place with everyone serving as each other's support system." After six weeks of IAT treatment, he was told by the doctors there that his cancer was under control and that he could return home, taking with him a six-month supply of serum. After three and a half months of IAT, a CAT scan at his local hospital confirmed that the tumor had not grown and the cancer had not spread. Today, he says, he feels great and leads an active life. He gives himself daily injections of plasma protein fractions, which help to augment his immune system. However, he adds:

> One thing that does upset me is the fact that we supposedly live in a free country, but I had to leave my country to exercise my freedom of choice regarding the medical therapy I wanted and not what Big Brother Government says is

acceptable. This is not right. Everyone should be able to freely choose the type of medical therapy they want regardless of the type of illness.

After considerable research, both before and after treatment, I have come to the conclusion that my government, in particular the FDA and the National Cancer Institute, has violated my right to medical freedom of choice. I also feel that their war on cancer and excessively regulatory posture is fostering a medical monopoly which is not in the best interests of the American people.

Cancer patients need to know about alternative types of therapy, but not one medical doctor at my local hospital or at Mayo Clinic shared with me the option offered by Dr. Burton's therapy, or any other type of therapy. If you ask me, the medical quacks are those who claim to be professional medical people in our country but who deny their patients complete knowledge of all types of medical therapy.

My recommendation to any family stricken by cancer is to explore all possible options, and talk with patients who have undergone various forms of treatment. Don't simply rely on your family doctor or the cancer specialist in your area. Take time to do a little research. The time you spend may save your life.

Another advocate of IAT is Margaret Smith, who, without warning, suffered a massive hemorrhage from her bowel in May 1980. Three days later, emergency surgery led to a diagnosis of Stage III cancer of the transverse colon, an adenocarcinoma with extension through the colon wall and metastases to the pericolonic lymph node. Several nodules were found deep within the liver. The five-year survival rate for metastasized colon cancer is virtually zero in conventional medicine.

Margaret, a kindergarten teacher from Costa Mesa, California, underwent a colostomy, which created an artificial opening in her colon for the elimination of wastes. Her hospital oncologist recommended that she begin chemotherapy immediately, but she decided to postpone making the decision until after the colostomy was reversed. In June, another oncologist agreed to monitor her with the understanding that "when" (his word) the cancer came back, chemotherapy was all that he could offer, even though, as he admitted, chemotherapy is generally ineffective against advanced colon cancer.

Margaret began to cleanse her body with a vegan diet, avoiding all animal foods and drinking two or three glasses of carrot juice a day. She still drinks a combination carrot, celery, and apple juice, rich in beta-carotene, a precursor of vitamin A that the body converts to vitamin A. Beta-carotene stimulates the immune system by increasing the concentration of natural killer cells, the production of interferon by T-lymphocytes, and the anticancer activity of *monocytes* (large white blood cells). Beta-carotene is also a scavenger of oxygen *free radicals*, unstable toxic compounds that form continuously in the body and abet degenerative processes. Vitamin A and the carotenoids (including beta-carotene) act by different pathways to boost immune function. There is often a deficiency of vitamin A in the blood of cancer patients.

In July, Margaret's colostomy was reversed; but in December 1980, a routine test showed her CEA level to be above normal, and her oncologist recommended chemotherapy. (A CEA Assay monitors the presence of *carcinoembryonic antigen* in the blood serum. An antigen is a foreign substance, such as a virus or poison, that stimulates the production of antibodies. High CEA levels indicate the presence of various types of cancer.)

Refusing chemotherapy, Margaret went to the Bahamas and started Burton's Immuno-Augmentative Therapy. Told that Dr. Burton recommended a diet higher in protein than her vegetarian diet, she returned to eating a small amount of meat. For the next six and a half years, she gave herself daily shots of blood fractions and her condition steadily improved until her CEA Assay gave a normal reading. In 1987, Dr. Burton said that she could stop taking the shots, except during her twice-yearly "tune-ups," for which she revisited the clinic. Today, Margaret's health is excellent and her cancer is in remission. She follows a sensible diet emphasizing whole grains, legumes, cabbage, broccoli, and fruits and also takes supplements of vitamins E and C fortified with selenium and zinc, antioxidants that scavenge free radicals.

The IAT approach differs from orthodox immunotherapy, which gives generalized stimulation to the immune system. IAT is a two-step procedure consisting of an evaluation to measure the deficiencies of specific blood proteins, followed by serum-injection therapy to correct the imbalances. Dr. Burton believes that the body combats cancer every day and that a healthy immune system is capable of destroying abnormal cells in the same way it defends itself against other forms of disease.

The four blood-serum proteins isolated by Burton are thought to work in sequence to help combat cancer. One of the components, tumor antibody, "recognizes" the mutant cancer cells and either destroys them or reverts them to normal. These tumor antibodies are "alerted to the presence" of cancer cells by a protein produced by the tumor cells themselves—*tumor complement factor* (*TCF*). The debris caused by the tumor destruction goes to the liver, the body's "sanitation department," which processes and disposes of all the tumor waste materials. But if the liver becomes overburdened, a patient, in the most extreme case, could die of liver malfunction. So, to protect the body, a *blocking protein* temporarily stops tumor antibody, permitting the liver to complete its job. When the liver has eliminated the necrotic (dead) cancer cells, a *de-blocking protein* neutralizes the blocking protein, thus allowing tumor complement to call the antibodies back into combat. This four-part dynamic process works to destroy the tumor in a regulated manner.

Each patient's immune system is evaluated once or twice daily, five days a week. The blood-analysis data show the relative activity of the tumor cells and "tumor-kill" process and also allow daily monitoring of a person's responses to therapy. In this way, IAT becomes highly individualized, with every dosage based upon personal reaction rather than averaged or estimated.

The data are entered into a computer for analysis using a computer program developed empirically by Burton and his colleagues through seventeen years of experience. The computer calculation draws on clinical examination as well as blood analysis. Each therapeutic intervention is based on the most recent assessment of the patient's native immune capabilities, the status of tumor activity, the effects of the most recent therapy, and the accumulated effects of all previous therapy and response.

Following treatment, which usually lasts six to eight weeks, patients return home with a supply of serum and a computerized prescription to guide their therapy in the ensuing weeks or months. Scheduled checkups follow at the clinic to reassess the tumor activity and the prolonged effects of the therapy. Patients are strongly urged to continue their relationship with their family or attending physicians. "Over the years, we've been receiving much more cooperation from the patients' doctors," says Burton.

The Freeport, Grand Bahama, clinic is an outpatient facility, so patients must make arrangements for accommodations. Not everyone is accepted for treatment. A person must have had a formal diagnosis of cancer made by an accredited and recognized hospital. If a person's condition can be treated successfully by orthodox therapy, the person is strongly advised to undergo conventional treatment. IAT can be used as an adjunctive therapy with surgery, chemotherapy, or radiation to achieve the best results.

Surgery, considered a "pro-immune" technique, is most beneficial prior to treatment with IAT. Once the tumor bulk has been removed, the native immune mechanism, strengthened through immuno-augmentation, can destroy stray cancer cells remaining after surgery and help prevent secondary tumor growth.

Critics of the IAT approach fault it for lacking awareness of the roles diet, tobacco, and other environmental factors play in therapy. Arlin Brown, an advocate of alternative cancer therapies, suggests, "If you go to Dr. Burton's clinic, we recommend that you continue your other constructive therapies, especially a strong anticancer diet. The reason for this is that Dr. Burton is trying to gather more exact statistics on the efficacy of his method; and if the patient is using another method, then Dr. Burton won't know what is responsible for the patient's recovery. We must respectfully disagree with him in this regard. We feel that the patient's life is more important than the refining of Dr. Burton's statistics. In fact, it would be most enlightening if Dr. Burton were to add at least one more category of statistics to his research, namely, the combination of his immunotherapy and nutritional therapy. Patients could be given the choice of taking Dr. Burton's method alone or taking the optional combination treatment."[5]

Even though Dr. Burton does not recommend any special diet while following the IAT program, patients are encouraged to eat animal proteins. The injection components used in IAT work in conjunction with protein, and Burton maintains that certain immunoproteins are based on amino acids not readily obtainable from vegetable sources. Recommended protein foods include some red meat but mostly fowl, seafood, eggs, cheese, and nuts.

"To date I have not come across a truly efficacious anti-cancer diet," says Dr. Burton. "I.A.T. augments the patients' immune process. They must make these proteins from amino acids obtained from animal source. Macrobiotic diets, starvation diets, and coffee enemas deplete the immune mechanism."

Heavy alcohol consumption is strongly discouraged. If IAT is working, liquor consumption places an extra burden on the patient's liver as the organ works to rid the body of the alcohol as well as the breakdown products from the tumor destruction.

At one time, Burton asked patients to curtail cigarette smoking, but he found that this often creates severe stress. Since Burton emphasizes the role of stress and emotional factors in cancer, he now advises, "If an individual is suffering from anything other than lung cancer and uses smoking as a mental crutch, that person can go ahead and smoke. It's better than taking pain killers."[6]

Burton believes the mind plays an important role in cancer control. Stress depresses the immune system, and Burton holds that depressed immune-system function leads to cancer. "When patients get down on themselves, they're losers—it's over," he notes. Research studies confirm that the cancer patient who maintains a positive, determined attitude survives longer than the despondent, pessimistic patient.

Fifteen years after Burton took the bold step of opening a clinic in the Bahamas, immunology is creating a lot of excitement in the treatment of cancer. Orthodox doctors and scientists borrow freely from Burton's innovations without acknowledging the source. Today, the American cancer establishment shows no interest in giving Burton credit for his work, a quarter-century after his public demonstrations of rapid tumor shrinkage in animals astounded the medical and scientific worlds. Maybe the day will yet come when cancer patients will not have to leave the United States, "the land of the free," to avail themselves of the treatment of their choice.

Resources

Immuno-Augmentative
 Therapy Center
P.O. Box F-2689
Freeport, Grand Bahama
Phone: 809-352-7455

For further information on Immuno-Augmentative Therapy and details on treatment.

IAT Patients' Support Group
Mr. Frank Wiewel
P.O. Box 10
Otho, IA 50569-0010
Phone: 515-972-4444

For patient emotional support.

Reading Material

Diagnosis: Cancer—Prognosis: Life, by Jane Riddle Wright, Albright and Company (P.O. Box 2011, Huntsville, AL 35804; 205-539-3288), 1985. Also available from the Immuno-Augmentative Therapy Center (see above for address and phone number).

Gary Null's Complete Guide to Healing Your Body Naturally, by Gary Null (see Appendix A for description).

The Cancer Survivors and How They Did It, by Judith Glassman (see Appendix A for description).

The Cancer Industry: Unravelling the Politics, by Ralph W. Moss (see Appendix A for description).

"The Vendetta Against Dr. Burton," by Gary Null and Leonard Steinman, *Penthouse,* March 1986.

Immuno-Augmentative Therapy: Cancer Research and Treatment, Immuno-Augmentative Therapy Center (see page 70 for address and phone number). Patient booklet.

Immuno-Augmentative Therapy: Case Histories, Immuno-Augmentative Therapy Center (see page 70 for address and phone number). Patient booklet.

Chapter 7

LIVINGSTON THERAPY

Virginia Livingston, M.D., who died of heart failure in 1990 at the age of eighty-four, pioneered an immunological therapy based on her bacterial theory of cancer. Today her work is being carried forward by the Livingston Foundation Medical Center, an outpatient facility in San Diego run by her daughter Julie Anne Wagner. At the time of this writing, the clinic was undergoing a reorganization. Interested readers should contact the clinic (see the Resources section at the end of this chapter) for an update on its status.

In 1947, Dr. Livingston discovered a form-changing microbe that she believed to be the cause of most cancer in humans and animals. She later named this highly unusual bacterium *Progenitor cryptocides* ("hidden, ancestral killer"). Livingston repeatedly isolated this microorganism from virtually every cancer of humans and animals. She also demonstrated that it can cause cancer when injected into animals. She believed that Progenitor, present in everyone from birth and found in human sperm, is held in check by the immune system. But when immunity is weakened by poor diet, stress, surgery, toxins, or other debilitating factors, the dormant multiform microbe can multiply in overwhelming numbers, become invasive, and promote the growth of tumors. *P. cryptocides* has been found in very high concentrations in cancer patients.

What is so unusual about this bacillus is its apparent ability to change drastically in size and shape at different stages of its development. It can shrink to the minuscule size of a lethal virus. In Livingston's laboratory, filtered cultures of *Progenitor cryptocides,* containing no bacteria, were observed to transform back into bacterial-sized microbes. Using electron microscopy, she and her coworkers photographed what they identified as the submicroscopic, virus-like forms of the microbe.

Many or most conventional microbiologists deny the existence of such form-changing, or pleomorphic, germs. Pleomorphic bacteria adapt to changes in their environment by defensively losing their cell walls. They enter complicated life stages, interspersed among body tissues and organs, awaiting the proper conditions to revert to their original forms. These versatile germs have been dismissed as mere laboratory curiosities. Yet according to Raymond Brown, M.D., a former fellow at the Sloan-Kettering Institute for Cancer Research, "Pleomorphic organisms are demonstrable as the silent stage of a gamut of infections." He says that they "have been repeatedly found" in cancer, arthritis, multiple sclerosis, and other diseases of "undetermined" origin.[1]

The primary aim of the Livingston therapy is restoring the body's natural defenses by strengthening the immune system. The program includes vaccines, a largely vegetarian raw foods diet, gamma globulin, and vitamin and mineral supplements. Antibodies are given to reduce the danger of cancer microbes circulating in the blood and to shrink tumors. An *autogenous vaccine*—that is, a vaccine prepared from a culture of the patient's own bacteria—is also given, in conjunction with BCG (bacillus Calmette-Guérin), a weakened tuberculin vaccine that stimulates the immune system. Sometimes nonspecific vaccines, such as one containing mixed bacteria for use in respiratory infections and to boost general resistance, are also used.

In February 1990, California health officials ordered the Livingston clinic to stop using its autogenous vaccine, claiming that the vaccine had not been shown to be "safe and effective." Dr. Livingston's attorney told the media that the doctor "is offering a legitimate choice for people. There is no evidence [the vaccine] is harmful; there is no evidence it doesn't help." He added that Livingston would begin a fight to overturn the state's order and vindicate her approach. In fact, he said, the autogenous vaccine had been used for years, with hundreds of case histories of apparent effectiveness.

"We have literally thousands of people who receive the vaccine," Dr. Livingston told a congressional hearing on alternative cancer therapies in March 1990, three months before her death. "We have a very high remission rate, and our patients who are well now are very angry and upset that this has been taken away."

No complaints from patients prompted the California health officials' "cease and desist" order. Livingston was never contacted by the authorities before the order was handed down. "The prosecution of Dr. Livingston gives a good idea of what the California health department had in mind when its officials drafted the witch-hunting bill S.B. 2872," notes Ralph Moss, editor of *The Cancer Chronicles* newsletter,[2] referring to a repressive bill that would have allowed the state to seize the property of practitioners of alternative medicine. Violating the Fourteenth Amendment to the United States Constitution, the California bill specifically calls for "seizure without [due] process."

Support for the effectiveness of Livingston's autogenous vaccine comes from preliminary data in a clinical study undertaken by Vincent Speckhart, M.D., an oncologist, and Alva Johnson, Ph.D., a professor of microbiology at the Medical College of Hampton Roads, East Virginia Medical School. In work with forty patients, Dr. Speckhart found that the autogenous vaccine is useful in reversing immunosuppression in cancer patients. He reported a complete response in three patients, one with breast cancer, one with chronic lymphocytic leukemia, and one with malignant lymphoma. He also noted a partial response in a patient with malignant melanoma. He was quoted in a newspaper article as saying that four of the first six patients showed "rather dramatic" improvement, which included the shrinkage or disappearance of tumors.[3]

In her 1984 book, *The Conquest of Cancer* (see Resources), Dr. Livingston presented the case histories of many long-term survivors who benefited from her standard immunotherapy program, which included the autogenous vaccine. Among the patients who fully recovered were victims of advanced terminal breast cancer with metastatic cancer of the lungs, terminal cancer of the esophagus with liver metastasis, colon cancer metastatic to the liver and spine, nodular sclerosing Hodgkin's disease, breast cancer metastatic to the spine and hip, metastatic melanoma, widespread cancer of the abdomen with involvement of the ovaries, metastatic ovarian cancer, and cancer of the prostate with multiple metastases to the bone. Cases successfully treated by cooperating physicians using the autogenous vaccine and other components of the Livingston program are included in Livingston's 1972 book, *Cancer: A New Breakthrough* (see Resources).

How can pleomorphic cancer bacteria cause a malignancy? One possible answer explored by Livingston and her colleagues is that *Progenitor cryptocides* attacks the genetic "memory" in the nucleus of healthy cells, causing the cells to proliferate uncontrollably. Dr. Irene Diller, a microbiologist with the Institute for Cancer Research in Philadelphia, described cancer microbes as interfering with cell division in tissue cultures, producing binucleate cells and other abnormal processes that could lead to cancer.[4] Dr. Diller carried out her research with her husband, William Diller, a parasitologist at the University of Pennsylvania. By 1969, Livingston concluded that *P. cryptocides* causes infection, which lowers the immune response, thereby enabling cancer cells to multiply. Cancer, she stated, is an immune deficiency disease.[5]

Another possible mechanism came to light in 1974 with Dr. Livingston's extraordinary discovery that her cancer microbe, *P. cryptocides*, could secrete a growth hormone in the test tube nearly identical to a human hormone, *human chorionic gonadotrophin* (*HCG*).

The human placenta is coated with HCG, protecting the fetus from the mother's immune system. Livingston proposed that the secretion of this mammalian hormone by the cancer microbe protects the microbe *and* the cancer cells from destruction by the immune system. She called HCG "the hormone of life and the hormone of death." It is present as *choriogonadotropin* (*CG*) in sperm, the trophoblast (the outer layer of cells through which the developing embryo receives nourishment), the bone marrow, and cancer cells. Normal HCG controls the reproductive processes. But when HCG is not kept in check by antibodies, white blood cells, and dietary factors, it can build up uncontrollably and stimulate tumor growth, according to Livingston. She believed that the hormone secreted by *P. cryptocides* turns normal cells into cancer cells when their immune function is weak or essential nutrients are deficient.

Livingston's claim that bacteria could produce a human hormone in the test tube was labeled nonsense. But a few years after she made her discovery, her contention was confirmed by orthodox scientists at Rockefeller University, Princeton Laboratories, and Allegheny General Hospital in Pittsburgh. Hernan Acevedo, Ph.D., of Allegheny General Hospital, showed that all cancer cells, animal or human, contain CG. And in 1977, the fact that a lowly microbe produces CG was used to win government approval for genetic engineering.

Livingston found that *abscisic acid*, a plant hormone and vitamin A analog occurring in many foods, neutralizes the production of CG. She called abscisic acid "nature's most potent anti-cancer weapon," claiming that it stops cancer cells from multiplying. Animal experiments have shown that it is a potent antitumor agent.[6] Virtually all cancer patients entering the Livingston clinic reportedly have low levels of abscisic acid in their bodies.

Consequently, the Livingston anticancer diet emphasizes foods rich in abscisic acid such as carrots, mangoes, avocados, tomatoes, lima beans, and green leafy vegetables. According to Livingston, nearly all cancer patients lose their ability to break down vitamin A in their liver and make abscisic acid. Therefore, she recommended drinking carrot juice mixed with dried liver powder. The liver enzymes break down the vitamin A and form abscisic acid in the juice. "The powder does all the work for your liver," she wrote.

Much recent research shows that vitamin A is protective against the onset of cancer from carcinogens. For over a decade, scientists have used a group of vitamin A analogs called *retinoids* to force cancer cells to develop into normal cells. This is called differentiation therapy. Abscisic acid, a plant growth regulator, is one of the retinoids. It suppresses the growth of plants, causing seedlings to "go to sleep" in the autumn. Livingston believed abscisic acid also suppresses cancer microbes. Human abscisic acid, produced in the liver, breaks down vitamin A into retinoids, which in turn are thought to regulate CG and cancer microbes.

The Livingston anticancer diet emphasizes nonprocessed, fresh vegetables and fruits and whole grains. Foods should be raw or very lightly cooked to preserve the vitamins, minerals, and enzymes that help rebuild the body and raise immunity. Refined flour, white sugar, and all foods with empty calories are prohibited. Salt and high-sodium foods must be restricted, while potassium-rich fruits and vegetables should be emphasized. Most animal products are forbidden because they are often loaded with toxins, synthetic hormones, antibiotics, and pesticides that damage the immune system. Livingston pointed to a body of scientific evidence demonstrating that a vegetarian diet is best for human beings.

As patients begin to recover, they may eat some fish. But chicken, eggs, beef, and milk products are forbidden because Dr. Livingston's research led her to conclude that these foods are contaminated with *Progenitor cryptocides* and may transmit cancer to human beings.

Many chickens processed for human consumption have tumors, visible and invisible, but these tumors are missed by the inspectors on the production line due to rushed processing techniques and lax enforcement practices. Dr. Livingston believed that nearly 100 percent of chickens on American dinner tables have the active, pathogenic, viral form of the cancer microbe, which she held to be transmissible to humans. Animal husbandry expert Elizabeth McCulloch estimates that 40 percent of human cancers are caused by this pervasive cancer in chickens and eggs.

As early as 1911, Dr. Peyton Rous of the Rockefeller Institute demonstrated that 90 percent of the chickens sold in New York City contained sarcomas (cancers) caused by a microbe small enough to pass through a filter designed to catch bacteria. Viruses, which are much smaller than bacteria, could pass through the filter. Yet Dr. Rous, who won a Nobel Prize in 1926 for his work, did not conclude that this "tumor agent" was a virus. Scientists who came along later assumed Rous's tumor agent to be a virus. However, Dr. Livingston pointed out that a true virus needs living cells to survive, whereas the Rous tumor agent could be dried and stored at room temperature for months or even years, then injected into chickens *who all developed cancer.*

Livingston and her research team at Rutgers University spent several years growing the mysterious Rous tumor agent in culture media and studying it under the electron microscope. The group included Dr. Eleanor Alexander-Jackson, a Cornell University microbiologist, and the aforementioned Dr. Irene Diller. After dozens of experiments, they concluded that the Rous agent was in fact *Progenitor cryptocides*, the form-changing cancer microbe. It was shown to be transmissible to humans from beef and poultry. The results were published in what Livingston considered a landmark paper.[7]

Rous's Nobel Prize–winning work on tumor agent was confirmed in Britain by a number of researchers, including Dr. W. M. Crofton. A longtime investigator of pleomorphic microbes, Dr. Crofton was widely known for his use of autogenous vaccines in the treatment of cancer and infections.[8]

Livingston's theory of the transmissibility of pleomorphic cancer microbes holds far-reaching implications for public health. Livestock, often imprisoned in cramped, unhealthy quarters, are frequently fed chicken manure because of its high protein content. Thus, the hamburger or bacon you eat could be infected with *P. cryptocides,* according to Livingston's observations. Even drinking milk is risky, she believed, since 80 to 90 percent of cattle carry leukemia, as the cattle industry's own literature admits.

Livingston's views have been rejected or ignored by the American meat, dairy, and poultry industries. And her bacterial theory of cancer causation remains unacceptable to the medical orthodoxy even though a century of research underlies pleomorphism. The American Cancer Society added the Livingston vaccine to its Unproven Methods blacklist in 1968 despite the fact that it had never undertaken an investigation of Livingston's methods and never asked the National Cancer Institute to do so.

In Europe, though, Dr. Livingston's ideas on the transmissibility of cancer microbes are taken seriously. As nutritionist Gary Null points out, in Switzerland and Sweden, milk from leukemic cows is not permitted to reach the market since it is considered a serious risk to public health. "Such strictures have not been imposed in the United States," explains Null, "in part because the U.S. dairy industry simply doesn't believe, and no government authorities will test, Dr. Livingston's theories."[9]

A Vassar graduate, Virginia Livingston hardly fit the image of a "quack," which is how the medical establishment generally portrays practitioners whose ideas and methods do not fit the prevailing model. Born in Meadville, Pennsylvania, she received her medical degree in 1936 from New York University and was the first woman to be a resident physician in a New York City hospital. In a long, distinguished career, she was an associate professor of biological sciences at Rutgers University, director of the Laboratory of Proliferative Diseases at Presbyterian Hospital in Newark, New Jersey, and a microbiology professor at the University of San Diego. In 1971, she founded the medical center that bears her name. The clinic is still dedicated to cancer research and treatment building upon her discoveries.

Livingston observed the cancer microbe microscopically as an acid-fast (blue-, red-, or purple-stained) coccus or granule. Occasionally, large round forms of *P. cryptocides* can be identified. Observation is made by examining live, whole blood under a dark-field microscope, which offers an advantage over the examination of dead blood traditionally done by most clinical laboratories. In dark-field microscopy, the blood specimen is illuminated by a special condenser. Objects in the observation field show up as brightly lit bodies against a dark background. In contrast, it is impossible to see the live, moving microbes in dead blood that has been stained. The filterable, virus-like forms of *P. cryptocides* can only be seen using an electron microscope.

When Livingston identified *P. cryptocides* as the cancer microbe, she did not claim that her discovery was unique. In fact, she said this is the same microorganism that has been observed for over 100 years by various researchers.

The controversy over pleomorphic microbes can be traced back to a famous dispute between Louis Pasteur, the French chemist, and his chief rival, French microbiologist Antoine Béchamp. Pasteur believed *nonchangeable* microbes that invade the body are the primary cause of disease. (On his deathbed, however, he allegedly renounced this "germ theory.") Béchamp, a medical doctor, chemist, and professor at the University of Toulouse, put forth the "microzyma theory," postulating for all bacteria a common ancestor present in all living organisms. Through careful experiments, Béchamp found that all animal and plant cells contain microzymas (tiny molecular granules) that can evolve into bacteria under certain conditions and outlive the host organism. He believed that the form of any strain of bacteria is primarily determined by its environment and that microzymas can evolve into disease-producing forms through changes in the body's inner "terrain."

Although Béchamp's work won support and some confirmation among his contemporaries, influential, flamboyant Pasteur won out, and the idea of eternally unchanging germs became scientific doctrine. Béchamp's concept of pleomorphic microbes was pursued by Dr. Ernst Almquist (1852–1946), a Swedish bacteriologist and physician who had worked with Robert Koch of Germany. Nobel Prize–winner Koch, discoverer of the tuberculin bacillus, also noted (but never investigated) the pleomorphic phases of the typhoid bacillus.

German bacteriologist Guenther Enderlein developed a biologic treatment for cancer based on his six decades of observing pleomorphic microorganisms (see page 16). His therapy is used today in Europe and the United States.

In the 1930s, California researcher Royal Rife demonstrated that pleomorphic microbes are clearly visible in human cancer specimens at a microscopic magnification of 30,000 using a light microscope he invented. Rife was able to destroy the cancer microbe using a bioelectronic instrument in a noninvasive, painless treatment. (See page 268.)

Livingston's work in the culture of pleomorphic organisms from all types of cancer—and in the induction of cancer in animals using these organisms—was corroborated and paralleled by Florence Seibert, Ph.D., at the University of Pennsylvania. Because the standard light microscope cannot reveal pleomorphics in their smaller phase, Seibert and her associates utilized a density-measuring apparatus to prove their existence. Like Livingston, she maintained that a highly specific vaccine could be made from the cancer microbes of a patient and used to prevent the spread of the cancer to other parts of that patient's body.

Many other researchers have also demonstrated the existence of pleomorphic organisms implicated in cancer and other diseases. Nevertheless, most microbiologists continue to insist that "a coccus is a coccus is a coccus" and always remains so. The idea of a bacterium changing from a coccus to a rod, to a fungus, or to a virus-size form is completely unacceptable to them.

In her book *The Conquest of Cancer*, Livingston claimed a success rate of 82 percent in treating cancer and "over 90 percent" when counting patients for whom the therapy was of some benefit. These figures should be treated with healthy skepticism and caution. As pointed out elsewhere in this volume, 80 percent seems to be a favorite figure cited by alternative practitioners in support of their work. Dr. Jules Vautrot, in a recent review of Livingston's work, concluded that "overall success in remission of cancer is moderate through the use of her therapy."[10] Vautrot is president of the Cancer Federation, a California-based educational and research group open to alternative approaches, and a professor of health sciences at Chico State University.

A study published in April 1991 in the *New England Journal of Medicine* presented data to show that terminally ill cancer patients had the same median survival—fifteen months—whether they were treated by orthodox therapy or the Livingston protocol.[11] The news media used the study to caricature alternative therapies as worthless. But a very different interpretation is possible. As Dr. Jules Vautrot comments, "There are two conclusions that can be drawn from the article: 1) When cancer is extensive or advanced, poor results of treatment are forthcoming from both orthodox and unorthodox therapy, and 2) The 'unproven' remedy developed by Dr. Livingston matches orthodox remedies under the conditions of this study. It is a testimony to the perseverance of Dr. Livingston that in the evening of her life, her therapy judged to be 'unproven' by the American Cancer Society shows equal merit with orthodox therapy within the limits of this study."[12]

Most terminal patients, it should be noted, come to the Livingston Foundation Medical Center "after having been so heavily treated that their immune systems are all but destroyed, and their tumors are far advanced," to quote Dr. Livingston. The lethal effects of toxic chemotherapy and radiation undoubtedly make recovery more difficult for these patients. Because of this, the *New England Journal* study would have been more effective if the patients in question had been recently diagnosed with cancer. As John Steinbacher, executive director of the Cancer Federation, notes, "A study of dying patients seems to be rather counterproductive."

Resources

Livingston Foundation Medical Center
3232 Duke Street
San Diego, CA 92110
Phone: 619-224-3515

For further information on Livingston therapy and details on treatment.

Reading Material

The Conquest of Cancer, by Virginia Livingston-Wheeler with Edmond G. Addeo, Franklin Watts (387 Park Avenue South, New York, NY 10016; 800-843-3749), 1984.

Cancer: A New Breakthrough, by Virginia Wuerthele-Caspe Livingston, Livingston-Wheeler Foundation (3232 Duke Street, San Diego, CA 92110; 619-224-3515), 1972.

Gary Null's Complete Guide to Healing Your Body Naturally, by Gary Null (see Appendix A for description).

The Cancer Survivors and How They Did It, by Judith Glassman (see Appendix A for description).

The Cancer Industry: Unravelling the Politics, by Ralph W. Moss (see Appendix A for description).

Chapter 8

ISSELS' WHOLE-BODY THERAPY

A pioneer in alternative cancer treatment, Josef Issels, M.D., of Germany achieved remarkable remissions, even in advanced cancer patients, through a combination of therapies designed to shrink the tumor and repair the body's defense mechanisms. His "whole-body" approach included anticancer vaccines, a low-protein diet emphasizing organic raw foods, and fever therapy to stimulate immune function. In addition, he employed an arsenal of methods to rebuild the immune system and change the body's biochemistry so as to eliminate the "tumor milieu" that allowed the cancer to develop in the first place.

Among the methods Dr. Issels employed were detoxification, ozone-oxygen therapy, homeopathic remedies, liver-extract injections, and enzyme supplements. The sites of "focal infection," such as teeth and tonsils, were removed if infected, since Dr. Issels believed they release toxins into the system that lower resistance and trigger disease. Dr. Issels utilized very-low-dose chemotherapy, surgery, and radiation in combination with immunotherapy, although conventional modes of treatment were generally used as a lifesaving necessity. Issels' whole-body (or *Ganzheit*) program also included psychotherapy to deal with the emotional factors that he felt could hinder recovery.

Dr. Issels is now living in retirement in Florida. A "multimodality immunotherapy program" based on his methods is offered by Ahmed Elkadi, M.D., and colleagues at the Panama City Clinic in Panama City, Florida. This chapter will first describe the Issels approach as Issels practiced it and will then review the work of Dr. Elkadi.

An intuitive healer and penetrating clinician, Dr. Issels had a "proven record of success with terminal cancer patients [that] stands unparalleled in the history of medicine," writes Jack Tropp in *Cancer: A Healing Crisis*.[1] Whether or not this is an overstatement, many reputable observers found much to commend. Two independent studies—one at King's College Hospital in London, the other at the University of Leyden in Holland—confirmed that 16.7 to 17 percent of Issels' terminal patients led normal, cancer-free lives for at least five years. Their life expectancy upon admission had been less than one year. John Anderson, M.D., author of the first study (and a consultant to the World Health Organization), concluded, "I am of the considered opinion that this is a new approach to cancer treatment and appears to be a considerable improvement on what is usually offered. My overall opinion is that the Issels approach to the treatment of cancer is a unique and pioneering solution to a very difficult problem. He is undoubtedly producing clinical remissions in patients who have been regarded as hopeless."

In conventional medicine, "cure" means that the cancer patient has survived five years from the time of diagnosis, even if he or she is in horrendous condition. But Dr. Issels' statistics are based on different criteria altogether: not only is the patient alive at least five years after starting treatment, but he or she is well and free of any detectable signs of cancer. This makes the figures all the more impressive.

Far ahead of his time, Issels was boycotted and isolated by the German medical establishment, which spared no effort to suppress his innovative work. By 1958, the American Cancer Society had blacklisted him; it later formally condemned him by placing his therapy on the Unproven Methods list even though it had never observed his practice.

Finally, the German medical authorities leveled trumped-up charges of fraud and manslaughter against Issels, and in 1960, Issels was imprisoned in a cell block containing only convicted murderers. A judge told Issels' lawyer, "If we can convict Issels of fraud, we have a list of over 100 doctors we can also arrest—and then the internal cancer therapy is finished."[2] Dr. Issels was eventually acquitted of all charges. But his persecution "demonstrates that the European cancer establishment has been just as corrupt as its American counterpart and just as opposed to alternative cancer therapies which work," observes Barry Lynes in his excellent book *The Healing of Cancer*.[3]

To Issels, cancer is "a general disease of the whole body" rather than a local disease confined to the place where the tumor occurs. In his view, cancer is a chronic systemic illness and the tumor is merely a late-stage symptom "able to exist and grow only in a bed already prepared for it." This is the "tumor milieu"—the internal environment resulting from damage to organs and organ systems and metabolic disturbances that weaken the body's defense against malignancy.

The body constantly produces some cancer cells. In Issels' view, a healthy immune system can destroy these cancer cells and prevent them from multiplying. But when the body's chronic degeneration leads to a permanent inability to destroy cancer cells, a tumor can develop. This deteriorated condition is ideal for the proliferation of what Issels called "the live oncogenic [cancer-generating] agent," a microbe that feeds on toxic wastes concentrated in an unhealthy body. Issels believed this cancer-causing germ to be the same pleomorphic, or form-changing, microorganism observed by Dr. Virginia Livingston (Chapter 7) and other investigators.

The Issels program included immunization against the specific type of cancer being fought. Issels made vaccines from antigens that cause the body to produce specific antibodies. "This is really no more than an extension of the standard vaccination technique against any infectious disease," he wrote.[4] He also used a tumor-specific vaccine developed by Dr. Franz Gerlach, a Viennese microbiologist who worked at Issels' clinic. "It was also possible with this vaccine—a pool of mycoplasma—to achieve remission in malignant tumors of animals and human beings," reported Dr. Issels.[5] To produce this vaccine, cultures of tumor *mycoplasm*—tiny microorganisms implicated as the causative agents of disease—were obtained by ultrafiltration of tissue from malignant tumors. In addition, Issels used general immunotherapy to help destroy the tumor milieu. This included autovaccines prepared from extracts from a patient's infected teeth and tonsils, as well as other immune-boosting vaccines.

Dr. Issels maintained that the body has four closely interrelated defense systems and that the malfunctioning of any of them could contribute to a tumor milieu. One of these four defensive zones produces lymphocytes and antibodies, which most doctors regard as the whole of the immune system. But for Issels, the immune system also includes the detoxifying organs (the large intestine, skin, kidneys, and liver) and the epithelial tissue lining the body cavities, with its colonies of friendly bacteria. The fourth defense zone—the body's connective tissue—stores proteins, salts, and water and digests toxins and harmful microorganisms by capturing and binding them chemically. Whole-body therapy is aimed at restoring the integrity of all four of these defense systems.

Issels used conventional treatments such as surgery, chemotherapy, and radiation very circumspectly. He emphasized that such interventions must be complemented by immediate measures to stimulate the body's own immunological defense system. As he explained in a 1980 lecture, "In patients with a rapidly growing tumor who cannot expect immediate help from long-term immunotherapy, we combine this treatment with chemotherapy according to the morphology of the tumor. Thus we have been able to stop the growth by chemotherapy so that the following immunotherapy had time to act. . . . The combination of immunotherapy and chemotherapy seems today to be the most effective treatment of incurable patients on a wide basis. Thus many patients could be cured who would have died without any doubt if only one of these therapies had been used. By the whole-body immunological treatment alone or combined with chemotherapy, also inoperable tumors were reduced in size so that surgery could be performed. Blocked ureters or gallbladders could be freed, making it possible to continue treatment of patients who would otherwise have been lost."[6]

Issels was highly critical of orthodox medicine, in which "the patient gets too much chemotherapy, so much chemotherapy that the last defense mechanism is destroyed. You need two, three months to build up. Very sad, very bad," he said. "In thirty years there has been no improvement in the treatment of cancer. Because the way they go, by the official medicine, is wrong. It is *proven* that it's wrong. But they do it."[7]

Issels induced fever in patients while constantly monitoring them. Fever therapy, used in Europe for centuries, triggers a dramatic rise in the number of disease-destroying leukocytes in the bloodstream. It also causes the lymphocytes to produce a great deal of antibodies that destroy bacteria and toxins. Modern conventional medicine rejects fever therapy, viewing a fever as something to suppress with antibiotics. In contrast, Issels gave patients a "fever shot" once a month to raise the body temperature as high as 105°F, where it remained for a couple of hours. He induced active fever with the ethical drug Pyrifer, made from specially treated coli bacteria. He induced passive fever by means of hyperthermia: the patient was placed inside a cylinder containing electrodes that bombarded his or her body with ultra short waves.

In 1984, hyperthermia was approved by the FDA as a medical procedure to treat cancer (see Chapter 21). The rationale behind it, according to orthodox medicine, is that cancer cells are more sensitive than normal cells and cannot tolerate excessive heat.

Another method that Issels employed was ozone therapy. He used it to increase the oxygen supply to cells and destroy bacteria and viruses in the bloodstream. He administered a combination of medically pure ozone-oxygen to patients by drawing a volume of blood, combining it with an ozone-oxygen mixture, and reintroducing it into the patient's bloodstream. Many studies have demonstrated ozone therapy's direct anticancer effects (see Chapter 20).

Substitution therapy is Issels' term for measures designed to restore specific organs and rebuild the body. He prescribed organ extracts, including injections of liver and mesenchymal extracts, to repair damage to organs and improve their functioning. He also administered organ-specific RNA and DNA, proteolytic enzymes to destroy the protein coat surrounding tumors, as well as vitamins and minerals to strengthen the body's enzyme activity.

Dr. Issels also held diet to be critical to changing the body's biochemistry and reversing the tumor milieu. Like many other anticancer regimens, the Issels diet was rich in organically grown fruits, vegetables, and whole grains. Large quantities of juices, herbal teas, and water were recommended. Issels believed the cancer patient suffers fluid depletion and needs to be "rehydrated." Raw foods, he believed, should ideally make up one-half to two-thirds of the dietary intake. He said vitamin and mineral supplements should be taken, notably vitamins A, B complex, C, and E. Buttermilk and cottage cheese were permitted, but meat was to be avoided since it is difficult for advanced cancer patients to digest and is loaded with synthetic hormones, pesticides, nitrates, and antibiotics that place further stress on the body. Yogurt and supplements of *lactobacillus acidophilus*, a cultured milk product, were recommended to eliminate harmful intestinal flora that interfere with digestion. Tobacco, coffee, commercial tea, and alcohol were forbidden.

For Dr. Issels, the "elimination of all causal factors" that contribute to immune deficiency included the removal of infected teeth and tonsils. In a 1987 speech delivered in New York City, he also stressed the value of removing amalgam fillings and teeth whose dead pulp had been removed by root-canal treatment. Issels believed that infected teeth and tonsils impair the immune system. "I *do not* recommend that healthy tonsils and teeth be removed," he said, "but I believe that if they are diseased, they cause the body's natural resistance to be lowered, thus acting as an important contributory factor to tumor development. In these cases I insist on their removal."[8] He also claimed that toxins from infected tonsils could contribute to heart disease. Issels reported notable improvement in many patients following tonsillectomies.

While these techniques remain highly controversial even within the alternative cancer field, at least one component of Issels' recommendations has gained wide currency—the removal of metallic dental fillings, which, according to critics, spread toxins through the body, interfere with our innate bioelectric functioning, and cause disease. Even many healthy people have replaced metal fillings and dental amalgams with a plastic compound held to be nontoxic and safe. According to Dr. F. Fuller Royal, M.D., H.M.D., medical director of the Nevada Clinic in Las Vegas, "Metallic ions have been known to be toxic to cells since the late nineteenth century. It is not out of the realm of possibility that dental metals are related to an increase of cancer in the U.S. today through their influence on dedifferentiation in rapidly growing cells and through suppression of the body's immune system. Continuous exposure to small electric currents, as occurs with amalgams, is known to stress the endocrine glands, decrease the activity of the immune system and may enhance certain viruses and bacteria."[9]

In some countries—Sweden, for example—the potential hazards of placing toxic metals like mercury, nickel, and beryllium in the teeth have been acknowledged and appropriate action taken. As a first step in its effort to eliminate the use of amalgam in dental fillings, Sweden's Social Welfare and Health Administration has stopped the placement of amalgams in pregnant women in order to prevent mercury damage to the fetus. Research has linked the use of amalgam and alloy fillings and crowns with many diseases, including coronary artery disease, headaches, Meniere's disease, chronic fatigue syndrome, chronic immune deficiency syndrome, and various skin diseases.[10]

The American Dental Association (ADA) resolutely denies that metallic amalgam is harmful. In fact, the ADA has declared that the removal of amalgam from nonallergic patients because it is allegedly a toxic substance is "improper and unethical." But according to Dr. Fuller, "The ADA's position on amalgam fillings becomes ludicrous when one considers that dental practitioners are subject to rigorous and very detailed instructions from health authorities about how to handle dental amalgam, as for example to clean up every kind of small spillage, minute particles of amalgam in the sinks, in the sewage system, on the floor, etc. Furthermore, dentists are warned against every direct contact with the mercury in amalgams. Consequently, amalgam seems to be a highly poisonous compound! However, medical and dental authorities, apparently without any reservations at all, recommend that the same highly toxic amalgam should be inserted into the mouths of human beings! The ambiguity of such action lacks all common sense and has no parallel in all the other fields of medicine."

Issels knew how important it was to enlist the patient as a full-time partner in the struggle to get well. Instead of succumbing to lonely isolation and wallowing in depression, his cancer patients were routed out of their beds to do light mountain climbing in the Bavarian Alps surrounding the doctor's world-famous Ringberg Clinic. "Go climb a mountain," Issels encouraged his patients. The patients also participated in a daily exercise program that included jogging.

Go and Climb a Mountain was the title of a documentary film about Issels made by the British Broadcasting Corporation. The film's scheduled airing in March 1970 was cancelled under intense pressure from Britain's cancer establishment. After a public outcry, the documentary was finally shown in prime time to 14 million people in November 1970. This created an enormous public interest in Issels' therapy. Then Britain's medical orthodoxy sent a five-man team to Germany to investigate Issels' clinic. Two of the team members were outspoken opponents of Issels; only two members spoke German, and they weren't cancer specialists. Their biased report, full of inaccuracies, was published, not in any medical journal, but by the British government in a concerted effort to discredit Dr. Issels. In protest, the editor of *New Scientist,* a leading British journal, blasted the medical establishment for its "vicious intolerance of an unorthodox outsider." But the smear campaign succeeded in badly damaging Issels' clinic, which eventually had to close.

Since 1984, Dr. Ahmed Elkadi has been using a program based in part on Issels' therapy to treat patients with cancer, AIDS, lupus, and other chronic degenerative diseases associated with immune deficiency. His Panama City Clinic, located on Florida's gulf coast, has treated approximately fifty cancer patients. "About half of the patients improve, some with remissions," says Dr. Elkadi, who first visited Issels in 1981 at the latter's outpatient clinic in Bad Wiesee, Germany. "In most of our patients we have documented considerable improvement in immune functioning, which gives them a better chance of healing," Elkadi continues, emphasizing that his multimodality immunotherapy program (MIP) is not a cure. Yet, based on the results thus far, he expects a remission rate with advanced cancer patients "that will at least match the 17 percent rate obtained by Dr. Issels."

Dr. Elkadi, an Egyptian-born American citizen, is the director of the clinic and has served as an assistant professor of thoracic cardiovascular surgery at the University of Missouri School of Medicine. He earned his medical degree from Graz University in Austria and a doctorate in surgery from Vienna University. According to Dr. Issels, Dr. Elkadi "is very good. His program is a modified one because Dr. Elkadi has to comply with the regulations in the United States. He does his work very carefully."

The MIP protocol combines basic elements of Issels' therapy, including a largely vegetarian, natural-foods diet; supplements of pancreatic enzyme, tumor antigen, vitamins, and minerals; fever therapy once a week; psychotherapy; and regular exercise. Stress reduction is achieved with the help of counseling and biofeedback training. Patients also use guided imagery or visualization in an effort to enhance the immune system's defenses (see Chapter 29). Other elements of the MIP include vitamin C infusions, detoxification through coffee enemas (see pages 190 and 206), and acupuncture. Removal of infected teeth and tonsils is suggested, but the decision is up to the patient. "We mention that mercury in dental fillings may contribute to immune suppression," says Dr. Elkadi. "If hair analysis reveals the presence of high levels of mercury, then we will suggest a removal of mercury fillings."

A component of the program introduced by Elkadi is the use of the black seed, or *Nigella sativa*, known for centuries in the East as a healing seed. In 1959, the crystalline active ingredient, nigelone, was isolated from the oil of the black seed, Dr. Elkadi and his colleagues have published a number of studies on the immune-enhancing effects of *Nigella sativa*, which include boosting of natural killer cell activity and an increase of helper T-cells, white blood cells that stimulate antibody production.[11]

Cancer patients usually spend two to three months at Dr. Elkadi's ambulatory clinic, then follow a home maintenance protocol, possibly indefinitely. "We do not advise patients to abandon any conventional treatment modality to which they are responding and which is well tolerated," explains Dr. Elkadi. Some patients elect to discontinue their conventional treatment because it is ineffective or the toxic side effects are unbearable.

Another current practitioner of the Issels method is Dr. Wolfgang Woeppel, who is also highly recommended by Dr. Issels. Dr. Woeppel's clinic, the Hufeland Klinik, is located in Bad Mergentheim, Germany (see Resources).

Resources

Panama City Clinic
Ahmed Elkadi, M.D.
236 South Tyndall Parkway
Panama City, FL 32404
Phone: 904-763-7689

For further information on multimodality immunotherapy and details on treatment.

Hufeland Klinik
Wolfgang Woeppel, M.D.
Bismarckstrasse
Bad Mergentheim, Germany
Phone: 011 49 7931-8185

For further information on Issels' whole-body therapy and details on treatment.

Reading Material

Cancer: A Second Opinion, by Josef Issels, Hodder and Stoughton (P.O. Box 257, North Pomfret, VT 05053; 615-929-3111), 1975.

Dr. Issels and His Revolutionary Cancer Treatment, by Gordon Thomas, Peter H. Wyden (New York), 1973. Out of print; check your local library.

Gary Null's Complete Guide to Healing Your Body Naturally, by Gary Null (see Appendix A for description).

The Cancer Survivors and How They Did It, by Judith Glassman (see Appendix A for description).

"Immunotherapy in Progressive Metastatic Cancer—A Fifteen-Year Survival Follow-Up," by Josef Issels, *Clinical Trials Journal*, vol. 7, 1970.

Part Three

HERBAL THERAPIES

Herbs are Mother Nature's powerful pharmacopeia. Herbal medicine is probably the oldest form of treatment in the world. There were no synthetic medicines, or very few, 250 years ago, when hundreds of thousands of plant species were the main source of drugs for the world's people. Herbs and other plants are the direct ancestors of many of the most potent and effective modern drugs.

Penicillin is derived from a mold and is thus, in a sense, herbal or plant-based. The same is true of other antibiotics, since they are based mostly on substances produced by fungi. Many modern drugs are still closely related to their herbal origins—for example, digitalis comes from foxglove, and atropine, from belladonna. Medical history is full of examples of initial professional hostility toward folk remedies that eventually became valuable tools in conventional medicine, such as chinchona bark for malaria and May apple for cancer.

Nearly every ancient and aboriginal culture has used herbs for the prevention and cure of disease. Around 1500 B.C., the ancient Egyptians wrote the *Papyrus Ebers,* which lists over 700 herbal medicines. In the United States, herbal remedies were widely prescribed until the late 1800s, when the American Medical Association (AMA), a trade group of doctors committed exclusively to allopathic medicine, used its wealth and political power to restrict or stamp out alternative forms of treatment.

In treating cancer, natural healers around the world have used over 3,000 plants species. There is currently a large body of scientific literature on plants and herbs citing their anticancer activities in lab studies and humans. The herbal remedies for cancer that are popular in the United States at any given period represent a tiny fraction of the anticancer plants that have been culled almost at random from Mother Nature's vast botanic pharmacopeia.

Two modern anticancer drugs—vincristine sulfate and vinblastine sulfate—were developed after researchers at Eli Lilly and Company tested folk remedies in a cancer screening program and found that the Madagascar periwinkle, a perennial herb, showed anticancer activity in animals. The May apple is another example of an age-old cancer remedy yielding a modern "wonder drug." The Penobscot Indians of Maine used the rhizome (underground stem) of this flowering plant to treat cancer. The resin from May apple was specified in a nineteenth-century American materia medica to treat cancerous tumors. Recently, etoposide (or VePesid), a semisynthetic derived from May apple by Bristol-Myers, has proven effective in treating cancer of the testicles and small-cell cancer of the lungs.

There are many useful herbal remedies awaiting "discovery" among the thousands of folk medicines. Fewer than 2 percent of the potentially valuable plants in the tropics have been analyzed for therapeutic properties. NCI has had a cyclic interest in herbal remedies for cancer. It recently embarked on an extensive program of plant research, joining forces with ethnobotanists from leading organizations to search tropical forests globally for plants believed to have anticancer effects.

A new anticancer drug resulting from the NCI's screening program is taxol, a compound from the bark of the Pacific yew tree. Hailed as the most exciting new experimental anticancer drug in fifteen years, taxol demonstrated dramatic tumor-dissolving effects in about one-third of women treated for advanced ovarian cancer. In advanced breast cancer unresponsive to any other drug, 52 percent of the women given taxol in one recent study experienced drastic tumor shrinkage, according to the May 13, 1991, issue of the *New York Times,* and in three of the twenty-five women, the tumors disappeared. Taxol has also shown effectiveness against lung cancer and probably has other anticancer uses. But the developer, Bristol-Myers Squibb, is wrangling with the government, loggers, and ecologists over access to the dwindling supply of rare yew trees in the Pacific Northwest. According to the May 1991 issue of *Townsend Letter for Doctors,* taxol is in short supply, with the current stock sufficient to treat perhaps just 200 to 300 patients. Efforts to synthesize the drug are underway at ESCA-Genetic Corporation in California. NaPro, Inc., based in Washington and Colorado, says that its attempts to collect the branches and needles of yew trees have been hampered by the United States Forest Service and other government agencies, as reported in the Summer 1991 issue of *The Choice.*

Most of the research on the use of natural compounds to treat cancer and viral diseases is being done abroad. The Chinese government has funded an intensive study of traditional Chinese herbal medicine. One system widely used in Chinese hospitals, called Fu Zhen therapy, features ginseng, astragalus, and other herbs. Fu Zhen therapy has been found to increase the functions of T-cells, white blood cells that trigger antibody production and boost immune-system activity. The herbal therapies of Indian Ayurvedic medicine and Chinese medicine are covered in Part Seven of *Options,* which focuses on bioenergetic medicine.

The American "cancer industry"—the ACS, NCI, AMA, and the big pharmaceutical companies—pours billions of dollars into investigating *synthetic* compounds instead of undertaking large-scale research into time-honored herbal remedies that have demonstrated success. The reason for this is simple: it is much easier to patent a synthetic compound, and reap enormous profits from it, than to patent a natural compound readily harvested from Nature.

So the drug companies isolate a bioactive substance from a medicinal plant and make some molecular modifications in it; their synthetic product can then become proprietary, or exclusive. This way, the pharmaceutical giants can recoup the $125 million it costs to test a new drug and bring it to market.

If you and I could simply pick some weeds or herbs, brew them into a tea, drink the tea, and avoid or reverse a terrible disease, the drug companies and the doctors would watch their enormous profits evaporate. This is why the parameters of drug-industry science are totally regulated. We are told that the medical monopoly's restrictive regulations are necessary for two reasons: safety and efficacy. But substantial evidence for the effectiveness of some herbal cancer treatments (and other nontoxic alternative therapies) belies this rationale.

A synthetic pill contains an *isolated* chemical compound. Pharmaceutical scientists take one chemical from a plant, leaving behind the hundreds of other compounds and also all the minerals, vitamins, and fibers that accompany the one chemical in the live plant. "Each raw herb has a unique combination of chemicals in it. An herb's medicinal effect is the result of the synergistic activity—the working together—of all the chemicals that the herb contains," notes Dr. Laurence Badgley, M.D., author of the textbook *Energy Medicine.* By ingesting a synthetic chemical isolate containing molecular chains altered in the laboratory, we may well be depriving ourselves of the full healing effects of the herb from which the chemical came.

In treating cancer, herbs can support the body's process of ridding itself of malignant growths. Herbal remedies that work via the liver, enhancing its detoxifying activity, include burdock, blue flag, and yellow dock. Remedies known for their tonic and cleansing actions on the lymphatic system, such as echinacea and pokeroot, are also frequently used. Red clover, mistletoe, sweet violet, garlic, and kelp are among the plants commonly cited for their specific action in inhibiting tumor growth. Herbs are often one component in a holistic approach to cancer that embraces dietary changes and psychological reappraisal. Holistic medicine addresses the physical, emotional, mental, and spiritual factors in illness.

Part Three of *Options* focuses on five herbal treatments for cancer. The Hoxsey therapy, driven out of the United States after curing many patients, still flourishes just south of the border. Essiac, the Canadian Indian herbal remedy, is one of the most remarkable stories in all of medicine. Iscador, an extract of mistletoe, has been used medicinally over the centuries. Pau d'arco and chaparral are available at health-food stores.

Besides these five remedies, there is a whole tradition of herbal medicine, encompassing many approaches, for the treatment of cancer. It is still possible, though difficult, to find a medical herbalist who will treat cancer. People interested in pursuing this can find information, formulas, and leads in two books by naturopath Michael Tierra: *The Way of Herbs,* published in 1989 by Pocket Books (1230 Avenue of the Americas, New York, NY 10020; 800-223-2336), and *Planetary Herbology,* published in 1988 by Lotus Press (distributed by Lotus Light, P.O. Box 2, Wilmot, WI 53192; 800-548-3824). Another book providing some basic information on herbs and cancer is Jethro Kloss's *Back to Eden,* revised and published in 1988 by the Back to Eden Books Publishing Company (P.O. Box 1439, Loma Linda, CA 92354; 714-796-9615). Black and yellow herbal salves for skin cancers and breast tumors, derived from a formula used by American Indians, are discussed by Jane Heimlich in *What Your Doctor Won't Tell You,* published in 1990 by HarperCollins Publishers (10 East 53rd Street, New York, NY 10022; 800-242-7737). The salves, very painful to use, are said to draw the tumor out through the skin.

Another relevant book is *Cancer Salves and Suppositories,* by Ingrid Naiman and Susan Meares, published in 1992 by Bodhisattva Trust (1227 St. Francis Drive, Suite C, Santa Fe, NM 87501; 505-988-3111). It describes a variety of herbal salves and suppositories and includes formulas, comments from patients, and a resource guide. Finally, *The Layman's Course on Killing Cancer,* by Loren Biser, outlines an herbal self-treatment program based on the life work of medical herbalist John Raymond Christopher, who treated patients for cancer and other illnesses at his Salt Lake City clinic. Persons interested in the Christopher herbal program are strongly advised to first seek professional medical treatment and then to pursue the therapy (or any herbal therapy) under professional supervision. (For information on *The Layman's Course,* write to the University of Natural Healing, 355 West Rio Road, Suite 201, Charlottesville, VA 22901; 804-973-4400.)

Chapter 9

HOXSEY THERAPY

For over three decades, Harry Hoxsey (1901–1974), a self-taught healer, cured many cancer patients using an herbal remedy reportedly handed down by his great-grandfather. By the 1950s, the Hoxsey Cancer Clinic in Dallas was the world's largest private cancer center, with branches in seventeen states. Born in Illinois, the charismatic practitioner of herbal folk medicine faced unrelenting opposition and harassment from a hostile medical establishment. Nevertheless, two federal courts upheld the "therapeutic value" of Hoxsey's internal tonic. Even his archenemies, the American Medical Association and the Food and Drug Administration, admitted that his treatment could cure some forms of cancer. A Dallas judge ruled in federal court that Hoxsey's therapy was "comparable to surgery, radium, and x-ray" in its effectiveness, without the destructive side effects of those treatments.

But in the 1950s, at the tail end of the McCarthy era, Hoxsey's clinics were shut down. The AMA, NCI, and FDA organized a "conspiracy" to "suppress" a fair, unbiased assessment of Hoxsey's methods, according to a 1953 federal report to Congress. Hoxsey's Dallas clinic closed its doors in 1960, and three years later, at Hoxsey's request, Mildred Nelson, R.N., his long-time chief nurse, moved the operation to Tijuana, Mexico.

The Bio-Medical Center, as the clinic is now called, treats all types of cancer, with Nelson overseeing a staff of fully licensed medical doctors and support personnel. The records indicate that many patients, some arriving with late stages of the disease, have been helped and even completely healed of cancer by the nontoxic Hoxsey therapy, which today combines internal and external herbal preparations with a diet, vitamin and mineral supplements, and attitudinal counseling.

The medical orthodoxy labeled Harry Hoxsey "the worst cancer quack of the century." His herbal medicine was denigrated as worthless, simply "a bottle of colored water" containing extracts of useless backyard weeds. FDA officials would go to patients' houses, intimidate them, tell them they were being duped by a quack, and take away their Hoxsey medicines. The American Cancer Society added the Hoxsey therapy to its blacklist of Unproven Methods in 1968, using its customary phraseology about the lack of any evidence that the treatment works.

Yet no representative of the ACS has ever visited the Bio-Medical Center or scientifically tested the Hoxsey remedies. Hoxsey repeatedly urged the AMA and NCI to conduct a scientific investigation of his formulas, but his pleas went unanswered. Instead, his practice was outlawed, the FDA banning the sale of all Hoxsey medications in 1960. His therapy was driven out of the country by a close-minded medical fraternity that continues to view inexpensive, nontoxic herbal medicine as a direct competitive threat.

Today we know that Hoxsey's plant-based remedies contain naturally occurring compounds with potent anticancer effects. According to eminent botanist James Duke, Ph.D., of the United States Department of Agriculture, all of the Hoxsey herbs have known anticancer properties.[1] All of them are cited in *Plants Used Against Cancer*, a global compendium of folk usage of medicinal plants compiled by NCI chemist Jonathan Hartwell. Furthermore, Duke noted, the Hoxsey herbs have long been used by Native American healers to treat cancer, and traveling European doctors picked up the knowledge and took it home with them to treat patients.

Hoxsey treated external cancers with a red paste made of bloodroot (*Sanguinaria canadensis*)—a common wildflower—mixed with zinc chloride and antimony sulfide. The rootstock of bloodroot, a spring-blooming flower, contains an alkaloid, sanguinarine, that has powerful antitumor properties. North American Indians living along the shores of Lake Superior used the red sap from bloodroot to treat cancer. Drawing on Indian lore, Dr. J. W. Fell, working at Middlesex Hospital in London in the 1850s, developed a paste made of bloodroot extract, zinc chloride, flour, and water. Applied directly to a malignant growth, Dr. Fell's paste generally destroyed it within two to four weeks. In the 1960s, various teams of doctors reported the complete healing of cancers of the nose, external ear, and other organs using a paste made of bloodroot and zinc chloride—a mixture virtually identical to Hoxsey's.[2]

The American Medical Association condemned Hoxsey's "caustic pastes" as fraudulent in 1949, even though a prominent Wisconsin surgeon, Dr. Frederick Mohs, in 1941 had used a red paste identical to Hoxsey's to fix cancerous tissue that he surgically removed under complete microscopic control.[3]

Medical historian Patricia Spain Ward reported "provocative findings of antitumor properties" in many of the individual Hoxsey herbs when she investigated the Hoxsey regimen in 1988 for the United States Congress's Office of Technology Assessment.[4] The basic ingredients of Hoxsey's internal tonic are potassium iodide and such substances as licorice, red clover, burdock root, stillingia root, barberis root, pokeroot, cascara, prickly ash bark, and buckthorn bark. Ward noted that "orthodox scientific research has by now identified antitumor activity" in most of Hoxsey's plants.

For example, two Hungarian scientists in 1966 reported "considerable antitumor activity" in a purified fraction of burdock. Japanese researchers at Nagoya University in 1984 found in burdock a new type of *desmutagen,* a substance that is uniquely capable of reducing mutation in either the absence or the presence of metabolic activation. This new property is so important, the Japanese scientists named it the *B-factor,* for "burdock factor."[5]

Hoxsey himself believed that his therapy normalized and balanced the chemistry within the body. Like many other holistic healers, he considered cancer to be a systemic disease, not a localized one. Cancer, he wrote, "occurs only in the presence of a profound physiological change in the constituents of body fluids and a consequent chemical imbalance in the organism." His herbal medicines are intended to restore the original chemical balance to the body's disturbed metabolism, creating an environment unfavorable to cancer cells, which cease to multiply and eventually die.[6] The herbal remedies are said to strengthen the immune system and to help carry away wastes and toxins from the tumors that the herbal compounds caused to necrotize. While this theory may be inexact, current research appears to be vindicating Hoxsey, or at least showing that his method merits a thorough, unbiased investigation by the medical orthodoxy.

Mildred Nelson was first introduced to the Hoxsey approach in 1946, when her mother, Della Mae Nelson, underwent the Hoxsey therapy for cancer. Mildred, a conventionally trained nurse from Jacksboro, Texas, believed Hoxsey was a quack, so she went to Dallas to try to talk Della Mae out of her foolishness. Instead, she ended up taking a job at Hoxsey's clinic as a nurse. Her mother recovered and is alive and well today. Mildred's father was also treated by Hoxsey for a recurrence of cancer in the eye socket, having had one cancerous eye removed earlier. He became cancer-free and remained so until his death in 1957 from meningitis.

According to Hoxsey's autobiography, *You Don't Have to Die* (see Resources), his family's healing saga began in 1840 when Illinois horse breeder John Hoxsey, his great-grandfather, watched a favorite stallion recover from a cancerous lesion on its leg. The horse, put out to pasture to die, grazed on one particular clump of shrubs and flowering plants and healed itself. John Hoxsey picked samples of these plants, experimented with them, and formulated an herbal liquid, a salve, and a powder. He used these medications to treat cancer, fistula, and sores in horses that breeders brought from as far away as Indiana and Kentucky. The herbal formulas were handed down within the family, and Harry's father, John, a veterinary surgeon, began quietly treating human cancer patients. From the age of eight, Harry served as his father's trusted assistant. After years on the road as an itinerant healer, he opened the first Hoxsey Cancer Clinic in Dallas in 1924.

Thus began a protracted battle pitting Harry Hoxsey, an ex-coal miner and Texas oilman whose family traced its lineage to Plymouth Colony, against the American medical establishment. Hoxsey was arrested more times than any person in medical history, usually for practicing medicine without a license. But no cancer patient ever testified against him. On the contrary, his patients would gather at the jail in a show of support, hastening his release. Senators, judges, and some doctors endorsed his anticancer treatment. Although the colorful, flamboyant healer fit the stereotyped image of a quack, legions of supporters, once gravely ill with cancer, said they owed their lives and continued well-being to him.

Finally, in 1954, an independent team of ten physicians from around the United States made a two-day inspection of Hoxsey's Dallas clinic and issued a remarkable statement. After examining hundreds of case histories and interviewing patients and ex-patients, the doctors released a signed report declaring that the clinic

> ... is successfully treating pathologically proven cases of cancer, both internal and external, without the use of surgery, radium or x-ray.
>
> Accepting the standard yardstick of cases that have remained symptom-free in excess of five to six years after treatment, established by medical authorities, we have seen sufficient cases to warrant such a conclusion. Some of those presented before us have been free of symptoms as long as

twenty-four years, and the physical evidence indicates that they are all enjoying exceptional health at this time.

We as a Committee feel that the Hoxsey treatment is superior to such conventional methods of treatment as x-ray, radium, and surgery. We are willing to assist this Clinic in any way possible in bringing this treatment to the American public.[7]

But the treatment was denied to the American public. In 1924, according to Hoxsey's autobiography, Dr. Malcolm Harris, an eminent Chicago surgeon and later president of the AMA, had offered to buy out the Hoxsey anticancer tonic after watching Hoxsey successfully treat a terminal patient. Hoxsey would get 10 percent of the profits, according to the offer, but only after ten years. The AMA would set the fees, keep all the profits for the first nine years, then reap 90 percent of the profits from the tenth year on. The alleged offer would have given all control to a group of doctors including AMA boss Dr. Morris Fishbein.

Hoxsey refused the offer, or so he claims. The AMA denies that any such incident ever occurred. In any event, two things are certain: The "terminal" cancer patient, police Sergeant Thomas Mannix, fully recovered and lived another decade. And Morris Fishbein became a powerful, relentless enemy of Hoxsey.

Another opponent was Assistant District Attorney Al Templeton, who arrested Hoxsey more than 100 times in Dallas over a two-year period. Then, in 1939, Templeton's younger brother, Mike, developed cancer. He had a colostomy, but the cancer continued to spread; his doctors told him nothing more could be done for him. When Mike secretly went to Hoxsey and was cured, Al Templeton had a change of heart. The once-hostile prosecutor became Hoxsey's lawyer.

Esquire magazine sent reporter James Burke to Texas in 1939 with the aim of doing an exposé that would discredit Hoxsey as a worthless, dangerous quack. Burke stayed six weeks, became a strong supporter of Hoxsey and later his publicist, and filed a story entitled "The Quack Who Cures Cancer." *Esquire* never published it.

In 1949, Morris Fishbein, long-time editor of the *Journal of the American Medical Association* (*JAMA*), wrote an attack on Hoxsey that was published in the Hearst papers' Sunday magazine supplement, read by 20 million people. In the piece, entitled "Blood Money," Fishbein, the influential "voice of American medicine," portrayed Hoxsey as a malevolent charlatan and repeated many of the unsubstantiated charges that he had been printing for years in *JAMA*.

Hoxsey sued Fishbein and the Hearst newspaper empire for libel and slander. It seemed a hopeless David-versus-Goliath contest, but Hoxsey won. Although his monetary award was just two dollars, he achieved a stunning moral victory. Fifty of his patients testified on his behalf. The judge found Fishbein's statements to be "false, slanderous and libelous." And Fishbein made astonishing admissions during the trial, such as that he had failed anatomy in medical school and had never treated a patient or practiced a day of medicine in his entire career. Even more shocking, *Dr. Fishbein admitted in court that Hoxsey's supposedly "brutal" pastes actually did cure external cancer.*

The leader of America's "quack attack" was now on the defensive. Critics charged the AMA with being a doctor's trade union, setting national medical policy to further its own selfish interests. The United States Supreme Court agreed that the AMA had conspired in restraint of trade. Dr. Fishbein was forced to resign.

In 1953, the Fitzgerald Report, commissioned by a United States Senate committee, concluded that organized medicine had "conspired" to suppress the Hoxsey therapy and at least a dozen other promising cancer treatments. The proponents of these unconventional methods were mostly respected doctors and scientists who had developed nutritional or immunological approaches. Panels of surgeons and radiation therapists had dismissed the therapies as quackery, and these promising treatments were banned without a serious investigation. They all remain to this day on the American Cancer Society's blacklist of "Unproven Methods of Cancer Management."

By this time, the Hoxsey clinic in Dallas had 12,000 patients and Harry Hoxsey was contemplating running for governor of Texas, a post that would enable him to appoint the state medical board and thereby get an impartial investigation into his therapy. Hordes of Hoxsey's patients flooded Washington, D.C., demanding medical freedom of choice. Hoxsey threatened to picket the White House with 25,000 cured patients. But the FDA and other federal agencies mounted a massive legal and paralegal assault. A therapy with the potential to help cancer sufferers was hounded out of the country.

When Mildred Nelson moved the clinic to Mexico in 1963, Hoxsey stayed in Dallas in the oil business. In 1967, he developed prostate cancer. He took his own tonic, but ironically, it didn't work for him. Although surgery is fairly routine for prostate cancer, he refused to have it, fearing that the Dallas doctors would take their revenge on him on the operating table. Hoxsey spent his last seven years as an invalid, dying in isolation, nearly forgotten. He was buried around Christmas in 1974, without an obituary or tribute in the Dallas newspapers.

The Bio-Medical Center in Tijuana, a glass-walled mansion within sight of the United States–Mexico border, is an outpatient clinic only. Patients who arrive before 9 A.M. are seen without an appointment. They are given a complete workup, including a physical examination, lab tests, and X-rays, and have their clinical history taken. Patients are advised to bring existing medical records from other hospitals and facilities. After their appointment, which usually lasts one full day, sometimes longer, patients return home with enough Hoxsey medications and supplements to last several months. They are encouraged to make a follow-up visit after three to six months.

The herbal tonics, salves, and powders given are adjusted to suit the specific needs of each patient, taking into account his or her general health, the location and severity of the cancer, and the extent of previous treatments for it. The Hoxsey therapy is reportedly effective in alleviating pain in many cases.

Dietary specifications include the total avoidance of pork, vinegar, tomatoes, carbonated drinks, and alcohol. The forbidden foods are thought to work against the therapeutic action of the medicine. Patients are also told not to consume bleached flour or refined sugar and to ingest very limited amounts of salt. Supplements include immune stimulants, yeast tablets, vitamin C, calcium capsules, laxative tablets, and antiseptic washes. Patients are counseled to adopt a positive mental outlook and to assume complete responsibility for their own health. The clinic also offers chelation, immunotherapy, and homeopathy, as well as chemotherapy in extremely serious, life-threatening cases.

The types of cancer said to respond best to the treatment include lymphoma, melanoma, and external (skin) cancer. The clinic's patient brochure includes case histories of patients successfully treated for breast, cervical, prostate, colon, and lung cancers.

In 1965, Margaret Griffin of Pittsburgh was given one year to live by her conventional doctors. She had been having blackouts, and X-rays revealed that she had two tumors around her aorta. Exploratory surgery confirmed the existence of the tumors and also uncovered lesions in the right lung, a blockage of the superior vena cava, and metastases to the lymph glands. Thirty doses of cobalt radiation failed to arrest the growing tumors and made Margaret feel worse. As time went on, her face became puffy, she experienced difficulty breathing, and she felt that she was going steadily downhill.

Margaret decided to fly to Dallas to try the Hoxsey therapy. After visiting the clinic, she took four teaspoons per day of the herbal tonic for several months and followed the prescribed diet. She noticed no improvement, however, and was having serious doubts about the therapy's value. But after ten months on the regimen, her breathing improved, her strength returned, and she sensed a dramatic overall improvement. When she called her family doctor for a checkup, he refused to see her "because you didn't believe in my diagnosis." Subsequent X-rays taken by a different doctor indicated that the two tumors and related conditions were gone.

Margaret continued to take the Hoxsey tonic until 1979, when she went off it for a five-year period. In 1984, she had a build-up of fluid in her right lung. Surgery revealed a recurrence of the tumor blocking the superior vena cava. Margaret went back on her Hoxsey regimen, and her lung problem cleared up. X-rays taken in 1989 showed no sign of cancer, and today, more than twenty-five years after she was given a year at most to live, Margaret is alive, healthy, and active.

"Mildred Nelson is a totally dedicated healer," says Margaret. "The medical community should pay homage to her. I told Mildred that I wish we could clone her. The world needs her."

Approximately 80 percent of the patients seen at the Bio-Medical Center benefit substantially from the treatment, according to Nelson. No full-scale independent studies have ever been done to evaluate this claim, however. In an informal tracking survey, Steve Austin, a naturopath from Portland, Oregon, and colleagues followed approximately thirty-five Hoxsey patients. They were able to stay in touch with twenty-two of them either for five years or until death. Austin, who teaches at Western States Chiropractic College in Portland, visited the Bio-Medical Center in 1983 and asked patients walking through the doors if they would be willing to participate in his survey. He then kept in touch with them through annual letters.

Of the twenty-two patients, eleven had died by the end of the five years and eleven were still alive. Among the survivors, three said their condition was deteriorating, but eight claimed to be totally cancer-free. All eight of the cancer-free survivors had previously been diagnosed in the states by medical doctors.

Austin, who plans to publish his findings, emphasizes that his case studies should be considered very preliminary. His sample was small, and it is possible that many of the twenty-two patients were in the very late stages of cancer. Also, a number of the patients may have failed to take their medicine or to stay on the recommended diet.

"The outcome—8 out of 22 5-year survivors—suggests that the results were better than chance, especially since one of the 8 had late-stage melanoma and another had lung cancer," says Austin. "I was a skeptic about the Hoxsey program. Initially, it felt pretty hokey to me. But

Mildred Nelson told me, 'Everything is open here. Go out there and talk to any of the patients. They all know somebody who has been cured by the treatment.' When I mingled with the patients and spoke to them, Mildred's statement turned out to be true, though our results certainly do not suggest a substantial benefit in 80 percent."

Mildred Nelson has said that if she cannot find a health professional whom she feels she can entrust to run the clinic and fill her shoes, the Hoxsey therapy may one day die with her. That would be a tragic end to the Hoxsey saga. Meanwhile, cancer patients who are interested in Hoxsey's methods but cannot afford the trip to Mexico can avail themselves of at least part of the regimen. Three herbal distributors sell products that are apparently identical to the Hoxsey internal tonic formula, or very nearly so. The herbal capsules sold by one of these distributors reportedly requires only supplemental potassium iodide; the other two distributors' products—one, a blend of herbal tinctures— are said to be virtually identical to the Hoxsey tonic formula.

It should be emphasized that none of these distributors is in any way connected with the Bio-Medical Center, and none claims that its product is useful in treating cancer. The quality of these Hoxsey-like herbal mixtures and the results for people who use them are unknown. Furthermore, taking only the herbal component of the therapy and neglecting the other aspects of the program could weaken the overall effect. If a cancer patient wishes to pursue a Hoxsey-like protocol without a trip to Mexico, it is strongly recommended that he or she do so under the direction of a qualified physician or holistic practitioner. For more information about resources for these herbal products or for practitioner referrals, contact the Center for Advancement in Cancer Education (see page xvi for the address and phone number).

Resources

Bio-Medical Center
P.O. Box 727
615 General Ferreira
Colonia Juarez
Tijuana, Mexico 22000
Phone: 011 52 66-84-9011
       011 52 66-84-9081
       011 52 66-84-9082
       011 52 66-84-9376

For further information on Hoxsey therapy and details on treatment.

Reading Material

You Don't Have to Die, by Harry Hoxsey, Milestone Books (New York), 1956. Out of print; check your local library.

The Cancer Survivors and How They Did It, by Judith Glassman (see Appendix A for description).

"Does Mildred Nelson Have an Herbal Cure for Cancer?" by Peter Barry Chowka, *Whole Life Times,* January–February 1984.

"The Troubling Case of Harry Hoxsey," by Ken Ausubel, *New Age Journal,* July–August 1988.

Other Material

Video: *Hoxsey: When Healing Becomes a Crime* (originally entitled *Hoxsey: Quacks Who Cure Cancer?*), 1987. Ninety-six minutes. An excellent, very moving documentary on the Hoxsey therapy, covering its history, the Bio-Medical Center, and the politics and economics of cancer. Produced and directed by Ken Ausubel and coproduced by Catherine Salveson, R.N., it premiered at the Margaret Mead Film Festival in New York and was shown on cable television. Available from Realidad Productions (P.O. Box 1644, Santa Fe, NM 87504; 505-989-8575).

Chapter 10

ESSIAC

Essiac, a harmless herbal tea, was used by Canadian nurse **Rene Caisse** to successfully treat thousands of cancer patients from the 1920s until her death in 1978 at the age of ninety. Refusing payment for her services, instead accepting only voluntary contributions, the Bracebridge, Ontario, nurse brought remissions to hundreds of documented cases, many abandoned as "hopeless" or "terminal" by orthodox medicine. She aided countless more in prolonging life and relieving pain. Caisse obtained remarkable results against a wide variety of cancers, treating persons by administering Essiac through hypodermic injection or oral ingestion.

The formula for the herbal remedy was given to Caisse in 1922 by a hospital patient whose breast cancer had been healed by an Ontario Indian medicine man. Essiac came within just three votes of being legalized by the Canadian parliament in 1938. Over the years, many prominent physicians voiced their support for the efficacy of Caisse's medicine. For example, Dr. Charles Brusch—a founder of the prestigious Brusch Medical Center in Cambridge, Massachusetts, and a former physician to President John F. Kennedy—declared that "Essiac has merit in the treatment of cancer" and revealed that he cured his own cancer with it. In a notarized statement made on April 6, 1990, Dr. Brusch testified, "I endorse this therapy even today for I have in fact cured my own cancer, the original site of which was the lower bowels, through Essiac alone."

Despite such support, Rene Caisse lived under the constant threat of persecution and harassment by Canadian authorities. Today, Essiac is unapproved for marketing in the United States and Canada. However, Resperin Corporation of Ontario provides Essiac to patients in Canada under a special agreement with the Canadian Health and Welfare department, which permits "emergency releases of Essiac on compassionate grounds" while still deeming it "an ineffective cancer treatment." Another company reportedly has the authentic formula for the herbal remedy in Caisse's handwriting, plus eight of her formula variations for specific cancers, including cancer of the prostate. It recently made Essiac available through various distributors. A number of herbal distributors claim to sell the original Essiac tea. Prospective users should carefully weigh the background of all vendors and examine all claims with caution.

Rene Caisse refused to publicly divulge the precise Essiac formula during her lifetime, fearing that a monopolistic medical establishment would either try to discredit the formula or use it to reap enormous profits. Also, she wanted Essiac safe for immediate use on suffering cancer patients, but medical experts demanded prior testing on lab mice. Caisse repeatedly offered to reveal the exact formula and method of preparation if the Canadian medical authorities would first admit that Essiac had merit in the treatment of cancer. But the doctors and politicians argued that they realistically couldn't give any such endorsement until they first knew what was in the herbal mixture. The result was a stand-off.

The principal herbs in Essiac include burdock root, turkey rhubarb root (Indian rhubarb), sheep sorrel, and slippery elm bark. Burdock root, a key active ingredient, is also a major ingredient of the Hoxsey herbal remedy (see Chapter 9). As discussed in the chapter on the Hoxsey therapy, two Hungarian scientists in 1966 reported "considerable antitumor activity" in a purified fraction of burdock.[1] In addition, as also discussed, Japanese scientists at Nagoya University in 1984 discovered burdock contains a new type of desmutagen, a substance uniquely capable of reducing cell mutation either in the absence or in the presence of metabolic activation. So important is this property, the Japanese researchers named it the B-factor, for "burdock factor."[2] Another herb in Essiac, turkey rhubarb root, was demonstrated to have antitumor activity in the sarcoma-37 animal test system. Herbalists, however, believe that the synergistic interaction of herbal ingredients contributes to their therapeutic effects. They point out that laboratory tests on a single, isolated compound from one herbal formula fail to address this synergistic potency.

Through her work with cancer patients, Caisse observed that Essiac broke down nodular masses to a more normal tissue, while greatly alleviating pain. Many patients would report an enlarging and hardening of the tumor after a few treatments. Then the tumor would start to soften. People also frequently reported a discharge of large amounts of pus and fleshy material. Masses of diseased tissue were sloughed off in persons with breast, rectum, and internal cancers. After this process, the tumor would be gone.[3]

Caisse theorized that one of the herbs in Essiac reduced tumor growth while other herbs acted as blood purifiers, carrying away destroyed tissue as well as infections related to the malignancy. She also speculated that Essiac strengthened the body's innate defense mechanisms, enabling normal cells to destroy abnormal ones as Nature intended.

Even if a tumor didn't disappear, Caisse maintained, it could be forced to regress, then surgically removed after six to eight Essiac treatments, with much less risk of metastasizing and causing new outbreaks. "If there is any suspicion that any malignant cells are left after the operation," she stated, "then Essiac should be given once a week for at least three months, supplying the body with the resistance to a recurrence that is needed."

She wrote, "In the case of cancer of the breast, the primary growth will usually invade the mammary gland of the opposite breast or the auxilla, or both. If Essiac is administered either orally or by hypodermic injection, into the forearm, the secondary growth will regress into the primary mass, enlarging it for a time, but when it is all localized it will loosen and soften and can then be removed without the danger of recurrence."[4] Caisse spoke from personal experience, having administered thousands of Essiac injections to gravely ill patients, always under the supervision of a physician.

In 1983, Dr. E. Bruce Hendrick, chief of neurosurgery at the University of Toronto's Hospital for Sick Children, urged Canada's highest health officials to launch "a scientific clinical trial" of Essiac. In a letter to the Canadian Minister of Health and Welfare, Dr. Hendrick reported that eight of ten patients with surgically treated tumors of the central nervous system, after following an Essiac regimen, had "escaped from the conventional methods of therapy including both radiation and chemotherapy."[5] Yet today, patients in Canada must go through a bureaucratic maze that makes it difficult or impossible for them to receive Essiac therapy.

The story of Essiac began in 1922, when Caisse, a surgical nurse working in a Haileybury, Ontario, hospital, noticed an elderly patient with a strangely scarred, gnarled breast. When Rene asked the woman, who was nearly eighty, what had happened, the woman replied that some thirty years earlier, she had developed a growth on her breast and an Indian friend had offered to heal it with herbal medicine. This woman and her husband then went to Ontario, where doctors confirmed the diagnosis of advanced cancer and told her the breast would have to be surgically removed. Opting instead to take her chances with the Indian herbal healer, the woman returned to his mining camp and drank the brew daily. Her tumors gradually shrank, then disappeared. Over two decades later, when Caisse stumbled across her in the hospital, she was still totally cancer-free.

Caisse asked the woman for the herbal recipe. "My thought was that if I should ever develop cancer, I would use it," Caisse later wrote.

In 1924, Caisse's aunt, Mireza Potvin, was diagnosed with advanced cancer of the stomach and was told she had six months at the most to live. Remembering the Indian brew, Rene asked her aunt's physician, Dr. R. O. Fisher of Toronto, for permission to try it on her dying relative. Dr. Fisher consented, and Rene gathered the herbs to brew the tea. After drinking the herbal concoction daily for two months, Mireza Potvin rallied, got well, and went on to live another twenty-one years.

Soon Caisse and Dr. Fisher teamed to treat cancer patients who had been written off by their doctors as terminal. Many of these patients, too, showed dramatic improvement. Working nights and weekends in Toronto in her mother's basement, which Rene had converted into a laboratory, she and Dr. Fisher experimented on mice inoculated with human cancer. They modified the combination of herbs to maximize efficacy. It was at this point that Rene named the herbal treatment Essiac (her name spelled backwards).

One of Rene's first cases was a woman who had cancer of the bowel complicated by diabetes. In order to avoid further problems, the patient stopped taking insulin in 1925. Under Essiac therapy, the woman's tumor at first became larger and harder, almost obstructing her bowel. Then, as she continued her Essiac injections, the tumor softened, got smaller, and disappeared. Oddly enough, the woman's diabetes also disappeared during the course of Essiac treatment.

Dr. Frederick Banting, world-famous as the codiscoverer of insulin, reviewed this case in 1926. According to Caisse, Dr. Banting concluded that Essiac must have somehow stimulated the pancreatic gland into normal functioning, thus clearing up the diabetic condition. If this reported result is true, Essiac would appear to have potential in the treatment of diabetes.

Nine doctors petitioned the Canadian federal health department in 1926, urging that Caisse be allowed to test her cancer remedy on a broad scale. In their signed petition, they testified that Essiac reduced tumor size, prolonged life in hopeless cases, and showed "remarkably beneficial results," even where "everything else had been tried without effect."

In response, Ottawa's Department of Health and Welfare sent two investigating doctors armed with official papers to arrest Nurse Caisse or restrain her from practicing medicine without a license. When Rene explained to them that she was treating only terminal cases and accepting only voluntary contributions, the two interrogators backed off. One of them, Dr. W. C. Arnold, was so impressed by Caisse's clinical reports that he persuaded her to continue her experiments with mice at the Christie Street Hospital in Toronto. In that series of tests, mice implanted with human cancer responded to Essiac injections by living longer, their tumors regressing.

In 1935, the Town Council of Bracebridge turned over to Rene Caisse—for one dollar-per-month rent—the old British Lion Hotel for use as a cancer clinic. Over the next seven years, Caisse treated thousands of patients in this building, which had been repossessed by the village for back taxes. This unique arrangement came about after Dr. A. F. Bastedo of Bracebridge referred a terminally ill patient with bowel cancer to Caisse. Dr. Bastedo was so impressed by the patient's recovery, he persuaded the town council to make the hotel building available to Rene.

Shortly after the clinic opened, Caisse's seventy-two-year-old mother, Friselde, was diagnosed with cancer of the liver, inoperable because of her weak heart. One of Ontario's top specialists, Dr. Roscoe Graham, said she had only days to live. Rene began giving daily injections of Essiac to her mother, who had not been told she had cancer. After ten days of treatment, Friselde Caisse began to recover. She regained her full health, with diminishing doses of Essiac, and lived another eighteen years before passing away quietly from heart disease.

"This repaid me for all of my work," Rene reflected years later, "having given my mother 18 years of life which she would not have had. [It] made up for a great deal of the persecution I had endured at the hands of the medical world."[6]

After word of Caisse's impressive results spread to the United States, a leading diagnostician in Chicago introduced her to Dr. John Wolfer, director of the tumor clinic at Northwestern University Medical School. In 1937, Wolfer arranged for Rene to treat thirty terminal cancer patients under the direction of five doctors. Rene commuted across the border to Chicago, carrying her bottles of freshly prepared herbal brew. After supervising one and a half years of Essiac therapy, the Chicago doctors concluded that the herbal mixture prolonged life, shrank tumors, and relieved pain.

Dr. Emma Carson, a Los Angeles physician, spent twenty-four days inspecting the Bracebridge clinic in 1937. A skeptical investigator who originally intended to stay in Bracebridge for just a couple of days, she scrutinized the clinical records and examined over 400 patients. In her detailed report, Dr. Carson wrote:

> Several prominent physicians and surgeons who are quite familiar with the indisputable results obtained in response to "Essiac" treatments . . . conceded to me that the Rene M. Caisse "Essiac Treatment" for Cancer is the most humane, satisfactory and frequently successful remedy for the annihilation of Cancer "that they had found at that time" . . .
>
> I also visited, examined and obtained data at patients' homes where they were pursuing their business vocations as ably as if they had never experienced the afflictions of Cancer. They declared their restoration to normalcy was indisputably due to Miss Caisse's "Essiac" treatments. . . . They emphatically declared "were it not for Miss Caisse's Essiac remedy for Cancer, they would have departed from this earth" . . .
>
> As I examined each patient regarding intervening progress during the preceding week and recorded notes of indisputable improvements . . . I could scarcely believe my brain and eyes were not deceiving me, on some of the most seriously afflicted cases. . . .
>
> The vast majority of Miss Caisse's patients are brought to her for treatment after Surgery, Radium, X-Rays, Emplastrums, etc., has failed to be helpful, and the patients are pronounced incurable. Really the progress obtainable and the actual results from "Essiac" treatments and the rapidity of repair was absolutely marvelous and must be seen to convincingly confirm belief.

Another independent investigator of the Bracebridge clinic was Dr. Benjamin Guyatt, a University of Toronto curator and anatomy professor. After making dozens of inspections of the clinic during the 1930s, Dr. Guyatt summarized his findings as follows:

> The relief from pain is a noticeable feature, as pain in these cases is very difficult to control. On checking authentic cancer cases, it was found that hemorrhage was readily brought under control in many difficult cases. Open lesions

of lip and breast responded to treatment. Cancers of the cervix, rectum, and bladder had been caused to disappear. Patients with cancer of the stomach, diagnosed by reputable physicians and surgeons, have returned to normal activity.

. . . The number responding wholly or in part, I do not know. But I do know that I have witnessed in this clinic a treatment which brings about restoration, through destroying the tumour tissue, and supplying that something which improves the mental outlook of life and facilitates reestablishment of physiological functions.[7]

Supporters of the Bracebridge nurse presented a bill to the Ontario parliament in 1938 to allow Caisse to treat cancer patients with Essiac free from the constant threat of arrest to which she had been subjected. Over 55,000 people signed a petition supporting the bill, including patients, their families, and many doctors. The bill failed to pass by three votes.

This set the stage for the creation of the Royal Cancer Commission, which many believed was a judicial farce. Comprised of six orthodox physicians with expertise in surgery, radiation, and diagnostics and led by an Ontario Supreme Court justice, the commission was charged with an impartial investigation of alternative cancer therapies. Public hearings opened in March 1939.

Even though 387 of Caisse's patients showed up to testify, only 49 were allowed to be heard. One after another, patients and ex-patients testified that Rene Caisse had restored them to health and saved their lives after they had been given up as dead by their orthodox doctors.

Annie Bonar testified that her diagnosed uterine and bowel cancer had spread after radium treatments until her arm had swelled to double its size and turned black. Weighing ninety pounds the night before she was to have the arm amputated, she opted for Essiac therapy instead. After four months of the herbal treatment, her arm was back to normal and she had gained sixty pounds. A series of X-ray exams revealed she was cancer-free. The Royal Commission, however, listed Annie Bonar's case as "recovery due to radiation."

Walter Hampson, another patient of Caisse who testified, had cancer of the lip, diagnosed by a pathologist. Refusing radium, he underwent Essiac therapy and was restored to normal. Despite the fact that he had never had an operation (other than the removal of a tiny nodule for analysis), the commission classified his case as "recovery due to surgery." These examples could be multiplied many times.

In addition to misattributing recoveries, the Royal Commission also labeled numerous cases as "misdiagnoses," even though the patients had been diagnosed as definitely having cancer by two or more qualified physicians. Using duplicitous tactics like these, the commission was able to conclude that "the evidence adduced does not justify any favourable conclusion as to the merits of 'Essiac' as a remedy for cancer. . . ."

In 1942, a disheartened Rene Caisse, fearing imprisonment due to her medical work, closed her clinic. Over the next thirty-odd years, she continued to treat cancer patients in great secrecy from her home. Documents indicate that she was under surveillance by Canada's Health Department during the 1950s.

At the age of seventy, in 1959, Caisse was invited to the Brusch Medical Center in Massachusetts, where she treated terminal cancer patients and laboratory mice with Essiac under the supervision of eighteen doctors. After three months, Dr. Charles Brusch, eminent physician to the New England elite, and his research director, Dr. Charles McClure, concluded that Essiac "has been shown to cause a decided recession of the mass, and a definite change in cell formation" in mice. "Clinically, on patients suffering from pathologically proven cancer, it reduces pain and causes a recession in the growth; patients have gained weight and shown an improvement in their general health. . . . Remarkably beneficial results were obtained even on those cases at the 'end of the road' where it proved to prolong life and the quality of that life. . . . The doctors do not say that Essiac is a cure, but they do say it is of benefit."

The Sloan-Kettering Institute for Cancer Research tested one of the herbs in Essiac, sheep sorrel, between 1973 and 1976. Caisse sent a quantity of the herb to Sloan-Kettering, along with detailed instructions on how to prepare it as an injectable solution. On June 10, 1975, Dr. Chester Stock, a Sloan-Kettering vice president, wrote to Rene: "Enclosed are test data in two experiments *indicating some regressions in sarcoma 180 of mice treated with Essiac*" (emphasis added).[8] Despite these promising results, the tests ground to a halt when Rene was horrified to learn that instead of boiling the herb, as she had instructed, the scientists were *freezing* it.

In 1977, Rene sold the formula for Essiac to the Resperin Corporation, a Canadian company. Resperin's tests on Essiac, though initially encouraging, dragged on for years. Patients in Canada seeking Essiac through the government must first find a physician who will sponsor them and submit the appropriate official form. The physician should contact the Health Protection Branch of the Canadian Health and Welfare department to arrange to purchase the product from Resperin Corporation. The physician's request should roughly read: "I have a patient who has (type of cancer) affecting (body parts or organs). I request permission to treat the patient with Essiac on an emergency basis." The physician should mail the request to the Health Protection Branch, Bureau of Human Prescription Drugs, Director's Office, c/o Emergency Drug Division, Tower B—Second Floor, 355 River Road, Place Vanier, Vanier, Ontario K1A 1B8. Many doctors are reluctant to do this, however, fearing establishment pressure or ridicule. Even if the necessary forms are submitted, permission to use Essiac is not always granted.

A report issued in 1982 by the Health Protection Branch of the Canadian Health and Welfare department finds that "no clinical evidence exists to support claims that Essiac is an effective treatment for cancer." This blanket condemnation ignores sixty years of clinical documentation and observational evidence as well as laboratory studies. The report says:

> In 1982, 112 physicians who had received Essiac under these circumstances, were asked to submit case reports. Seventy-four responded on 87 cancer patients. Of these, 78 showed no benefit.
>
> Investigation of the nine remaining cases revealed that the cancer was progressing (four cases), the patient had died (two cases) or that the disease had stabilized (three cases).
>
> Of this last group, all the patients had previously undergone some form of cancer treatment which could have stabilized the disease.

The report does not explain why only 74 of the 112 physicians responded. Were the other 38 doctors perhaps afraid to submit responses favorable towards Essiac, fearing orthodox ridicule and peer pressure?

It is also not clear whether the 78 patients that "showed no benefit" experienced a reduction in pain or an improvement in appetite. These important components of cancer care are generally not counted as a benefit in such studies.

Were any of the 87 patients, all severely ill, given intramuscular injections of Essiac, as Rene Caisse so often administered in advanced cases? Critics of the report say that *no* patients were given intramuscular injections.

Was the herbal mixture prepared correctly, or were the herbs possibly frozen and damaged, as was done at Sloan-Kettering? Were the oral doses given frequently enough? Neither answer is known.

In three cases, "the disease had stabilized." What does this mean? Had the cancer stopped growing? If so, that is highly significant.

What about the four cases where the "cancer was progressing," plus the two cases where the "patient had died"? Why are these counted among the "remainder" rather than among those that "showed no benefit"? Doesn't that mean they *did* show some benefit, and if so, what were the benefits? The report does not say.

Even a casual analysis of these poorly run trials illustrates the bias that pervades much of the research purporting to be objective and scientific.

Gary Glum, biographer of Rene Caisse, calls the Canadian government report an outright deception. He says that some of the people listed in the report as "dead" were actually alive and well and that a number of them showed up on Caisse's doorstep in 1978, the first year of the study, to thank her profusely for having saved their lives. Glum views the report as one more attempt by Canada's medical orthodoxy to discredit Essiac.

A Los Angeles chiropractor, Glum spent three years researching Caisse's story. In his biography of the nurse, *Calling of an Angel* (see Resources),[9] published in 1988, Glum says he obtained the formula for Essiac from a woman who had achieved total remission of her cancer after treatment by Rene. This woman, according to Glum, was given the Essiac formula in writing by Caisse. The unidentified woman, as Glum tells it, tried to alert the world to the efficacy of Essiac in treating cancer, and in the late 1970s, she took her case as far as the Michigan Superior Court but was then constantly harassed by FBI (Federal Bureau of Investigation) and FDA officials.

Glum says that he later verified the authenticity of the Michigan woman's formula with Mary McPherson, an Ontario woman who was Caisse's close friend. McPherson lived and worked alongside Caisse for many years, after the Bracebridge nurse cured McPherson's mother of cancer in the 1930s. McPherson confirmed by telephone that she did in fact meet with Glum and that his formula was indeed correct, although there were variations that Rene occasionally used.

Glum's critics contend that the formula Glum gives in an instruction sheet accompanying his book is inaccurate. They charge that it is missing at least one key ingredient and is drastically off in the ratios of the various herbs. The critics allege that Glum's version of Essiac is not the true Essiac and that it is potentially harmful to patients.

Glum steadfastly denies this. He points out that he put himself at great personal and legal risk to divulge what he maintains is the correct formula. He asserts that he is the only person in the alternative cancer field who has openly publicized the exact details of a purported cancer cure, unlike others who keep the details of their therapy secret, or proprietary. Thousands of copies of Glum's book were seized and held at the United States–Canada border by Canadian authorities, who say the book is advertising of an unapproved drug. The book was finally allowed into Canada through the strenuous efforts of a high-ranking Canadian politician, yet thousands of confiscated books have still never been released, according to Glum.

Glum says he paid the unidentified woman $120,000 for the Essiac formula and insists that he will never recover the money. He claims that his formula is identical to the Essiac tested by medical researchers in the Soviet Union and China when Resperin officials were attempting to interest the medical establishments there in a cancer cure.

According to Glum, the herbal potion prepared by following the instructions supplied in his book has helped many cancer and AIDS patients get well. Some AIDS patients taking the herbal tea report that drastically low T-cell counts have risen to normal.

Sheila Snow, who coauthored a pivotal 1977 article on Caisse for Canada's *Homemaker's* magazine, believes that Glum's version of Essiac "is the recipe Rene used in the 1930s when she prepared the remedy in her Bracebridge clinic for hundreds of patients, and quite conceivably the one passed along to the Resperin Corporation for its clinical studies." In a July 1991 article on Essiac in the *Canadian Journal of Herbal Medicine,* Snow gives the exact recipe and preparation instructions presented by Glum. In her opinion, "We owe a large debt of gratitude to Dr. Glum for having the courage to take on this enormous responsibility—no small task!—at great personal financial expense, time and energy."

Dr. Charles Brusch, cofounder of the Brusch Medical Center where Rene worked in 1959, reported in a letter dated August 3, 1991, "I have been taking this [Essiac] myself since 1984 when I had several cancer operations, and I have every faith in it. Of course, each person's case is different as well as each person's own individual health history. . . . Someone may respond in a week; someone else may take longer, and whether or not someone is cured of cancer, the Essiac has been found to at least prolong life by simply strengthening the body."

Brusch went on to note that "I was given the true original formula by Rene when she worked with me in my clinic." He added that he passed along this authentic formula to Canadian radio producer-broadcaster Elaine Alexander of Vancouver, who had been following the Essiac story for twenty years and had interviewed on her program many cancer patients who had been cured through Essiac. Documents indicate that in November 1988, Brusch transferred Caisse's herbal formula to Alexander, who then arranged to have the product manufactured and sold through a distributor. Alexander's Essiac is offered strictly as a nutritional product, under a different brand name, with the manufacturer making no claims regarding its reputed value in treating cancer.

Alexander points out that the method of preparation, the precise ratios of the ingredients, and the correct dosages are all crucial to Essiac's efficacy. She says that Caisse continually improved on Essiac over the years through experimentation and that she believes Glum's version of Essiac may be "an early, primitive version" of a formula Caisse later strengthened and perfected. Alexander further claims that the various "specious facsimiles" of Essiac on the market can be quite dangerous.

Testimonials from cancer patients who achieved complete remission or considerable improvement using Essiac are obtainable from Elaine Alexander. These remarkable letters document cases of the last fifteen years and encompass many types of cancer, including pancreatic, breast, and ovarian cancer; cancers of the esophagus, bile ducts, bladder, and bones; and lymphoma and metastatic melanoma.

Muriel Peters of Creston, British Columbia, one of the people who wrote to Elaine Alexander to describe her experience with Essiac, was diagnosed in 1981 with a malignant tumor the size of an orange on her coccyx, the triangular bone at the base of the spine. She underwent surgery a week later. The surgeons told her, "We got it all," but according to Muriel, "By the time they had found the tumor, it had begun to flare up the spine among the nerve endings, so they could not cut there." She had twenty-nine radiation treatments following the surgery. In September 1982, sensing numbness in her lower abdominal area, she went to the Cancer Clinic in Vancouver and was told by a head surgeon that the tumor had spread to her spine and was inoperable, and nothing more could be done.

When her brother-in-law mentioned a man with cancer who had been given three months to live but was cured "somewhere down South," Muriel Peters followed up the lead. One month later, she visited the Bio-Medical Center in Tijuana, Mexico, and began the Hoxsey herbal therapy. Within three months, sensation returned to her lower abdomen, but this was followed by "three months of excruciating pain which no pills could relieve." She then began taking Essiac in liquid form, which she obtained from the Resperin Corporation through her doctor. After twelve days, the pain subsided. "From then on I was on my way up."

For the next year and a half, Muriel took Essiac daily. She also remained on the Hoxsey regimen, which consisted of an herbal tonic, vitamin supplements, and a special diet stressing fresh vegetables, greens, and fruits. "I felt the two complemented each other," Muriel explains. "Without the diet and the vitamins, I really doubt if either of the tonics would have been quite enough. The body has to rebuild what the cancer has broken down, therefore healthy foods are needed by the body to reconstruct itself."

About a year after she started her dual Essiac-Hoxsey program, Muriel returned for tests to the Vancouver Cancer Clinic. Incredulous, the attending doctor told her, "For reasons unknown there have been notable changes in your body."

"When the doctor left the room," recalls Muriel, "the attending nurse asked me what I was doing to bring about these changes, and I only said, 'I'm on a diet and vitamins.' The nurse asked, 'On your own?' I replied, 'No, by doctors directing.' She then said, 'Well, as long as you're not going to Mexican quacks, as many are doing.'"

A complete medical checkup in September 1989 found Muriel Peters cancer-free and in excellent health. At sixty-eight, she reported, "I'm the healthiest person in British Columbia. I love life and living. . . . I have learned what life is all about." X-rays and blood tests in January 1991 confirmed her to be in complete remission, nine years after she was diagnosed with inoperable, "hopeless" cancer.

Elaine Alexander says she met a Vancouver physician who, in 1990, had spoken with an oncologist at Canada's Health Protection Branch in Ottawa. This physician, according to Alexander, was told by the government oncologist, "It is known, at this office, that Essiac is effective against brain tumors, especially brain stem tumors." Critics of Essiac will no doubt dismiss this story as a self-serving fabrication. Yet Gary Glum has a remarkably similar story. He recalls a man who telephoned him to say that his two-year-old daughter had been diagnosed with an inoperable, advanced brain tumor and was given just weeks to live. The man, according to Glum, was calling to thank him for writing Caisse's biography, through which he had learned about Essiac. His daughter had been saved by the herbal remedy and, at age five, was in perfect health.

Are these stories just a singular coincidence? Glum and Alexander do not speak to each other. Their relationship, if anything, is one of rivalry, each party feeling that he or she possesses the "correct" Essiac formula. So it is ridiculous to suggest that they "compared notes" in order to concoct similar accounts of Essiac's reported efficacy in treating cancer.

It is more likely that Caisse experimented with her basic recipe over the years and that some of the contemporary products purporting to be Essiac reproduce major variants of her formula. Confirming this theory would require exhaustive detective work beyond the scope of this book. Readers are urged to thoughtfully evaluate any and all claims. Caution is advised since a number of the purported versions of Essiac on the market today do not even contain the principal herbs, instead substituting one or more incorrect ingredients.

The Canadian herbal remedy developed by Rene Caisse is not being recommended in this chapter as a "magic bullet" for all cancers. There is no hard evidence on what percentage of Caisse's patients survived five years or more. Nor is there any reliable statistical evidence on the efficacy of contemporary Essiac or Essiac-like herbal formulas. Despite the dramatic, near-miraculous cures Caisse undoubtedly achieved, an unknown percentage of patients under her care succumbed to their disease, perhaps too severely ill to be treated.

The world has become an infinitely more polluted place since the 1920s and '30s, when Caisse did her pioneering work. Carcinogenic, toxic chemicals and radioactive isotopes that pollute our water, air, and food also reside permanently in the cells of our bodies, weakening our natural immunity and possibly making the remission of cancer more difficult. For these reasons, combining Essiac with nutritional and other approaches may make the most sense.

Resources

Elaine Alexander
6690 Oak Street
Vancouver, British Columbia
V6P 3Z2
Canada
Phone: 604-261-1270

ESSIAC International
Mr. T.P. Maloney
Suite 2211
1081 Ambleside Drive
Ottawa, Ontario
Canada K2B 8C8
Phone: 613-820-9311

Reading Material

Calling of an Angel, by Gary L. Glum, Silent Walker Publishing (P.O. Box 92856, Los Angeles, CA 90009; no phone number), 1988. Can also be ordered directly from the author at P.O. Box 80098, Los Angeles, CA 90080; 213-271-9931. Includes an instruction sheet for a purported recipe for Essiac.

The Treatment of Cancer With Herbs, by John Heinerman, BiWorld Publishers (Orem, Utah), 1984. Out of print; order photocopies directly from the author at P.O. Box 11471, Salt Lake City, UT 84147; 801-521-8824.

"Could Essiac Halt Cancer?" by Sheila Snow Fraser and Carroll Allen, *Homemaker's,* June–July–August 1977.

"Old Ontario Remedies—1922: Rene Caisse ESSIAC," Sheila Snow, *Canadian Journal of Herbalism,* July 1991.

Chapter 11

MISTLETOE (ISCADOR)

Mistletoe, a semiparasitic plant once held sacred by Germanic tribes, the Celts, and Druid priests, has been used medicinally over the centuries. In 1920, Iscador, an extract of the European mistletoe, was proposed as a cancer remedy by Austrian thinker and biologic researcher Rudolf Steiner (1861–1925), the founder of Anthroposophy, a spiritual philosophy and movement. Since 1963, Iscador has been a key component in the cancer therapy offered by the Lukas Klinik in Arlesheim, Switzerland. It can also be administered totally outside the context of Anthroposophical care.

Steiner suggested, without any proof, that mistletoe was a possible treatment for cancer, basing his hunch on an analysis of the plant's unusual characteristics. Subsequent studies have demonstrated that mistletoe extract enhances immune-system activities that ward off or inhibit tumors. For example, it stimulates the thymus, the chief regulator of cellular immune reactions. It also increases the number of *granulocytes*, which are the scavenger white blood cells that consume invading antigens, and enhances *phagocytosis*, the white blood cells' ability to ingest and destroy other cells or foreign material. Iscador elevates the number of immunocompetent white cells and activates natural killer cells capable of spontaneously destroying tumor cells.[1]

Mistletoe extract also contains biologically active proteins (*lectins*) and other substances that have exhibited powerful antitumor action in animal and cell-culture experiments. In cancer patients, Iscador therapy—usually as an adjunct to conventional treatment, but sometimes on its own—has produced a slowing of tumor growth, occasional regression of tumors, and, in some cases, remission, even in "hopeless" or "terminal" cases. Proponents of Iscador claim that it is the only well-known cancer drug with a double-barreled effect—the destruction of cancer cells combined with a stimulation of the body's natural defenses. One theory holds that mistletoe proteins have a direct effect on DNA's genetic code, preventing the "translation" of the gene segments responsible for accelerated, uncontrolled cell division.

Despite a growing international medical literature in support of Iscador's anticancer properties, the mistletoe extract is blacklisted by the American Cancer Society. The ACS condemnation is based on an evaluation of the literature undertaken by Dr. Daniel Martin, a surgeon who has been an outspoken opponent of unorthodox therapies, and Dr. Emil Freireich, a pioneer of chemotherapy who was on record as an opponent of nonconventional cancer treatments. The two doctors found that the seventeen positive clinical and scientific papers sent to them on Iscador constitute "no evidence" of efficacy.[2]

While Iscador is not widely used in the United States, some American physicians incorporate it in their practice. American doctors can legally order Iscador directly from European manufacturers, even though the extract is not approved for sale in the United States. A handful of physicians in the United States who practice an Anthroposophically extended medicine include mistletoe as part of their therapeutic protocol. American patients can elect to travel to Europe for Iscador treatment. Mistletoe therapy is available at clinics, at hospitals, and in private practices in Switzerland, Germany, the Netherlands, the United Kingdom, Austria, and Sweden.

Iscador has been used mainly as an adjunct to surgery, radiation, and chemotherapy. The best results have been obtained in the treatment of solid tumors both before and after surgery and radiotherapy. Clinical trials at the University Hospital in Munich and in Basel, the Wien-Lainz Hospital in Vienna, and the Lukas Klinik have shown that Iscador therapy improves the survival rates for cancers of the cervix, ovaries, vagina, breast, stomach, colon, and lung as well as other locations.

Preoperative mistletoe therapy is given for ten to fourteen days prior to surgery. Its aim is to help prevent metastatic spread of the cancer due to the surgical intervention. Postoperative treatment is ideally begun immediately after surgery or radiotherapy. It is continued for a number of years, with a gradual reduction in dosage and an increase in the intervals between courses of injections. This follow-up treatment reportedly reduces the risk of recurrence after surgery or radiation.

Iscador is usually administered by subcutaneous injection at or near the tumor site. In some instances, it is given orally, such as with primary tumors of the brain and spinal cord. A typical course of treatment consists of fourteen injections given in increasing concentrations. In postoperative care, injections can be administered by a nurse or a relative, or by the patients themselves, with a progressive reduction of doses. Thus patients can look after themselves, as diabetics do, and need only see a doctor for occasional checkups.

Over the decades, Iscador has proven to be generally free of side effects, though many patients experience a moderate fever on the day of the injection and, in some cases, inflammation around the injection site, temporary headache, and chills. Very rarely, a local or general allergy develops, with skin reaction, shivering, bronchospasm, or shock, which may require discontinuation of the treatment.

Many cancer patients given Iscador therapy experience reduced pain, relief of tiredness and depression, better sleep, improved appetite with weight gain, and elevation of hemoglobin and red-blood-cell levels. Where Iscador therapy does not bring remission, it improves quality of life and may extend life.

The best responders to Iscador are carcinomas of the bladder, genitals, and digestive tract, and melanomas, according to Dr. Rita Leroi, who for many years was the supervisor of the Lukas Klinik. She says, "Breast cancer in women is a somewhat difficult field; for these, our best results are in the postoperative phase, whereas the present tumor is often refractory. A similar situation arises for inoperable lung carcinoma where we cannot boast of more than a somewhat longer life expectancy, whereas results with operable lung carcinoma are especially good."[3]

In treating inoperable tumors, prolonged Iscador therapy sometimes results in a better demarcation between the tumor and its neighboring tissues. This makes surgery possible and sometimes leads to the arrest of the tumor growth or even an occasional regression. When Iscador is used concurrently with chemotherapy, hormone therapy, or radiation, it often alleviates the undesirable side effects of these conventional treatments. But the best results with inoperable cancers have been obtained with tumors of the bladder, stomach, intestine, and genital organs, as well as skin cancers. The growth of bone metastases is often retarded. However, the results are not as good in treating inoperable cancers of the breast, lungs, or esophagus.

Iscador is also used to treat cancers of the bone marrow, connective tissue, and blood-forming organs, specifically lymphomas, sarcomas, and leukemias, although it is less effective with these cancers than with the solid carcinomas. Leukemia does not usually respond well to mistletoe therapy. Anthroposophical physicians also recommend mistletoe extract for what they consider precancerous states, such as ulcerative colitis, cervical erosion (such as dysplasia), a chronic gastric ulcer, abnormal growth of breast tissue (proliferative mastopathy), and Crohn's disease (chronic inflammatory bowel disease).

Rudolf Steiner believed that mistletoe preparations could correct the imbalance between the body's "form-giving forces," which create structure and find expression in the immune system, and its "cellular forces," which regulate cell division and growth. In Anthroposophical medicine, the form-giving tendencies hinder the development of tumors, but when these individualizing, formative forces are critically weakened, cellular growth gains the upper hand and, if unchecked, can lead to cancer. Factors believed to disrupt the formative forces include environmental carcinogens, impurities in the daily diet, poisons such as alcohol and tobacco, and chemical or genetic damage to the embryo.

Beyond the physical, cancer is viewed by Anthroposophical medicine as a disorder that generally has its roots at the level of soul and spirit. "Severe strokes of fate, failure of life-plans, unsatisfactory conditions of life etc. weaken the immune system . . . depressing the form-giving principle," according to Rita Leroi, M.D.[4] Dr. Leroi also says, "The essence of cancer lies . . . in a certain paralysis and disintegration of the higher principles, a process beginning on the level of spirit, trickling down gradually into the soul and the physical body."[5] As the formative forces weaken and lose their ability to keep cells performing their specialized functions, the cells become autonomous and selfish. "The cancer cell falls back into its own individual life—it no longer puts itself into the services of a higher organ or organism—it becomes egotistic," explains Anthroposophical physician Friedrich Lorenz.[6]

Just as the cancerous growth acts autonomously, rebelling against the ordering principles of the organism, so, in the realm of soul and spirit, a parallel process takes place in thinking, feeling, and willing, according to Anthroposophical medicine. "When thinking separates itself from feeling and willing and carries on its own, separate activity, then it also separates itself out of the reality of its proper purpose," writes Lorenz. "Thoughts become icy-cold and without love."[7]

Feeling, if no longer guided by thinking and will, leads to selfish desire, greed, and addiction, emotional or physical. Willing, if not imbued with life-filled thoughts or true feelings, becomes a destructive force. "In our day and age, we are surrounded by these phenomena world-wide—the same tendencies which manifest themselves in cancer as a tumor," states Lorenz.

Steiner predicted the anticancer properties of mistletoe extract, which he named Iscador, through an intuitive understanding of the plant's striking botanical characteristics. Unlike other plants, which align themselves with either the Sun (through heliotropism) or the Earth (through geotropism), "mistletoe is a self-willed plant in that it behaves as if the Earth were not there," says Leroi. A bushy plant that grows on trees, drawing off the water and mineral salts it needs, the European mistletoe "grows in any direction which happens to suit it, sideways, downward, any direction where it finds room to build up its own inner space."[8] Mistletoe also goes its own way with respect to time: it produces berries all year long, and it flowers in the winter. Mistletoe has no real roots but penetrates the tree's wood with sinkers, wedge-shaped rudimentary organs.

Steiner described mistletoe as a survivor of an ancient epoch in the Earth's evolution, a time before the surface of firm mineral ground had formed. In his scenario, there was a soft primeval mass with islands that supported the growth of plants at a developmental stage somewhere between our present-day plants and animals. Steiner believed mistletoe to be such an "animal-plant," left behind from the "Old Moon period" of the Earth. He spoke of mistletoe's "insane aristocracy," its tendency to do everything by its own rhythms, in its own time. "Just so is the tumor a manifestation of forces that work in an insane way in the human organism," observes Leroi. "But mistletoe conquers the tumorous tendency with its own rhythmically built-up formation, and with its exaggerated flowering impulse in which differentiation, subduing mere growth, is evident. This dynamic power to overcome tumor growth, conveyed to patients by injection of a suitable preparation, has a healing effect."[9]

Iscador, a fermented extract of the whole mistletoe plant, is manufactured by a method designed to enhance the plant's formative forces. Part of the processing takes place in a centrifuge, which blends saps extracted from plants in summer and in winter "to create a unity." The mistletoe used to produce Iscador grows on various host trees: oak, apple, elm, pine, and fir. "Iscador M" refers to preparations made from mistletoe grown on apple trees and is used to treat women with cancer. "Iscador P," from pine trees, is for both men and women. Different preparations are chosen according to the patient's gender and the location of the primary tumor.

Some types of mistletoe extract are combined with minute quantities of various metals, such as silver, mercury, and copper, thought to enhance the activity of Iscador on specific organs and systems. For example, an Iscador preparation with copper is used for primary tumors of the liver, gallbladder, stomach, and kidneys. Metals are added in exceedingly diluted concentrations, for instance, one-hundredth of a milligram of copper per one hundred milligrams of mistletoe. (In contrast, the dietary Recommended Daily Allowance for copper is two milligrams.)

The European mistletoe (*Viscum album*) is a different plant from the American mistletoe (*Phoradendron flavescens*). The herb should be taken only under proper supervision. The berries are poisonous and should not be eaten. Persons with heart trouble should be careful when using mistletoe, since it raises the blood pressure and speeds up the pulse. Mistletoe extract should never be taken at the same time as any prescription medicine containing a monoamineoxidase inhibitor; the mixture will cause serious side effects.

In Anthroposophical medicine, cancer is not so much a tragedy as an opportunity to undergo inner spiritual change and find new direction. For Steiner, the patient is a being of body, soul, and spirit who has the capacity for wrestling with the illness and even growing through it. The Anthroposophical physician enters into dialogue with patients to help them solve personal problems and gain insight into their destiny and their illness. Patients are encouraged to see the cancer not as a punishment but as a springboard for a change of mind and heart, allowing new impulses and new possibilities to be nourished. In Dr. Leroi's words, "We endeavor to help patients realize that their soul and spirit are an indestructible, God-given integral whole, and that they can grow inwardly because of their illness, even if it were to lead to disintegration of the physical body."[10]

At the Lukas Klinik, Iscador is part of a program encompassing diet, herbs, and therapies that use art, music, and movement. Artistic activities like painting, clay modeling, creative speech, and color therapy lift the patients out of their fixed habits and help them unblock their creative faculties. Eurythmy, involving rhythmic exercises, allows the soul to "breathe freely" again; group eurythmy is intended to help "introverted and self-centered cancer patients . . . learn hereby to take notice of other people and to move along with them in a common rhythm," according to Dr. Leroi.[11] Physical therapy includes oil massage as well as heat in various forms, such as hot baths with oils or herbs "prescribed in order to activate the warmth organism." Heat therapy not only boosts the immune response but is also valued by Anthroposophical healers for creating warmth believed to permeate the entire disease process at all levels.

The vegetarian diet recommended by the Lukas Klinik consists of organic, fresh fruits and vegetables, whole grains, juices, salads, olive and sunflower oils, some butter, sour milk, yogurt, and light cheeses. Foods to be avoided include tomatoes (held to be carcinogenic), mushrooms, hardened fats like margarine, and refined sugars. Alcohol and cigarettes are taboo. Patients should follow a light diet, with small meals taken at regular intervals and fairly frequently.

Fifty years of research on Iscador's antitumor and immune-enhancing properties support Rudolf Steiner's original insight, even though his goal—a complete disintegration of the tumor—has only been achieved to a limited extent. A 1990 study found that in cultures of human cells, a mistletoe lectin (protein) increased the production of *tumor necrosis factor–alpha*, a hormone secreted by immune cells that destroys cancer tissue. This lectin also boosted the production of interleukin-1 and *interleukin-6*, important mediators of immune response.[12]

Resources

Lukas Klinik
CH-4144 Arlesheim
Switzerland
Phone: 011 41 61-701-3333

For further information on mistletoe and details on treatment.

Physicians Association for Anthroposophical Medicine
P.O. Box 269
Kimberton, PA 19442

For a list of Anthroposophically oriented physicians in the United States.

Mercury Press
241 Hungry Hollow Road
Spring Valley, NY 10977
Phone: 914-425-9357

For books and booklets on Anthroposophy and Anthroposophical medicine.

Anthroposophic Press
R.R. 4, P.O. Box 94 Al
Hudson, NY 12534
Phone: 518-851-2054

For books on Anthroposophy and Anthroposophical medicine.

Reading Material

The Mistletoe Preparation Iscador in Clinical Use, by Rita Leroi, M.D., Society for Cancer Research (Research Institute Hiscia, CH-4144, Arlesheim, Switzerland; 011 41 61-701-2323), 1987.

Directions for the Use of Iscador in the Treatment of Malignant Conditions, written and published by the Society for Cancer Research (Research Institute Hiscia, CH-4144, Arlesheim, Switzerland; 011 41 61-701-2323), 1986. Written specifically for medical practitioners and pharmacists; not intended for patients.

An Anthroposophical Approach to Cancer, by Rita Leroi, M.D., Mercury Press (see page 126 for address and phone number), 1982.

Cancer: A Mandate to Humanity, by Friedrich Lorenz, M.D., Mercury Press (see page 126 for address and phone number), 1982.

Anthroposophically Oriented Medicine and Its Remedies, by Otto Wolff, M.D., Mercury Press (see page 126 for address and phone number), revised edition, 1989.

Anthroposophical Medicine: Spiritual Science and the Art of Healing, by Victor Bott, M.D., Healing Arts Press (One Park Street, Rochester, VT 05767; 800-445-6638), 1984.

Iscador: Compendium of Research Papers 1986–1991, edited by Paul W. Scharff, M.D., three volumes, Mercury Press (see page 126 for address and phone number), 1991.

Chapter 12

PAU D'ARCO

Pau d'arco is a popular herbal remedy for cancer sold in health-food stores. Available in the form of tea bags as well as capsules and loose powder, it is also known as lapacho, ipe roxo, and taheebo. The herbal tea is prepared from the inner bark of various species of a large South American tree that flowers a vibrant pink, purple, or yellow. This tree is the Tabebuia tree, native to Brazil and Argentina.

In South America, pau d'arco is widely used as a treatment for cancer and illnesses such as colds, flus, fevers, malaria, infections, syphilis, gonorrhea, and at least one kind of lupus. The tree also grows in India, where it is used for similar complaints. Supporters of pau d'arco say that it builds up immunity to disease, combats infection, and eliminates pain and inflammation. According to the late Jonathan Hartwell—biochemist, researcher for the National Cancer Institute, and author of the definitive *Plants Used Against Cancer*—pau d'arco tea has been used in folk remedies for cancers of the pancreas, esophagus, intestines, head, lung, prostate, and tongue; Hodgkin's disease; leukemia; and lupus erythematosus. One species of Tabebuia, *T. serratofolia*, is traditionally used in Colombia to treat cancer.

In the United States, word-of-mouth reports and written testimonials from cancer patients link tumor regression or remission to drinking pau d'arco tea. A recent case of a cancer sufferer apparently cured through pau d'arco was reported by biochemist Wayne Martin in the Winter–Spring 1991 issue of *Cancer Victors Journal*. The patient had surgery to remove a cancerous bladder but then developed a rectal metastasis and was given a series of radiation treatments. At the same time, he drank a lot of pau d'arco tea. He appears to be in complete remission, and since "the radiologists seem to have very little success in treating rectal cancer or metastases . . . this patient presumes that drinking taheebo tea had much to do with his remission." Martin has also received fragmentary reports of breast cancer patients doing well on taheebo tea.[1]

Bill Wead, whose 1985 book, *Second Opinion*, focuses on pau d'arco as a cancer treatment, had on file "literally hundreds of testimonies as to the efficacy of Lapacho." His book presents a number of case histories of cancer patients who attribute their recovery to the herbal medication.

However, "there is very strong evidence that once a remission has occurred, it is necessary to continue drinking the tea," according to Wead. He observed that in "a few" cases where remission had occurred after drinking pau d'arco, the cancer later returned. In some of these cases, the recurrence came only after the person stopped drinking the tea. Wead also emphasized that pau d'arco does not work for everyone.[2] There is no reliable statistical data on pau d'arco's efficacy against cancer or on its long-term effects, positive or negative. But an impressive body of laboratory evidence plus a handful of clinical studies indicate that *lapachol*, an organic compound present in the tea, has strong antitumor properties as well as antibiotic and antimalarial action.[3]

Given the promising reports of cancer patients benefiting from pau d'arco and the provocative scientific evidence that its components have antitumor action, why aren't the National Cancer Institute and the nation's medical research centers rushing to test this remarkable herbal tea, which might yield a safe, inexpensive cancer cure?

The NCI sponsored a single Phase I study of oral doses of lapachol over twenty years ago. Nineteen patients with advanced tumors and two patients with leukemia in relapse were given oral doses of lapachol ranging from 250 to 3,750 milligrams per day. Although the study was designed to measure only toxic and pharmacologic effects of the drug, the researchers found that one patient with metastatic breast cancer had a regression in one of several bone lesions. However, they also found that high oral doses of lapachol (1,500 milligrams or more per day) produced undesirable side effects such as nausea, vomiting, and a tendency to bleed. In addition, the investigators said they could not achieve therapeutic blood-plasma levels of lapachol without encountering anticoagulant effects and toxicity. On this basis, NCI concluded that lapachol was unfit for human use in treating cancer, and the drug's Investigational New Drug status was cancelled in 1970.

There are several things wrong with NCI's rush to judgment, however. First, the amount of lapachol consumed by drinking pau d'arco tea is much less than the high doses administered in this clinical trial. As Kathi Keville points out in the July 1985 issue of *Vegetarian Times,* "Toxicity of pau d'arco is very low. It produces nausea and anti-coagulant effects on the blood only in very high doses." In fact, even as the NCI dismissed lapachol as too toxic for use in human beings, United States Department of Agriculture (USDA) studies indicated that pau d'arco tea has less toxicity than coffee.

Second, according to the main author of the clinical study, Dr. J. B. Block, "Lapachol exhibited antitumor activity . . . with little toxicity noted by patients and no myelosuppression, hepatic or renal toxicity." Dr. Block and colleagues at the Harbor-UCLA Medical Center called for a re-evaluation of lapachol, noting that its anticoagulant effects may be inhibited simply by administering vitamin K.[4] This combination has proven effective in laboratory studies.

Third, the National Cancer Institute made the mistake of isolating a single component of pau d'arco—and then, on the basis of a test with that one substance, concluded that the herbal medicine is worthless. More recent studies in Scotland indicate that *some twelve different quinones* (aromatic compounds) in the pau d'arco bark synergistically interact and are more therapeutically effective than isolated lapachol.[5] As every herbal healer knows, each medicinal plant may contain a whole spectrum of biologically active substances that work in concert. By testing for one isolated type of activity in a laboratory setting, investigators overlook the value of a wide range of plant substances with powerful therapeutic properties demonstrated in the people who use the herbal remedy.

Here is a brief summary of a few of the studies done on pau d'arco worldwide:[6]

- Nine patients were given oral doses of lapachol for twenty to sixty days or longer. One complete tumor regression and two partial tumor regressions occurred. One patient had hepatic adenocarcinoma; another had basal cell carcinoma of the cheek with metastases to the cervix; and the third had ulcerated squamous cell carcinoma of the oral cavity.[7]

- The life span of leukemic mice treated with a lapachol derivative for nine days increased 80 percent over a control group.[8]

- West German scientists investigating pau d'arco for antitumor effects found that nine constituent compounds have dose-dependent immunomodulating effects on human immune-system cells. This suggests that the ability of pau d'arco compounds to destroy cancer cells may be at least partly due to stimulation of the immune system.[9]

- Extracts of pau d'arco (rather than lapachol alone) killed cancer cells in culture and reduced the occurrence of lung metastases in mice following surgery to remove tumors. Five times as many mice survived in the group given pau d'arco compared with the control group.[10]

- Lapachol was shown to have significant activity against Walker 256 carcinoma, especially when administered orally to animals implanted with this tumor.[11]

- Lapachol was found to be an excellent antitumor agent and antibiotic.[12]

Pau d'arco came to public attention in 1967 when the respected Brazilian magazine *O Cruzeiro* headlined the lead article in its March 18 issue, "Positive Cases Prove Discovery of a Cure for Cancer." The article described cancer victims who were cured by taking the herbal tea, as investigated by a Sao Paulo botany professor, Walter Acorsi. In tracking down the recovered patients, Professor Acorsi discovered that a number of doctors had been treating cancer patients successfully with lapacho tea. This included doctors working in the municipal hospitals of San Andrea, Brazil. Soon Acorsi himself was besieged by people asking for lapacho. He was amazed to see tumors shrink, pain diminish, and even hopeless cases show remission.

Much of the early clinical work on pau d'arco was done by Dr. Theodoro Meyer, an award-winning Argentine botanist, who made an extract from various lapacho inner barks in 1966 and gave his herbal medicine to doctors in hospitals. He died in 1972 after years of frustrated efforts to convince the medical establishment of the value of pau d'arco.

With the publication of the *O Cruzeiro* article, news of pau d'arco spread to neighboring countries. In Tucuman province along the Argentine Andes, Dr. Prats Ruiz, a general practitioner, successfully treated two children with leukemia who were not expected to live. One of them, five-year-old Maria Adela Vera, had leukemia-like symptoms, and doctors told her parents that her outlook was bleak.

Maria's steadily worsening cytological picture revealed a low erythrocyte count of 3 million and a platelet count of 60,000 on July 15,

1967. (Erythrocytes are red blood cells, and platelets are very small cells in the blood needed for clotting.) The hospital doctors, as a last resort, suggested to the girl's parents that they try Dr. Ruiz's clinic. After ingesting pau d'arco teas and elixirs for one week, the little girl greatly improved. On July 21, a blood analysis revealed that her erythrocyte count had gone up to 3.8 million and her platelet count to 120,000. By August 5, her platelet count had increased to 135,000, and even though she caught the flu in August, she recovered without complications and continued to improve until, by September, a blood analysis showed 4.2 million erythrocytes and 160,000 platelets. Maria was discharged from the clinic and taken home by her parents, with her apparent leukemia-like symptoms gone.[13]

As enthusiasm for pau d'arco intensified, so did the orthodox medical community's attempt to stifle interest in it. Soon after the *O Cruzeiro* article ran, signs were posted in the San Andrea hospital announcing that pau d'arco was no longer available. The hospital had originally promised the journal full documentation of its cancer cases, but hospital authorities were now prohibited from speaking further. Despite this, *O Cruzeiro* reporters were able to locate many people throughout Brazil who were willing to testify to lapacho's therapeutic effects.

Drinking pau d'arco tea soon became fashionable in holistic health circles in the United States, Canada, Australia, Germany, Japan, and Italy. But as pau d'arco became big business, cheap imitations using the wrong tree species flooded the marketplace worldwide.

According to Varro Tyler, Ph.D., author of *The New Honest Herbal*, some of the pau d'arco herbal teas marketed in the United States do not come from the Tabebuia species at all, even though they are labeled "lapacho colorado" or "lapacho morado." Instead, the packaging says they come from the bark of *Tecoma curialis,* a closely related member of the same plant family. Tyler, dean of Purdue University's School of Pharmacy, feels that the substitution most likely makes little difference because the therapeutic constituents, if any, are probably similar. He notes that the woods of various species of Tabebuia commonly contain from 2 to 3 percent to about 7 percent of lapachol, a napthoquinine derivative, and states that it is reasonable to assume this compound is also present in the bark. A critic of alternative therapies, Tyler deems the use of pau d'arco unwise because of its "lack of proven effectiveness" and its "potential toxicity."[14]

A recent analysis of the bark of specimens of the Argentine *Tabebuia impetiginosa* tree and other species collected for commercial purposes detected only trace amounts or no measurable amounts of lapachol.[15] According to Bill Wead's *Second Opinion,* Professor Walter Acorsi, in his research, discovered that out of over 250 varieties of the *Bignoniaceae* (the family to which the tree belongs), only one provides the purple lapacho bark that yields what seems to be a highly effective anticancer tea. This tree is the *Tabebuia impetiginosa* of Argentina. Others have identified the *Tabebuia heptaphylla* tree of Brazil as another reliable source of pau d'arco.

For the prospective user of pau d'arco, a good rule of thumb is: Let the buyer beware. "I have a feeling the market is loaded with fake pau d'arco," says biochemist Wayne Martin. Read the product label, brochure, or instructions carefully to see from which plant the tea comes. You might want to contact the vendor to see whether there are any testimonials on file from people who benefited from the use of the product, or if any such people are known. Some vendors may be reluctant to talk openly, but others may have such information available. You might also consider having the product tested by a laboratory to determine whether it contains lapachol and, if so, how much.

Most of the pau d'arco users whom Wead interviewed took drops of concentrated tea under the tongue every fifteen minutes to a half hour besides drinking up to eight cups of tea a day. They discontinued the drops once they experienced a purging or improved appetite and strength, but they all continued to drink the tea. Even after an apparent remission had occurred, all of Wead's interviewees felt strongly that it was necessary to continue drinking at least four cups of tea daily.

Bill Wead died of a heart attack in 1991. According to his brother Tim Wead, Professor Acorsi gave Bill the following guidelines concerning pau d'arco:

- Do not boil the tea in a tin pot or kettle. Ideally, a glass pot should be used. Stainless steel is acceptable.
- The packaging material of the tea should not be made of plastic.
- Pau d'arco in pill form is of little or no value.

Wayne Martin claims that if all cancer patients at an early stage of their disease practiced self-medication with pau d'arco tea, the cancer death rate would greatly decline. He says that the action of pau d'arco appears to be similar to that of warfarin sodium, an anticoagulant drug. (An anticoagulant is a substance that delays or prevents the clotting of blood.)

Warfarin sodium has been used in treating advanced cancer with some success. Clinical trials suggest that oral warfarin sodium has the ability to slow down tumor growth rate. According to this line of thinking, warfarin-like anticoagulants inhibit the formation of *fibrin,* the protein coat that surrounds and protects malignant tumors. Fibrin is believed to induce *angiogenesis,* the development of a vascular network providing blood and nourishment to a new cancer colony. In the Winter–Spring 1991 issue of *Cancer Victors Journal,* Martin reviews a number of experimental and clinical studies suggesting that warfarin-like drugs help prevent cancer from metastasizing.[16] He speculates that pau d'arco also has this action.

Resources

Pau d'arco is available at many health-food stores and through herbal distributors.

Reading Material

Second Opinion: Lapacho and the Cancer Controversy, by Bill Wead, Rostrum Communications (Vancouver), 1985. Available from the Cancer Control Society (see page xv for address and phone number).

The New Honest Herbal, by Varro Tyler, George F. Stickley Company (Philadelphia), second edition, 1987. Out of print; check your local library. A cautionary view of herbal therapies.

Chapter 13

CHAPARRAL

Chaparral, a dark olive green plant native to the southwestern United States and Mexico, has been widely used as a treatment or adjunctive remedy for cancer. Also known as creosote bush and greasewood, the hardy shrub grows abundantly even in the driest, hottest desert regions. For centuries, Native Americans have brewed the leaves and stems of chaparral to treat a host of illnesses, including cancer, venereal disease, arthritis, rheumatism, tuberculosis, colds, stomach disorders, and skin infections. In folk medicine, chaparral has been used for leukemia and cancers of the kidney, liver, lung, and stomach.

Persons with cancer taking only chaparral tea have claimed remission or shrinkage of tumors, as reported in various magazine articles. Chaparral is also used by persons with AIDS for its immune-stimulating properties. Commonly available in health-food stores, the herb can be taken as a tea, tincture, capsule, or pill.

Besides containing immune-stimulating *polysaccharides*, chaparral has as a key ingredient *nor-dihydroguaiaretic acid* (*NDGA*), which has been shown to have powerful antitumor properties. NDGA inhibits electron transport in the *mitochondria*, or "energy-producing factories," within cancer cells, thereby depriving tumors of the electrical energy they require to exist.[1]

NDGA is also a potent inhibitor of *glycolysis*, the breakdown of sugars and other carbohydrates by enzymes. The work of Nobel Prize–winning biochemist Otto Warburg indicates that cancer cells live by fermenting sugar in anaerobic (airless) reactions. NDGA is a strong inhibitor of both anaerobic and aerobic glycolysis. Dean Burk, Ph.D., outlined a possible mechanism of action for NDGA based on Warburg's work, suggesting that chaparral may actually reorient the fermentation process of cancer cells.[2] Burk performed experiments with NDGA at the National Cancer Institute. His research showed that in laboratory cultures, "this is a very active agent against cancer," in the words of Dr. Charles Smart of the University of Utah Medical Center.

Modern science lends support to the Indians' faith in the healing virtues of chaparral. To a curious visitor, a Pima Indian of Arizona once said, "This plant cures everything. It is what nature gave us."[3] The Mexicans call the creosote bush *gobernadora* ("governess") because chaparral reputedly governs the body, reversing all manner of ailments. This belief in chaparral's therapeutic powers is shared by many Native American tribes, who use the herb to treat everything from the common cold to bladder stones to cancer. Chaparral is recognized in current herbal medicine as "one of the best herbal antibiotics, being useful against bacteria, viruses, and parasites," writes naturopath Michael Tierra in *The Way of Herbs*.

Until 1967, NDGA was a common additive in baking mixes, candies, oils, lards, frozen foods, vitamins, and various pharmaceuticals. An antioxidant, it kept these items from spoiling by preventing the growth of bacteria. It is a powerful scavenger of free radicals, the reactive chemicals that form continuously in the body and have been shown to damage cells.[4]

Chaparral is an incredibly resourceful plant. It luxuriates in blistering, dry areas where few animals or plants can survive. Its taproot reaches five or six feet into the earth, and with its large network of root laterals meshing up to fifty-five square yards of soil, the plant gets its full share of water even in the lightest shower. Nature has provided chaparral with a protective varnish on its tiny leaves to lock in the precious stores of water. And the bush secretes a substance that prevents plant seeds—including many of its *own* seeds—from germinating around it. This method of botanical birth control, called allelopathy, is achieved through chaparral's strong growth-inhibiting properties, which may be chemically related to its tumor-inhibiting action.

Chaparral caught the interest of the medical profession when Ernest Farr, an eighty-seven-year-old Mormon temple worker from Mesa, Arizona, came to the University of Utah Medical Center with a malignant melanoma, a deadly form of skin cancer, on his right cheek and neck. After three operations to remove it, the recurring growth returned a fourth time, and in October 1967, the doctors advised Farr to have another surgical excision and a radical neck dissection. He refused and, in November, began treating himself with chaparral tea, which he made by steeping the dried leaves and stems in hot water (approximately seven to eight grams of leaves per quart of water). He drank two cups of this tea daily and took no other medication.

By February 1968, the facial lesion had shrunk to the size of a dime and the neck mass had disappeared. When Farr returned to the university medical center in Salt Lake City in September 1968, the lesion on his cheek was the size of a tiny pimple, two to three millimeters in diameter. Farr had gained twenty-five pounds and was in excellent health.[5]

Farr lived to be ninety-six. According to testimony by Kathlyn Windes of Tempe, Arizona, he died of the same melanoma, which recurred after the conventional doctors treating him at that time refused to let him have chaparral. Kay Windes got Farr's story on a cassette tape. She also obtained a shorter version in his own hand-writing in which he describes his method of drying chaparral at home. On the tape, Farr tells how a woman with cancer of the neck and breast healed herself by drinking chaparral tea twice a day. This woman, who worked on a cattle ranch, was alive and well forty-five years after her recovery.[6]

Galvanized by Ernest Farr's dramatic recovery, University of Utah scientists in 1969 to 1970 tested chaparral tea and NDGA on fifty-nine cancer patients with advanced incurable malignancy. Some patients drank two to three glasses of chaparral tea per day, while others received oral doses of pure NDGA (250 to 3,000 milligrams per day). Four patients had tumor remissions. One of the four was Farr, who was included in the study. Another patient had advanced melanoma. The third, who had a regression lasting two months, had choriocarcinoma spread to the lungs. And the last, who had a temporary regression, had widespread lymphosarcoma. Another melanoma patient experienced a 95 percent regression, following which the remaining growth was removed by surgery. Also, 27 percent of the patients showed "subjective improvement" during their treatment with chaparral tea or NDGA.[7]

Dr. Hugh Hogle, a University of Utah physician, one of the authors of the NCI-sponsored study, in 1970 informed the American Cancer Society of a fact he had not previously presented in any of his reports: one of the four patients manifesting "significant regression" remained in remission for four months before suffering a relapse.[8] Yet, in a 1972 letter that Dr. Hogle wrote to a woman in California who had requested information about chaparral, he stated that the longest regressions had lasted "only two and one half months."

Medical anthropologist John Heinerman, in his book *The Treatment of Cancer With Herbs,* points out a number of inconsistencies in the University of Utah study. Heinerman suggests that the university medical team became "somewhat upset" at the media publicity spotlighting its work as a potential cancer cure. "The full story about the abrupt halt in the chaparral research done at the University of Utah Medical Center . . . will never be fully known," concludes Heinerman.

An elderly Amish man cured himself of terminal cancer by taking fifteen chaparral tablets a day, according to a June 27, 1979, story by William McGrath, a columnist for *The Budget,* an Ohio newspaper serving the Amish-Mennonite community. In his book, Heinerman tells how a leukemia sufferer from Oakland, California, arrested his cancer by going on a "chaparral cleansing program." The man's daily regimen included double-strength chaparral tablets, comfrey, and Nectar D'Or liquid minerals.

A woman diagnosed with cancer of the cervix at the University of Oregon Medical School gynecology clinic was advised to have either a hysterectomy or a cave biopsy of the cervix. Doctors told her that her condition would not respond to any form of therapy. But she refused surgery and instead began taking powdered herb combinations in capsule form twice a day, one capsule of chaparral once a day, and ginseng tea. The combination capsules included chaparral leaves, blood-root, red clover blossoms, burdock root, echinacea root, goldenseal root, comfrey leaves, ginseng root, and greater celandine, along with smaller quantities of fourteen other herbs. A Pap test of her cervical cells taken one month later showed no evidence of cancer.[9]

Tom Murdock, founder of Nature's Way, a well-known herb company, reported that chaparral helped his wife's breast cancer go into remission when conventional medical treatment failed. After Lavoli Murdock's recovery, Tom began selling the desert shrub; chaparral thus helped start the family's herbal business.

A formula for chaparral tea as a cancer remedy is given by Arlin J. Brown in *March of Truth on Cancer.*[10] Brown's recipe is as follows:

> Put 4 ounces in a 2-quart bottle and add 1 cup of boiling water. Steep for about 10 minutes and then fill to about 1 inch from the top with boiling water. Put on tight-fitting lid, set in the sun for 2 days, and strain. Drink 3 cups a day.

Brown, who runs the Arlin J. Brown Information Center dispensing information on alternative cancer therapies, advises that patients who drink chaparral should take a good iron supplement. "If you take chaparral for a few years without an iron supplement, it will destroy the blood-forming organs in the body," he says. Laboratory tests and clinical experience with the desert herb indicate that it is nontoxic, generally has no side effects, and is compatible with medication.

Even though there are known cases of people who brought their cancer into remission on chaparral alone, Brown strongly advises against such a regimen. "To take only chaparral tea, or pau d'arco, or Essiac, or whatever is not enough. A person with cancer needs an intensive program combining detoxification and immune enhancement. Chaparral taken alone might help in some early cases of cancer, but it's by no means a total therapy. You need to detoxify the body—through vegetable and fruit juices, herbs, blood purifiers, and other measures such as colonic irrigations or coffee enemas. Then you need immune enhancement by going on a proper diet and taking immune-boosting supplements. Only through such a program can cancer patients maximize their chances of preventing a recurrence."

Herbalist Michael Tierra has outlined a therapeutic anticancer program combining diet and detoxification. In *The Way of Herbs*, Tierra specifies an herbal formula that he believes can aid the body in detoxifying itself. This formula emphasizes "the most powerful blood purifiers in the herbal kingdom," chaparral and echinacea, and also includes red clover blossoms, cascara sagrada, astragalus, ginseng, and other herbs. Another anticancer herbal formula featuring chaparral, echinacea root, pau d'arco, and red clover blossoms is given in Tierra's *Planetary Herbology*, which attempts to synthesize Western herbal medicine and traditional Chinese and Ayurvedic systems. Recognizing that cancers and tumors are "difficult to treat," Tierra sets forth a balanced diet for the cancer patient based on whole grains, beans, and fresh vegetables, and excluding red meat and (usually) dairy foods.[11]

Chaparral tea has a strong, resinous odor and an unpleasant taste. The Mexicans call the herb *hediondilla*, "little bad smeller." For this reason, many people prefer to use chaparral in tablet form. Several types of chaparral tablets are commercially available. The best are those in which the pure, powdered plant leaves have been compressed into tablets without the use of coatings, binders, fillers, excipients, or flavorings.

Another variation on chaparral therapy is Jason Winters Herbal Tea. Jason Winters, a former stunt man, reportedly healed himself of terminal cancer after cobalt treatments failed to reduce the size of a large tumor on his neck. He claims to have eliminated the tumor himself in three weeks by drinking a tea made from chaparral, red clover (a principal ingredient of Hoxsey herbs), and the root of a certain white flower from Singapore that he dubbed herbaline. Winters has never divulged the identity of this flower, supposedly because if he did, the plant might soon become very scarce.

Winters calls himself Sir Jason (he was knighted in Malta), and the front cover of one of his books describes him as "a combination of James Bond, Marco Polo, and Ponce de Leon." His marketing organization seems to be promoting Jason Winters Herbal Tea as something of a cure-all for whatever ails you besides cancer. Despite the puffery, however, cancer and leukemia patients have reportedly recovered or derived benefit from the tea's use.[12] Those interested in learning more about Sir Jason's quest for personal health could start with his book *Killing Cancer* (Vinton Publishing, Mound, Minnesota), available in health-food stores.

Scientific research on chaparral has continued sporadically. Recent studies by microbiologist Emiliano Mora at Auburn University have demonstrated that an extract of chaparral kills malignant cancer cells in test tubes. In experiments dating back to the 1960s, NDGA had significant growth-inhibiting activity against some animal tumors, though not against others. Despite the intriguing results obtained with chaparral in the laboratory and the known cases of cancer remission, the resourceful desert shrub remains condemned on the American Cancer Society's Unproven Methods blacklist. But chaparral, an incredibly adaptive plant, may outlive even the ACS's condemnation.

Resources

Chaparral is available at many health-food stores and through herbal distributors.

Reading Material

The Treatment of Cancer With Herbs, by John Heinerman, BiWorld Publishers (Orem, Utah), 1984. Out of print; order photocopies directly from the author at P.O. Box 11471, Salt Lake City, UT 84147; 801-521-8824.

Part Four

NUTRITIONAL THERAPIES

For decades, the cancer establishment insisted that diet has no effect on cancer. Those who pointed to a link between nutrition and cancer were dismissed as food faddists. But in 1982, the National Academy of Sciences (NAS) reversed itself in a 472-page report that said the typical American diet—high in animal protein, saturated fat, and sugar—was strongly associated with the majority of cancers. Long-term eating patterns were linked to the onset of 60 percent of cancers in women and 30 to 40 percent of cancers in men, according to hundreds of medical studies reviewed by the NAS panel. The NAS report set forth dietary guidelines urging drastic decreases in meat, poultry, egg, dairy, and refined-carbohydrate intake, coupled with a greater consumption of whole cereal grains, vegetables, and fruits.

In 1984, the American Cancer Society came out of its ivory tower and issued dietary guidelines very similar to those of the NAS. The combined recommendations of these two organizations include the following:

- Cut down on total fat intake. Eating less fat reduces the odds of developing breast, colon, and prostate cancer.
- Eat more high-fiber foods such as vegetables, fruits, and whole-grain cereals. These types of foods help reduce the risk of colon cancer.
- Include dark green, red, and orange vegetables and fruits, which are naturally rich in vitamins A and C.
- Include cruciferous vegetables such as cabbage, broccoli, and Brussels sprouts since they contain compounds that may help prevent cancer of the gastrointestinal and respiratory tracts.
- Be moderate in the consumption of salt-cured, smoked, and nitrite-cured foods. They have been linked to stomach and esophageal cancer.

Diet is additionally listed as a means of "primary cancer prevention" in the 1990 edition of the American Cancer Society publication *Cancer Facts and Figures.*

All the main features of the cancer-preventive diets recommended by the NAS and ACS have been central to the therapeutic anticancer diets prescribed for decades by alternative health practitioners. Common sense suggests that if poor nutrition can cause cancer, ideal nutrition may be able to reverse or slow it. But the medical establishment does not recognize nutrition as a *treatment* for cancer. It dismisses such therapies as quackery. As William Dewys, ex-associate director of the National Cancer Institute's chemoprevention program, said, "The nutritional therapies do a leap of logic in saying that if diet has a role in preventing cancer, then the same diet has relevance in terms of treatment. There is no solid evidence for that."

Hundreds of recovered cancer patients who got well on nutritional therapies are living evidence that diet *can* help cure cancer. People who brought their cancer into remission on such programs are simply dismissed by the medical orthodoxy as "anecdotal evidence." In the eyes of the ACS, they do not exist.

Nutritional therapies are used to attempt to eliminate the physiological or biochemical factors supporting the growth of cancer cells. When these conditions no longer exist in the body, proponents contend, the tumor will die. Many nutritional therapies include detoxification measures to rid the body of poisons, external and internal. External toxins come from cooked and refined foods, food additives, preservatives, pesticide residues, and drugs and synthetic growth hormones force-fed to animals before they are cruelly slaughtered. The internal source of toxins in the body are the waste products of metabolism, which are best cleansed from the cells with raw fruits and vegetables or their juices.

Most anticancer diets share certain features: they are largely vegetarian; they avoid or limit animal products; and they emphasize vegetables, fruits, and whole grains, especially fresh, organically grown foods. Meat is avoided because it has been implicated as a cause of cancer for several reasons. It contains chemical carcinogens, harbors transmittable cancer viruses, lacks fiber, has a high fat content, and has high levels of the hormone prolactin. An example of toxic meat is charcoal-broiled steak, two pounds of which contains as much benzopyrene as the smoke from *600 cigarettes.* When mice are fed the carcinogen benzopyrene, they get stomach cancer and leukemia. Another example is meat fat. When meat fat is heated, another carcinogen—methylcholanthrene—is formed. Even tiny doses of this substance increase cancer susceptibility.

About 70 percent of pork products have added nitrites, as do many other meat products, to protect against botulism-like germs. Animal corpses turn a sickly gray-green color after several days, so the meat industry tries to mask this discoloration by adding nitrites, nitrates, and other preservatives to make the meat look red. Many of these substances have repeatedly been shown to be carcinogenic. Furthermore, the nitrites in meat combine with amines found naturally in innumerable foods, producing deadly carcinogenic agents called nitrosamines.

"Meat animals" bred for slaughter on the factory farms that dominate American agriculture are force-fed chemical feed mixtures, injected with synthetic hormones to stimulate growth, and stuffed with appetite stimulants, antibiotics, sedatives, and other chemicals. The toxic residues from these noxious substances are present in your hamburger and pork chop. Many of these substances have been found to be cancer-causing; in fact, many animals die from these drugs before they can be led to slaughter.

Meat-eaters face another danger. Many animals are infected with diseases that are undetected—or simply ignored—by the meat producers and inspectors. Often, if cancer or tumors are present in one part of an animal's body, the cancerous part is cut away and the rest of the body is sold as meat. But cancer microbes from the tumors may be present in the rest of the animal's body. Worse yet, the tumors themselves are sometimes euphemistically labeled "parts" and incorporated into mixed meats such as hot dogs. Tumors are quite common in factory-farm animals. Cancer viruses in animal tumors can be transmitted from one species to another. For example, in 1974, it was found that chimpanzees fed from birth with milk from leukemic cows died of leukemia in the first year of life. There seems to be no valid scientific reason why the human species should be an exception to this form of cancer transmission.

The bacteria in meat-eaters' intestines reacts with digestive juices to produce cancer-causing chemicals within the body. This may explain why bowel cancer is widespread in meat-eating areas like the United States and Europe while it is extremely rare in more vegetarian countries such as India. Many studies have demonstrated that bacterial action converts bile acid in the human intestine into carcinogens. For example, certain types of clostridia (a bacteria found in the gut) are able to metabolize a bile acid, deoxycholic acid, converting it to the powerful carcinogen 20-methlycholanthrene. The key point to remember is that diet directly affects both bile acids and intestinal bacterial flora. Consumption of meat fat increases the production of such carcinogens. Vegetarians produce much less deoxycholic acid than do meat-eaters.[1]

Eating meat and animal fats promotes high levels of prolactin, a pituitary hormone that helps to start milk formation and lactation in women. High prolactin levels stimulate mammary tumor growth in animals. When humans switch from a meat diet to a vegetarian diet, their prolactin levels are cut nearly in half.[2]

Meat, poultry, dairy products, and eggs provide 100 percent of our dietary cholesterol and antibiotic and hormone additives. These foods are also our primary sources of saturated fats and pesticides. Studies show that by avoiding all meat, eggs, and dairy products, you can cut your risk of a heart attack by 90 percent.

Women who eat meat daily get nearly 4 times as much breast cancer as women who eat it less than once a week.[3] A woman's risk of breast cancer rises dramatically with her intake of meat, eggs, butter, and cheese. One out of every ten American women will develop breast cancer.

For men, the risk of fatal prostate cancer is 3.6 times higher among those who eat meat, cheese, eggs, and milk daily than among men who seldom or never eat these products. This worldwide pattern was confirmed by a twenty-year study at California's Loma Linda University involving over 6,500 men.

Cervical cancer, like breast cancer, is most prevalent among women whose diets are high in fat, particularly animal fat. Uterine cancer shows exactly the same relationship: the more fat a woman eats, the higher her risk.

Ovarian cancer reveals a similar pattern. Women who eat eggs three or more days per week are 3 times as likely to develop fatal ovarian cancer than women who eat eggs less than one day per week. This finding emerged from a twenty-year study published in the *Journal of the American Medical Association* on July 19, 1985.

Colon cancer is also closely correlated worldwide to a diet high in meat and animal fat and low in fiber.

Cancer patients considering one of the nutritional therapies, or another therapy that has a dietary component, should realize that a balanced vegetarian diet is not only completely safe and nutritionally adequate, it is also more healthful than an animal-based diet. Studies have repeatedly shown that vegetarians have a much lower incidence of cancer, heart disease, atherosclerosis, diabetes, obesity, and other degenerative conditions that take a heavy toll on lives each year. Vegetarians also live longer than meat-eaters. A study of a large group of vegetarians—the Seventh-Day Adventists—revealed that their rates of nutrition-related cancers (colon, rectum, intestine, and so forth) were 50 to 70 percent lower than for the general population.[4]

The all-too-common SAD (Standard American Diet) consists of 40 to

45 percent fat, mostly animal fat from meat and other products. The SAD, an unhealthy, cancer-causing diet, features chemically grown, chemically treated, processed, bleached, refined, sugared, salted, artificially colored and flavored, and almost totally devitalized "food." It contains a dangerous excess of protein. A person eating the meat-based SAD gets twice as much protein as he or she needs, even by conservative government standards. Diets with high levels of animal protein and fat are closely correlated with the most prevalent cancers in the United States. Excess protein is also linked to kidney stones, diabetes, osteoporosis, obesity, and excessive vitamin losses.

Most Americans have been brainwashed into believing that they must eat regularly from the so-called Four Basic Food Groups—meat, milk, vegetables and fruit, and bread and cereal. This scheme was concocted in 1956 by the United States Department of Agriculture working closely with the meat and dairy industries to beef up sales of meat and dairy products. In fact, the Four Basic Food Groups were preceded in the 1930s by the Twelve Food Groups. And in 1992, the Agriculture Department concocted a Food Guide Pyramid, which created five basic food groups by adding a new "essential" category—fats, oils, and sweets! In April 1991, the Physicians' Committee for Responsible Medicine (PCRM), a nonprofit organization with 10,000 members, presented a New Four Food Groups of grains, vegetables, legumes (beans, peas, and soy products), and fruit. PCRM physicians point out that meat and milk are health-depleting foods and recommend a vegetarian way of eating. Among the PCRM doctors who announced the New Four Food Groups were Denis Burkitt, discoverer of twenty-seven diseases including Burkitt's lymphoma, and T. Colin Campbell, a Cornell University nutritional biochemist.

"We're basically a vegetarian species. We should be eating a wide variety of plant foods and minimizing our intake of animal foods. The goal ought to be a diet made up of 80 to 90 percent plant foods, at a minimum," says Dr. Campbell, summarizing the findings of the China Health Project, a massive study undertaken by Cornell University, Oxford University, and two Chinese academies. Begun in 1983, this ongoing research project tracking the eating habits of 6,500 Chinese is the most comprehensive and rigorous study ever done on the relationship between diet and health. Participants who ate the most meat and cholesterol had the highest rates of cancer. The ideal percentage of fat intake was found to be 15 to 20 percent, perhaps less, *not* the 25 to 30 percent of all calories now recommended by the United States government-agribusiness complex. The study also confirmed that eating a lot of protein, especially animal protein, is closely linked to cancer and chronic diseases.

In a study recently released by the German Cancer Research Center in Heidelberg, vegetarians were found to have a more active immune system, with their white blood cells twice as effective against tumor cells as those of meat-eaters. The researchers surmised that either vegetarians harbor more natural killer (NK) cells to attack cancer cells or their NK cells are simply more powerful. The vegetarians in the study also had higher blood levels of carotene, the precursor of vitamin A, known to have antitumor properties.[5]

Part Four of *Options* focuses on three anticancer dietary regimens: wheatgrass therapy, macrobiotics, and the Moerman diet popular in Europe. It also touches on the raw foods diet and Natural Hygiene. Metabolic approaches to cancer treatment are covered in Part Five. It should be noted that many of the other therapies discussed in this book have a strong dietary (mostly vegetarian) component, for example, Livingston (Chapter 7), Issels (Chapter 8), and Iscador (Chapter 11).

People who decide not to pursue a dietary therapy should nevertheless give serious thought to incorporating nutritional changes into their lives no matter what therapy they choose. For a thorough look at meat-based and plant-centered diets and their effects on health, try John Robbins' *Diet for a New America* (Stillpoint Publishing International, Box 640, Meetinghouse Road, Walpole, NH 03608; 800-847-4014). Another very useful book is *Problems With Meat,* by John Scharffenberg, M.D. (Woodbridge Press Publishing Company, Box 6189, Santa Barbara, CA 93160; 800-237-6053).

Chapter 14

WHEATGRASS THERAPY

Wheatgrass, the grass grown from wheatberries (wheat seeds), is rich in chlorophyll, a substance nearly identical to the hemoglobin in human blood. Wheatgrass has sixty times more vitamin C than oranges, weight for weight, and eight times more iron than spinach, weight for weight. The sweet, green juice pressed from young, freshly cut wheat plants contains over 100 vitamins, minerals, and nutrients. It has all of the eight essential amino acids, plus eleven other amino acids, polypeptides (amino-acid chains), and the bioflavonoids (compounds related to vitamins) believed to neutralize toxic substances in the blood.

Wheatgrass is a storehouse of enzymes vital to cell respiration, digestion, and blood cleansing. Filled with liquid oxygen, wheatgrass juice also contains a number of anticancer agents, among them abscisic acid, a natural substance that has caused tumors to shrink or disappear in animal experiments. It's also a good source of laetrile (called vitamin B17), believed by many to have anticancer properties.

Wheatgrass therapy was developed by Ann Wigmore and is now offered at several independent holistic centers around the country. This nontoxic, noninvasive treatment combines the use of wheatgrass juice with a diet of organically grown, totally raw foods. Emphasis is on sprouted grains, nuts and seeds, fresh uncooked fruits and vegetables, fermented foods (to prevent harmful bacteria from growing in the intestinal tract), and greens such as buckwheat and sunflower. Exercise, aerobics, visualization, attitudinal change, and enemas (including wheatgrass enemas) for detoxification are other key elements of the program.

Wheatgrass therapy has been used for a wide range of acute and chronic degenerative diseases. In treating cancer and other conditions, the aims are to rebuild the body through good nutrition and detoxification and to restore the natural immune system so the body can mend itself. "The body of the cancer patient must heal itself in the same way any body rebounds from a cut, bruise, or common cold," says Ann Wigmore, founder of the Hippocrates Health Institute (now the Ann Wigmore Foundation) in Boston. "The body must replace the lost cells with new cancer-free ones." Wheatgrass juice, it is claimed, helps to detoxify the body, eliminate dead tissue, and nourish the system. A nutritional program combining wheatgrass and "live" foods (that is, uncooked foods—with enzymes and nutrients undamaged) is said to create optimal immune functioning, enabling the whole organism to reverse the cancer.

Wheatgrass therapy has brought about striking recoveries from cancer. Yet many people in the alternative cancer field do not consider it a primary therapy. They believe it might be most useful for early cancers and would recommend it, if at all, as a first-phase detoxification measure. Their feelings are that it might be effective against early, localized tumors but that it is just not strong enough for more advanced forms of cancer.

There may be some truth in this assessment. However, I was given newspaper clippings about, and testimonials by, long-term survivors from the five wheatgrass therapy centers I contacted. Staff at one of the five centers could recall no full remissions of cancer since 1986. Their best success story was a woman who succumbed to severe liver cancer after five years. She reportedly lived much longer and with much less pain than she would have on conventional treatment alone. Personnel at another well-known center could not provide me with recent cases of long-term remission, though they did present evidence of patients who had received substantial benefit from the therapy over the last two or three years.

The apparent scarcity of long-term survivors could be explained, at least partly, by poor documentation and lack of follow-up. Persons with cancer typically do a two- or three-week residential program at one of the centers, then go home to follow the regimen on their own. Some clients, but not all, return for periodic visits. Some undoubtedly go off the diet; some may recover but fail to keep in touch with the health center. "We're into helping people, not into statistics—we're just not into the documentation," a woman at the Health Institute of San Diego said. She said that her institute has many cases of long-term cancer survivors but that it does not give out names in order to respect clients' privacy.

Eydie Mae Hunsberger, the best-known long-term survivor who used the wheatgrass protocol, recovered from a fairly early cancer.

In her book *How I Conquered Cancer Naturally*[1] (see Resources), she tells how her husband found a lump the size of a quarter in her breast in 1973. After a mammogram was taken, a surgeon advised her that the standard procedure was to take a biopsy in the operating room and send the suspect tissue to the lab while the patient was kept under anesthesia. If the lump proved malignant, a radical mastectomy would be performed at once. The surgeon told her that if she had malignant cancer, she had an 80 percent chance to live one year and a maximum life expectancy of five years. He set up an appointment for Eydie Mae to be admitted to the hospital in three days.

Deciding against radical surgery, Eydie Mae with great difficulty found a doctor who agreed to perform a lumpectomy. After removal of the growth, which proved malignant, she was put on an immuno-therapy program. But she had severe allergic skin reactions to the antibiotics, and she began "to feel like a pin cushion" from all the injections. Several months later, she discovered four new lumps under her right arm in the lymph glands and two more "located right under the surgeon's incision line."

After hearing about wheatgrass therapy, Eydie Mae resolved to go on the program. She and her husband, Arn, spent two weeks at the Hippocrates Health Institute (Ann Wigmore Foundation) in Boston's Back Bay district. When she went back to her San Diego doctor, the lumps were smaller, and after continuing the wheatgrass program for several months, her doctor pronounced her in "ideal condition." Eydie Mae, who died in 1984 after a bicycle accident, lived a vigorous, healthy life. She never underwent the physical and emotional trauma of mastectomy or the insidious side effects of chemotherapy or radiation.

In February 1989, David Jones of Vancouver was diagnosed with an incurable, Grade IV, non-Hodgkin's lymphoma. Completely paralyzed for three weeks, he entered the hospital in a wheelchair. Diagnostic tests, including a myelogram, disclosed that a three-inch-long lymphomatic tumor wrapped around his spine had invaded his spinal column. The cancer had spread to his blood and bone marrow. In March, doctors surgically removed the cancer from around his spine, and they strongly recommended that he undergo intensive radiation and chemotherapy to combat the remaining cancer in his lymph nodes, bone marrow, and blood. "Even if I agreed to the orthodox treatment, I was given a maximum of two years to live," says David.

Four days after the operation, David walked out of the hospital with a cane, to the dismay and astonishment of the doctors. "I had begun wheatgrass therapy on my own in January," explains David.

"After I refused the conventional treatment and told the hospital that I intended to heal myself through a wheatgrass and raw foods approach, the doctors talked about me in a derogatory fashion like I was some kind of mental patient. They said that, at best, I had a 20 percent chance of survival for two years."

A vegetarian in his teens, David, at age twenty-eight, had gone back to "a beer and barbecue style of eating, with lots of steaks, processed foods, junk food—in other words, the standard American diet." Physically active as a carpenter, soccer player, and skier, he was shocked when his rapidly spreading cancer disabled him completely. "I knew I had been abusing my body, and I knew I had to get back to a sensible diet to give my body a chance of recovery." Within a year of beginning the wheatgrass therapy, he was swimming and riding bikes up mountains. In mid-1990, he made two trips to the Ann Wigmore Foundation in Boston, where he learned the finer points of a therapy he had essentially taught himself by reading Ann Wigmore's *The Wheatgrass Book* (see Resources). In August 1990, his orthodox doctors were amazed to find no trace of cancer, and subsequent X-rays and blood tests confirmed him to be in remission.

"I give much credit to the neurosurgeon who helped save my life, but I know that I did the right thing for me in refusing radiation and chemo," says David, who is writing a book about his experience entitled *A Warrior in the Land of Disease.* "You don't get well by pouring juice down your throat. Wheatgrass therapy is a complete lifestyle, involving what and how you eat, the way you think and feel about yourself." Along with the organic diet, he now practices yoga, meditation, and breathing exercises. "Some of Ann Wigmore's ideas and methods may sound weird or funny at first glance," he adds, "but I think she has all the answers. She recognizes that Nature herself is the final healer. The Earth is in a desperate situation right now, and Ann's natural method of healing is one part of the solution."

Drinking wheatgrass as a dietary supplement has been popular in parts of Europe since 1925, but Ann Wigmore, born in Lithuania in 1909, first introduced the wheatgrass habit to the United States in the 1960s. She learned the techniques of natural healing from her grandmother, the town healer, who raised her on a diet of grass, herbs, roots, goat's milk, and a bread made of rye meal and straw. During World War I, Ann was trapped with her grandmother and several other people in an orchard cellar. They survived on the roots in the cellar and the grasses that Ann's grandmother would sneak out at night to gather.

Emigrating to the United States at the age of sixteen, Ann became a doctor of divinity and metaphysics. She adopted the all-American diet—high in meat, animal fats, and sugar, and low in fiber, fresh fruit, and vegetables—and she got sick. Remembering her grandmother's survival foods, she cured herself of gangrene and, later, she claims, of cancer of the colon.

Ann settled in Boston in the late 1950s and wrote a column for the *Natural Health Guardian,* a nutritional magazine. In 1960, she was awarded a degree as a naturopathic doctor from a French school. Determined to find out why certain grasses seem to have therapeutic properties, she contacted G. H. Earp Thomas, a soil scientist in New Jersey who helped agriculturists around the world in improving grasses. According to Ann, "Dr. Earp Thomas isolated over one hundred elements from fresh wheatgrass and concluded that it is a complete food." She then carried out feeding experiments with newborn chicks. After a few weeks, the chicks receiving wheatgrass along with their regular chick food "had grown twice as large as the others. They were more alert and had feathered out better." Groups of kittens and rabbits fed in similar fashion showed comparable results. "I knew, then, that I had been entrusted with a precious secret to help people."[2] She founded the Hippocrates movement in Boston in 1963, naming it after "the father of medicine," the Greek physician Hippocrates, whose byword was: "The body heals itself. The patient is only Nature's assistant."

The "live foods" component of wheatgrass therapy predates Wigmore's institute by many decades. Naturopathic health centers in India and many other countries have treated cancer patients with a diet of raw vegetables and fruits grown in organic soils free of synthetic fertilizers, pesticides, and chemicals. In Denmark, medical doctor Kristine Nolfi brought her malignant, fast-growing breast cancer under control in the 1940s through a raw foods diet, to which she applied the term "live food." Dr. Nolfi became the chief physician of a sanatorium, Humlegaarden, in Humlebaek, Denmark, where she treated patients with cancers of the breast, rectum, intestine, abdomen, stomach, lung, and brain.

"Patients suffering from cancer have generally suffered for many years from gastric catarrh and constipation. Cancer is the final stage in an over-acid and degenerated organism," wrote Dr. Nolfi. Her views are echoed today by the wheatgrass therapy movement in the United States. Dr. Nolfi also believed, "If cancer is discovered at an early stage, consistent consumption of raw vegetables and fruits may in many cases keep it in check, even for a considerable number of years. . . . If cancer is discovered at a later stage, consistent consumption of raw vegetables and fruits may certainly help to relieve pain and lengthen life, but it cannot ordinarily preserve life."[3]

Wheatgrass (not used in Dr. Nolfi's original regimen) contains concentrated chlorophyll, the green, proteinous pigment found in plants. When Ann Wigmore consulted with Earp Thomas, the soil scientist identified chlorophyll as the element in wheatgrass that made Ann's chicks, kittens, and rabbits so vibrantly healthy.

The chlorophyll molecule, as German scientist Richard Willstaeter observed in the early twentieth century, is almost identical to the hemoglobin molecule in human blood. The only major difference between them is that the central atom in hemoglobin is iron; in chlorophyll, it is magnesium. Just as hemoglobin carries oxygen to the cells in humans, chlorophyll carries oxygen to plant cells. According to Laurence Badgley, M.D., chlorophyll ingested by humans is beneficial to the entire body, its healing effect a "natural principle." Dr. Badgley, a specialist in natural immune-enhancing therapies, states that many germs invading the human body prefer to grow in tissues having a poor supply of oxygen. The chlorophyll from wheatgrass juice helps improve blood circulation, better nourishing the cells. It provides protective oxygenation, a defense against anaerobic bacteria.

Otto Warburg, the Nobel Prize–winning German biochemist, performed experiments in the 1930s to show that cancer cells cannot thrive in the presence of oxygen. Warburg believed that cancer is a process of cell mutation caused by oxygen deprivation at the cellular level. He held that any effective cancer therapy must increase the oxygen content of the blood. His claim that cancer cells multiply in an oxygen-poor environment seems relevant today, when we know that smoking, air pollution, lack of exercise, poor breathing, and high protein and fat consumption can starve the body of up to 25 percent of its available oxygen.[4]

Yoshihide Hagiwara, M.D., a Japanese scientist who advocates the use of grass as medicine, theorizes that chlorophyll—the "blood" of plants—is transformed into human blood when consumed by people. He speculates that the magnesium ion in chlorophyll is replaced inside the body with an iron molecule, making new blood. Dr. Hagiwara reasons that since chlorophyll is soluble in fat particles— and since fat particles are absorbed directly into the blood via the lymphatic system—chlorophyll can also be absorbed this way.[5]

Japanese scientists working along with Hagiwara found that enzymes and amino acids in young grass plants deactivated the cancer-causing and mutagenic effects of 3,4 benzyprene, a substance widely found in charcoal-broiled meats and smoked fish. Studies suggesting how chlorophyll helps to heal the body have been done by Tsuneo Kada, director of the Japan Research Center of Genetics. Kada and colleagues demonstrated that the juice of green plants inhibits chromosome damage, which is one of the links in the chain of events leading to cancer.[6] According to Kada, the enzymes in green grasses are efficient at detoxifying the body and neutralizing certain pollutants.

More evidence of green grass's remarkable restorative powers comes from Yasuo Hotta, a biologist with the University of California at San Diego. Hotta isolated a compound from young green barley grasses that reportedly has shown the ability to stimulate the production—and natural repair—of DNA and human sperm cells.[7] This compound has been provisionally named P4D1.

Impressive evidence that wheat-sprout extracts have anticancer action *in vitro* (in the test tube) emerged from a series of experiments conducted between 1978 and 1980 by Dr. Chiu-Nan Lai, a biologist with the University of Texas System Cancer Center, a part of the M. D. Anderson Hospital in Houston. Dr. Lai and her associates showed that extracts from the roots and leaves of wheat sprouts have a strong antimutagenic effect, that is, they decrease abnormal cell mutation. The wheat-sprout extracts also exhibited tumor-destroying action free of the usual toxicity of chemotherapy drugs. Dr. Lai speculated that wheatgrass's antimutagenic activity was due to some of its very minute trace elements (iodine, selenium, copper, arsenic, and platinum) interacting with the vitamins, minerals, and enzymes present.[8]

Extracts from wheat soaked overnight and sprouted showed no signs of inhibiting cell mutations in these experiments. "This means that the growing, vital energy of wheatgrass is more important than the sprouted seed," comments David Kingsley of the New Hippocrates Health Institute in Medford Square, Massachusetts.

Wheatgrass therapy for cancer victims begins with cleansing and detoxification of the body, often achieved through a three-day juice fast combined with enemas and colonics. During the fast, the person drinks wheatgrass juice; green drinks, extracted from sprouts and baby greens; vegetable juices high in mineral content; naturally sweetened lemon water; and Rejuvelac, a fermented wheatberry drink.

Rejuvelac, developed by Ann Wigmore over twenty-five years ago, is the liquid in which wheatberries were sprouted. The name comes from "*rejuve*nate" plus "*lac*tobacteria" since the drink contains friendly lactobacteria, which take up residence in the large intestine and repel harmful bacteria. This leads to a clean colon in which sludge cannot collect on the walls and disease-producing bacteria are unable to survive. Lactobacilli synthesize vitamin B12 and folic acid, two essential nutrients that help prevent anemia. Rejuvelac is full of fermentative enzymes that aid digestion. It is also rich in eight of the B vitamins as well as vitamins C, E, and K. Like other fermented foods, Rejuvelac can be considered "predigested." It contains protein that has already been broken down into amino acids that are easy to assimilate.

During the juice fast, both enemas with water and so-called *implants* (retention enemas) of wheatgrass juice are used once or twice daily to assist the cleansing process. Wheatgrass implants are wheatgrass-juice enemas taken deep in the bowel and retained for roughly twenty minutes. According to Ann Wigmore, "They are excellent for loosening hard fecal matter. The high magnesium content of wheatgrass is particularly effective for drawing out toxins from not only the colon but the liver and kidneys. Wheatgrass is also beneficial for supplying the body with missing nutrients because the soluble elements from wheatgrass juice can be absorbed by the portal circulation inside the colon. Most importantly, though, is the fact that you are introducing one of the most concentrated energies of the life force and sun into one of the most diseased areas of your body." Other alternative therapies that employ enemas as a detoxification measure are the Gerson therapy (Chapter 17) and the Kelley therapy (Chapter 18).

Wigmore claims that during a wheatgrass implant, a portion of the juice is absorbed into the portal circulation, which leads to the liver. Through this, she says, more chlorophyll goes directly to the liver than could otherwise reach it. The liver is the master organ of detoxification in the human body, performing hundreds of different functions, from cleansing the blood to storing nutrients. A few studies suggest that compounds in dietary grasses may stimulate liver function and prevent the depositing of fat on the liver. Through a combination of detoxification, sound nutrition, exercise, and positive outlook, the wheatgrass program aims to strengthen a flagging immune response, often associated with people who are ill with cancer.

Guests at a wheatgrass health center drink at least four ounces of wheatgrass juice a day. They are taught how to grow their own wheatgrass, how to press the juice, and also how to use the juice in enemas. Growing and harvesting wheatgrass is easy to do and can be done indoors. Wheatgrass is also available at some health-food stores. Although wheatgrass therapy can be done on one's own, the person with cancer who is serious about this modality would learn much from a stay at one of the wheatgrass institutes.

The raw foods diet that is integral to wheatgrass therapy is said to resemble the diet eaten by our human ancestors for millennia. Raw foods, organically grown with no pesticides, are rich in electrolytes, often missing in American diets. They provide abundant fiber, which aids in sweeping toxins from the body. Raw foods are mostly water and have no problem moving through the gastrointestinal system. They maintain all their vitamins and minerals and are living energy transferred to the body. Advocates of wheatgrass therapy claim that the vital energy locked in foods is weakened or destroyed by cooking, canning, and even, to some degree, freezing. A lot of research shows that vitamins, minerals, and other nutrients in foods are destroyed by cooking.

"The practice of cooking food destroys 100 percent of the enzymes in food," says Ann Wigmore. Enzymes are destroyed at around 115°F, hence the superior value of uncooked food. Enzymes, the catalysts of life, are essential to digestion, the growth and repair of tissues, and defense against infection and degenerative disease. When a person eats *cooked* foods, the body's enzyme-producing glands (stomach glands, pancreas, salivary glands, and intestinal glands) are repeatedly called upon to supply the enzymes necessary for processing the food. "Digestion of cooked foods uses up about 25 percent of our daily energy output," states Dave Kingsley. "When enzyme-rich foods are used, they reduce the body's workload and make more of this energy available for the healing process."

Chemotherapy destroys a good deal of the body's enzymes in a person already suffering from a lack of these enzymes, according to Wigmore. She holds that the lack of enzymes is a major contributing factor in the development of leukemia and other diseases. Some of the enzymes found abundantly in the raw foods diet are cytochrome oxidase, an antioxidant required for proper cell respiration; lipase, a fat-splitting enzyme; protease, a protein digestant; amylase, which facilitates the digestion of starch; transhydrogenase, an enzyme that aids in keeping the muscle tissues of the heart toned; pepsin, which helps in digesting protein and transforming it into amino acids used for energy and self-healing; and superoxide dismutase (SOD). Richly concentrated in cereal grasses, SOD has received a lot of attention in scientific circles for its role in slowing cellular aging and lessening the effects of radiation.

As generally practiced, the wheatgrass therapy diet is believed to be completely self-sufficient—no vitamin pills, supplements, or injections are required. In this respect, wheatgrass therapy differs from some other nutritional treatments for cancer such as the Gerson,

Kelley, and Moerman therapies. But a minority of wheatgrass practitioners do recommend supplements in certain circumstances. For example, vitamins A, C, and E may be recommended depending on the client's condition and special dietary needs.

The organic raw foods diet avoids the risk of cancer associated with high consumption of meat, dairy products, and eggs. The most prevalent cancers in the United States are closely correlated with a diet having lots of protein, lots of fat, and very little fiber. Furthermore, recent studies have found that nutritional factors "can have profound influences on . . . the development and manifestations of cancers"[9] and that "nutritional status plays a critical role in immunological defense mechanisms at a number of important levels."[10] In his paper "The Cancerostatic Effect of Vegetarian Diets," Tufts University researcher Dr. Eduardo Siguel recommends a low-protein diet high in complex carbohydrates and vegetables as the ideal way to strengthen the body's defenses against the growth of cancer cells. The diet he outlines is very similar to the organic diet of wheatgrass therapy and to other largely vegetarian anticancer diets such as macrobiotics, the Gerson diet, and the Moerman diet. Dr. Siguel posits that a "cancerostatic diet" starves cancer cells, which thrive more on animal-derived fatty acids. Apparently, plant oils yield short-chained fatty acids that have to be constructed into longer chains. Cancer cells are often weak cells and do better with the already-fashioned long-chain fatty acids received in an animal-based diet.[11]

"We don't cure anything. Instead we offer a lifestyle through which the body can rebuild and heal itself," says Brian Clement, director of the Hippocrates Health Institute in West Palm Beach, Florida. "People who are ill should not ignore what conventional medicine may have to offer. They should also give serious consideration to the evidence which shows that adopting the kind of diet we advocate can reverse disease."

A client who visited the Hippocrates Health Institute in the spring of 1988 had been diagnosed by his orthodox doctors two years earlier with lymphatic cancer spreading all over his body. As the man relates in a bylined article in the institute's newsletter, the oncologists had given him three months to live if he underwent chemotherapy. He began the chemo, but all his hair fell out, he broke out in blisters, and, he soon felt, his immune system was destroyed. Around that time, he heard about wheatgrass therapy. After thirty days of drinking wheatgrass juice, following the diet, meditating, and self-administering enemas, the client found his lymphatic system had become "completely clean." His lymph nodes returned to their normal size a short time later. The man was diagnosed again, and the doctor was "very amazed" to find that the cancer was in remission.

Marianne Dimetres of Southwick, Massachusetts, was diagnosed with advanced (Stage IV) uterine cancer in April 1988. Her doctors urged her to have surgery, but she refused; and in June, she spent three weeks at the Hippocrates Health Institute in Florida, where she began intensive wheatgrass therapy. "By the end of the visit, I felt much better than I'd felt in years," says Marianne, the mother of two small children. At home, she continued the regimen, supplemented with intravenous injections of vitamins A and C, through early 1991. She also became a patient of Emanuel Revici, M.D., receiving "guided lipid" medicines intended to correct the imbalances in her body's metabolism. (Dr. Revici's system is discussed in Chapter 4). Marianne also commenced group therapy with other cancer patients under Bernie Siegel's direction (see Chapter 29).

"I really believe that everything worked together," says Marianne. "The wheatgrass therapy was part of a program that turned my life around. It reduced the pain and pressure, and helped improve my bloodwork. I had lost my voice due to growths on my vocal chords, but the wheatgrass therapy helped me regain my voice within a few months."

Relenting to family pressure, Marianne underwent surgical operations in August and November of 1989 for removal of her uterus and part of her abdominal wall. "By the time I had the surgery," says Marianne, "the cysts in both ovaries were gone, and the cancer had receded dramatically. I was able to keep my ovaries and tubes." She attributes this to the combination of alternative approaches she adopted. Tests taken in late 1991 indicated that she is in total remission.

"I really do believe that conventional medicine has its place in treatment," says Marianne, "but I also strongly believe that you should have control of your own healing and the freedom to choose what's best for you. Getting well is not just a question of taking medicine. It's a life choice and involves one's body, mind, and spirit."

Describing her remarkable recovery, Marianne says, "I came to a place where I had to decide if I wanted to be terminal or not. Every cancer patient reaches this point. For me, the decision to live was a conversional experience. Cancer was the best thing that ever happened to me. It initiated a long learning process. Before I got sick, I was living my life skiing across the surface. When I got cancer, I came to realize what was important in life. My concerns now are for other people and the Earth."

Marianne, who is still "100 percent vegetarian," is studying art and psychology at Smith College. She runs four miles a day and does aerobics. She also walks barefoot across hot, live coals—fifty feet at a stretch in one recent public firewalking demonstration. She describes her firewalking ability as "an affirmation of faith . . . it comes from the faith that I discovered in learning to overcome cancer."

Another approach emphasizing raw foods that deserves mention is Natural Hygiene, a movement founded in the nineteenth century. It teaches people to stay healthy by living a life that is not hurtful to the body. Adherents generally eat organic, primarily uncooked foods, avoid smoking cigarettes and drinking alcohol, and pursue a lifestyle combining exercise, right thinking, and the elimination of stress. Herbert Shelton (1895–1985), a naturopathic physician who was one of the movement's leaders, ran a clinic in Texas where patients with cancer and other degenerative diseases were put on a fast in which only water was allowed.

Dr. Shelton believed that during a medically supervised fast, the body is compelled to use its reserves for food. Hence, tumors would be *autolyzed*, or dissolved, by cellular enzymes and absorbed into the circulation; still-viable nutrients would be used and the toxins eliminated, he said. Shelton claimed a high rate of recovery despite the late stage of some of his patients' cancers. Under Natural Hygienic care, he stated, tumors (not necessarily cancer) are often reduced to less than one-fourth of their original size. Dr. Shelton included a number of case histories in his book *Health for All*.[12]

Dr. Shelton's close associate—Virginia Vetrano, M.D., of Barksdale, Texas, who supervised the clinic for seventeen years—describes a man with skin cancer who fasted for fifty-two days and got well. Another skin cancer patient, she says, recovered after an eighteen-day fast. However, she warns, "skin cancer seems to be less malignant than other types." She also cautions, "Though some tumors may diminish in size while a person is fasting, they often increase in size, sometimes rapidly, after the fast. Nevertheless," she adds, "I kept a lady alive for ten years longer than the doctors said she'd live by fasting her once a year and keeping her on an all raw food diet between the fasts. She had a very malignant breast tumor."

Certainly, fasting is not for everyone. For many patients, it could be dangerous, depending upon the severity and extent of the malignancy, the person's physical strength, his or her mental outlook, and other factors. Many Natural Hygienists today tend to view fasting as an emergency measure in cases of severe illness like cancer. Their emphasis, instead, is on diet. A woman with breast cancer who recovered on a Natural Hygiene diet relates her experience in *Cancer*

Forum.[13] (For more information on Natural Hygiene or for a list of practitioners, contact the American Natural Hygiene Society, P.O. Box 30630, Tampa, FL, 33633; 813-855-6607.)

Resources

Ann Wigmore Foundation
196 Commonwealth Avenue
Boston, MA 02116
Phone: 617-267-9424

For further information on wheatgrass therapy and details on treatment.

Ann Wigmore Research and
  Educational Institute
P.O. Box 429
Rincon, Puerto Rico 00677
Phone: 809-868-6307

For further information on wheatgrass therapy and details on treatment.

Hippocrates Health Institute
1443 Palmdale Court
West Palm Beach, FL 33411
Phone: 407-471-8876

For further information on wheatgrass therapy and details on treatment.

New Hippocrates Health
  Institute
One Shipyard Way
Medford Square, MA 02155
Phone: 617-395-1608

For further information on wheatgrass therapy and details on treatment.

Health Institute of San Diego
6970 Central Avenue
Lemon Grove, CA 91945
Phone: 619-464-3346

For further information on wheatgrass therapy and details on treatment.

Creative Health Institute
918 Union City Road
Union City, MI 49094
Phone: 517-278-6260

For further information on wheatgrass therapy and details on treatment.

Reading Material

The Wheatgrass Book, by Ann Wigmore, Avery Publishing Group (120 Old Broadway, Garden City Park, NY 11040; 800-548-5757), 1985. Still the best general introduction to wheatgrass.

Be Your Own Doctor, by Ann Wigmore, Avery Publishing Group (120 Old Broadway, Garden City Park, NY 11040; 800-548-5757), 1982.

My Experiences With Living Foods: The Raw Food Treatment of Cancer and Other Diseases, by Kristine Nolfi, M.D., Health Research (P.O. Box 70, Mokelumne Hill, CA 95245; 209-286-1324), no date. Presents a raw-food approach without wheatgrass.

How I Conquered Cancer Naturally, by Eydie Mae Hunsberger with Chris Loeffler, Avery Publishing Group (120 Old Broadway, Garden City Park, NY 11040; 800-548-5757), 1992.

The Cancer Survivors and How They Did It, by Judith Glassman (see Appendix A for description).

Healing AIDS Naturally, by Laurence E. Badgley, M.D., Human Energy Press (1020 Foster City Boulevard, Suite 205, Foster City, CA 94404; 415-349-0718), 1987. Contains a chapter on wheatgrass therapy.

Rebuild Your Health With High Energy Enzyme Nourishment: Living Foods Lifestyle, by Ann Wigmore, Ann Wigmore Foundation (see page 159 for address and phone number), 1991. A detailed ninety-three-page manual with practical instructions.

Wheatgrass Therapy, by Sally Wolper, Wolper Publications (14134 Gladeside Drive, La Mirada, CA 90638; 213-921-8495), 1984. A useful fourteen-page booklet.

Improving the Immune System With Nutrition, by David Kingsley, New Hippocrates Health Institute (see page 159 for address and phone number), 1991. Manuscript. A synthesis of the scientific evidence supporting wheatgrass therapy. Also outlines a nutritional program.

Chapter 15

MACROBIOTICS

Macrobiotics is a nutritional system, a philosophy, and a way of life. It draws on Eastern wisdom with its understanding of complementary forces (yin and yang) embodying a universal principle. Macrobiotics holds that a change in diet can not only prevent cancer but may also reverse the cancerous process and eliminate the disease, even when conventional therapy is abandoned.

"Cancer is a disorder of the body's cells that results largely from improper diet," says Michio Kushi, a leader of the macrobiotics movement in the United States. Offering a common-sense alternative to the typical high-fat, low-fiber American diet associated with cancer and heart disease, the basic macrobiotic diet consists of 50 to 60 percent whole cereal grains; 25 to 30 percent vegetables; smaller amounts of soups, beans, and sea vegetables; plus occasional fish, seafood, seasonal fruits, nuts, seeds, and condiments. Chemically treated, highly salted, and highly processed foods are avoided, as is cooking with electricity. Prohibited foods include fatty animal products such as meat, poultry, eggs, and dairy items as well as fruit juices, canned and frozen foods, coffee and commercial tea, and refined sweeteners.

Many foods in the basic macrobiotic diet have been shown to reduce or inhibit cancer growth. For example, miso soup (made from fermented soybeans, cereal grains, and sea salt), when eaten daily, has been found to significantly reduce the frequency of stomach cancer in Japan. Shiitake mushrooms, used in a variety of macrobiotic dishes, have a powerful antitumor effect in mice. Common edible sea vegetables such as kelp, seaweed, and kombu cause regression of tumors in animals. Sea vegetables also inhibit the intestinal absorption of radioactive products and help decontaminate the body after exposure to radioactive materials. Cruciferous vegetables such as cabbage, broccoli, Brussels sprouts, cauliflower, and turnips, eaten frequently or daily in the macrobiotic diet, have recognized cancer-inhibiting properties.

Thousands of people have recovered from cancer and other chronic illnesses by using the macrobiotic approach. Others have done very poorly on the diet, and many have died. Cancer patients who follow macrobiotics as a therapy are advised to remain on the diet long after their disease is under control. The standard macrobiotic diet is much wider and more varied than the medicinal or recovery diet.

Michio Kushi, who heads the Kushi Institute in Massachusetts, has said that "only about 15 to 20 percent among my visitors . . . are able to get better. If they would come to me at an earlier stage of illness, or had greater family support, the percentage would be much higher."[1] Most cancer patients who try macrobiotics are in advanced stages of the disease, many declared medically terminal. They turn to macrobiotics after failing conventional treatments such as chemotherapy and radiation, which weaken the immune system.

"Only about half of my visitors have the physical and mental conditions strong enough to clearly understand the macrobiotic approach, which is to change their dietary and lifestyle patterns," Kushi explains. "Of these, half have the desire to change their way of life, but do not develop the proper understanding of the way of cooking to make themselves better. Or they may try the diet with a combination of various other programs which may even make them worse. Of the remaining quarter, some try successfully at first, but may lack family cooperation or the approval of their family doctor . . . so they may eventually return to their original way of life and become ill again."

Dr. Vivien Newbold, an emergency-care physician in Philadelphia, recently published a study of six patients with advanced, incurable cancer who used the macrobiotic approach of dietary and lifestyle changes to achieve complete regression.[2] Five of the patients achieved total remission for five years or more. One patient obtained remission after trying macrobiotics but failed to continue on the diet and died when the cancer recurred. In all six of the cases, the tumor regression could not have been due to any prior conventional treatment. The standard treatments that the patients had received were *palliative*, that is, the therapy given produces, at best, a temporary decrease in tumor size and a possible prolongation in life expectancy. "Conventional therapy has not resulted in any known cases of sustained regression or recovery from any of these cancers," comments Dr. Newbold.

One of the six patients, a sixty-one-year-old man, underwent exploratory surgery in 1982 and was found to have cancer of the pancreas metastasized to the liver. He began a macrobiotic diet in August 1982 and that month received a single course of chemotherapy, followed in September by a single dose of monoclonal antibodies. He found the chemotherapy debilitating and felt that it was not helping him, so he chose to discontinue all forms of conventional treatment and remain on the macrobiotic diet. A CAT scan done in June 1983 revealed no evidence of disease, and a subsequent CAT scan in December 1983 confirmed that the patient was cancer-free. As of this writing, a decade after his surgery, this man is very active, in excellent health, and still on a macrobiotic diet.

"This remission is especially noteworthy, as pancreatic cancers are usually rapidly fatal," observes Dr. Newbold. Four-fifths of patients diagnosed with pancreatic cancer die within six months.

Summarizing the results of her study, Dr. Newbold says, "The findings suggest that macrobiotics, by strengthening the patient's immune system and eliminating toxins from the diet, may aid patients with advanced stages of cancer who cannot be helped by medical means. Otherwise unexplained remissions continue to occur in patients who follow this diet. In view of the remissions of cancer and other serious diseases that have occurred in connection with the macrobiotic approach, the medical community would do well to investigate these phenomena seriously."

Dr. Newbold began her study after her husband was found to have terminal, medically incurable metastatic cancer of the colon in December 1983. In July 1984, her husband, who had gone on a macrobiotic diet, was feeling healthier than he had ever felt in his life, and a follow-up CAT scan revealed that about 70 percent of the cancer was gone. Excited by this remarkable development, Dr. Newbold called the American Cancer Society to share the information. According to her, the ACS director's response was, "It is of no interest to us." The National Cancer Institute responded in identical fashion. The article that she subsequently wrote detailing the remissions of the six medically incurable cancers was rejected by the *New England Journal of Medicine, The Lancet,* and the *Journal of the American Medical Association.* All three prestigious journals replied that the article was of insufficient interest to their readers.

Dr. Newbold asks:

> Does the medical profession really want to know if there is a possible way to cure cancer, or do they just want to keep funding a system that clearly has made next to no progress in the treatment of most cancers in the last fifty years? They

state repeatedly in their articles that a careful review of their literature reveals there are no documented cases of recovery using macrobiotics. . . . Of what use is a careful review of their literature if medical journals refuse to publish any cases indicating macrobiotics, or any other unconventional approach to healing for that matter, may have played an important role? Are our major scientific institutions made up of scientists who truly want to heal cancer? Isn't it strange that great institutions had no interest in reviewing the cases, going over the pathology slides, the x-rays and so on? Isn't it strange they had no interest in examining these patients carefully to look for the development of special antibodies that could help better understand regression of cancer? What kind of scientists do we have working in these major institutions?[3]

The erroneous notion that the standard macrobiotic diet is nutritionally inadequate persists in the medical community, according to Dr. Newbold. "I have seen it turn into tragic results on several occasions when patients with advanced cancer who had been doing well with macrobiotics went back to their doctors and were advised to add various foods to their diet, usually milk, meat, and poultry," she says. "I have seen many patients who were doing extremely well deteriorate rapidly and die after making such changes."[4]

The American Medical Association endorsed macrobiotics as nutritionally adequate in the 1987 edition of its *Family Medical Guide,* which states, "In general, the macrobiotic diet is a healthful way of eating." In 1984, a congressional subcommittee investigating various holistic diets concluded that the "macrobiotic diet appears to be nutritionally adequate. The diet would also be consistent with the recently released dietary guidelines of the National Academy of Sciences and the American Cancer Society in regard to possible reduction of cancer risks."

Recovery from advanced cancer using a macrobiotic approach requires tremendous commitment and a willingness to change, according to Dr. Newbold. "People with advanced cancer who are trying to recover through macrobiotics must realize that they're hoping for a miracle," she says. "The good news is that some people have succeeded." In her view, the majority of severely ill cancer patients who try macrobiotics fail because of a lack of family support and the isolation that patients experience as they attempt to cook for themselves and eat alone.

Despite the documented complete remissions of cancer patients, and despite the growing evidence of strong antitumor properties in macrobiotic foods, macrobiotics has not been accepted by the medical community. The American Cancer Society has placed macrobiotics on its blacklist of "Unproven Methods of Cancer Management." There is no evidence that any diet whatsoever "will influence the course of cancer once it starts," says Arthur Holleb, M.D., chief medical officer of the ACS. "You can improve your quality of life with a proper diet. You can reduce the risk of cancer. But it is dangerous to think that you can *cure* cancer with a diet."[5]

Interestingly, the American Cancer Society's official condemnation of macrobiotics as an unproven and probably dangerous method of cancer therapy was published in the same journal in which the ACS published its dietary recommendations for cancer prevention—just one month apart. In 1984, the ACS's nutritional recommendations called for cutting down on total fat intake; eating more high-fiber foods like whole-grain cereals, fruits, and vegetables; eating cruciferous vegetables; and eating foods rich in vitamins A and C. All of these dietary recommendations are features of the standard macrobiotic diet. The 1990 edition of *Cancer Facts and Figures,* published by the American Cancer Society, recognizes diet as a key component of "primary prevention" of cancer.

The popular misconception of the modern macrobiotic diet as an all-brown-rice regimen is partly due to George Ohsawa (1893–1966), a Japanese teacher who as a sixteen-year-old boy reportedly healed himself of incurable tuberculosis through a simple diet of brown rice, miso soup, sea vegetables, and other traditional foods. Ohsawa (pen name for Yukikazu Sakurazawa) developed an all-encompassing philosophy of harmony and balance with Nature that blended traditional Chinese, Japanese, and Indian thought and medicine with modern holistic perspectives. When Sakurazawa moved to Paris in the 1920s, he adopted "George Ohsawa" as his pen name and called his philosophy, and the diet that flowed from it, *macrobiotics* (from the Greek *macro,* meaning "large or great," and *bios,* meaning "life").

In his 1965 book *Zen Macrobiotics,* Ohsawa outlined ten stages of diet (designated −3 to +7), with each successive level reducing either the variety or percentages, or both, of certain foods. Diet Number 7 is 100 percent cereals, chiefly brown rice, plus small amounts of herb tea. Ohsawa regarded Diet Number 7 as the "highest" way of eating to treat illness. However, some followers of this rigid, deficient diet suffered serious health problems. Several adherents of Zen macrobiotics in the

United States were hospitalized, and one died. The woman who died was also taking drugs, and supporters of macrobiotics say that her understanding of proper practice was poor. The publicity surrounding these cases led to a lingering negative stereotype of the macrobiotic diet, even though contemporary proponents of macrobiotics disavow Ohsawa's dangerous dietary prescription and instead advocate a balanced, varied, nutritionally adequate regimen.

Ohsawa, who wrote over 300 books, classified food as being either expansive (more yin) or contractive (more yang), with the aim of promoting a balanced diet. The age-old yin-yang symbol, a circle with interlocking dark and light segments, represents the principle that everything is an interconnected part of a harmonious whole. The dark yin pole is feminine, passive, and expansive. The light yang pole is masculine, active, and constrictive. Each pole is defined by the other, and both are necessary to achieve integrated, harmonious balance. Macrobiotics sees everything in the world, not just food, as either yin or yang. Water, for instance, is yin; fire, yang. Ohsawa viewed health as the result of a proper balance of yin and yang factors in our daily diet and way of life. When the balance between these complementary forces becomes extreme or one-sided, he believed, sickness is the inevitable result.

Ohsawa maintained that the body's natural health will assert itself if you eat and live in harmony with the order of Nature. He did not claim originality for the simple, toxin-free diet he prescribed. On the contrary, he argued that it was practiced and described in ancient cultures around the world. When societies abandoned this healthy dietary practice, he felt, they declined and vanished, or else existed as a living corpse. To Ohsawa, cancer is a full-blown manifestation of egotistical thoughts and behaviors, a symptom of modern society's rampant opposition to the way of Nature.

Michio Kushi, who studied with Ohsawa, came to the United States from Japan in 1949. Along with Herman Aihara and other leaders in the macrobiotics movement, he preserved key elements of Ohsawa's system while incorporating a variety of new practices and ideas. Ohsawa's ten-stage dietary levels were replaced with the standard macrobiotic diet, which in practice is tailored to meet each person's highly individual needs, moods, and tastes.

Macrobiotic teachers and counselors encourage their patients to determine whether their condition is predominantly yin or yang or a combination of both. This diagnosis is based in part on the location of the primary tumor in the body. In general, tumors in the upper or peripheral parts of the body or in hollow, expanded organs are considered more yin. Examples include leukemia, lymphoma, Hodgkin's disease, and tumors of the esophagus, upper stomach, mouth (except the tongue), breast, skin, and outer regions of the brain. Tumors in the lower or deeper parts of the body or in the more compact organs are considered more yang. Examples are cancers of the colon, rectum, prostate, ovaries, bone, pancreas, and inner regions of the brain. Cancers thought to result from a combination of yin and yang factors include melanoma and cancers of the lung, bladder, kidney, lower stomach, uterus, spleen, liver, and tongue.

If a cancer is predominantly yin, a macrobiotic counselor will prescribe a diet that emphasizes yang foods. Conversely, if a cancer is more yang, it requires treatment with a predominantly yin diet. For a cancer caused by both extremes, a central, balanced way of eating is recommended. In all cases, extreme foods—those that are excessively yin or yang—should be strictly avoided, as these items caused the cancer to develop in the first place. By adjusting the diet to emphasize foods of a yin or yang nature opposite that of the cancer, a natural balance is thought to result, reversing the forces sustaining the malignancy.

According to Kushi, cancer is a means of self-protection for the body. A tumor is a localization of the abnormal cells that have developed as a result of excessive consumption of protein, fats, chemicals, and food additives. Cancer is the end stage of a long process. It's the body's healthy attempt to isolate toxins ingested over years of eating the modern unhealthy diet and living in an artificial environment. If we don't allow the excessive substances we consume to accumulate in localized areas and form tumors, we will find them spreading throughout the body, leading to a total collapse of vital functions and death by toxemia (poisoning). Cancer is the body's ultimate self-protection method.

From the macrobiotic standpoint, cancer is a symptom of modern society—our chemicalized agriculture; our unwholesome diet of processed, synthetic foods; our wanton pollution of the environment; our near-total divorce from Nature; and our preoccupation with short-term self-gratification at the expense of long-term health and well-being.

Beyond dietary guidelines, the macrobiotic system recommends a number of lifestyle changes. Getting regular exercise, developing a positive mental outlook, and using natural cooking utensils, fabrics, and materials in the home are strongly recommended. On the other hand, microwave cooking devices, electromagnetic radiation, excessive television watching, and chemical fumes should be avoided.

Patients are encouraged to accept that they are directly responsible for the creation of the disease through poor dietary habits, way of life, or patterns of thinking and feeling. Through self-reflection, patients examine those aspects of their lives that may have contributed to their illnesses, and they contemplate the larger scheme of Nature and their place in it. Self-reflection can take many forms, including prayer, meditation, and visualization.

Michio Kushi also recommends the following lifestyle changes:

- View everything and everyone you meet with gratitude . . .

- Please chew your food very well, at least fifty times per mouthful, or until it becomes liquid . . .

- To increase circulation, scrub your entire body with a hot, damp towel every morning or every night. If that is not possible, at least do your hands, fingers, feet, and toes.

- Initiate and maintain active correspondence, extending your best wishes to parents, children, brothers and sisters, teachers, and friends. Keep your personal relationships smooth and happy.[6]

A macrobiotic counselor will assess the patient's condition using traditional Oriental diagnostic methods. The patient is usually given a very precise diet, tailored to his or her particular needs and condition. This individualized diet often excludes many of the common foods in the basic macrobiotic diet while adding a number of specially prepared foods. Typically, the patient is evaluated every four to six weeks, and further adjustments are made to the diet as necessary.

Both the patient and his or her family are strongly encouraged to try to understand the importance of adhering to the dietary recommendations. Ideally, says Kushi, the patient should spend several days—preferably weeks—learning how to cook macrobiotically. Persons interested in cooking classes or health and dietary counseling can contact the Kushi Institute or One Peaceful World (see Resources).

In their 1983 book *The Cancer Prevention Diet* (see Resources), Kushi and coauthor Alex Jack encourage cancer patients not to combine the macrobiotic diet with surgery, radiation, or chemotherapy, except in immediately life-threatening circumstances such as an obstruction in the digestive tract. They point out that recovery may be more difficult as a result of the side effects and general weakening produced by orthodox methods. However, Kushi no longer opposes cancer patients' combining of the macrobiotic diet with conventional forms of treatment, leaving the decision to the patients and their families. There are many macrobiotic medical doctors around the country.

Dr. Terry Shintani, who practices general and preventive medicine in Hawaii and has studied at the Kushi Institute, believes that a patient should not blindly abandon conventional therapies. In *Doctors Look at Macrobiotics* (see Resources), Dr. Shintani, himself a follower of macrobiotics, advises patients to carefully weigh the risks and benefits of orthodox treatments and to consider complementary approaches.[7]

The types of cancer said to respond more readily to the macrobiotic diet include breast, cervical, colon, pancreatic, liver, bone, and skin. Cancers of the lung, ovaries, and testes are more difficult to treat macrobiotically. Cases considered medically terminal require the use of diet plus external applications such as a ginger compress, taro potato plaster, or buckwheat plaster. The methods for preparing these external applications are given in *The Cancer Prevention Diet.*

Mona Sanders, in the prime of her life at age thirty-seven, was diagnosed with an inoperable, Stage III brain tumor in August 1986, following an epileptic seizure and two surgical operations. The anaplastic astrocytoma was roughly the size of a small grapefruit. Mona, a vibrant woman who lives in the small town of Columbus, Mississippi, experienced nausea, vomiting, numbness in her right leg, and emotional trauma. Her doctors told her that she had only six to eighteen months to live and that chemotherapy could at best slow the tumor's growth. They predicted she would lose motor control and be confined to a wheelchair before death.

While contemplating macrobiotics as an option, Mona called the American Cancer Society hotline "to see if there was anything else I could do" besides the radiation and chemotherapy she was already receiving. The ACS volunteer's reply was, "Nothing. Good luck," and the line went dead.

In January 1987, Mona went to the Macrobiotic Learning Center in Brookline, Massachusetts, to learn cooking techniques, exercise, massage, home remedies, and methods to improve her mental outlook. Returning to Mississippi, she decided to discontinue chemotherapy after the third treatment and, with her family's support, continued her macrobiotic regimen "to heal my body and soul."

A CAT scan taken in April 1987, four months after Mona started macrobiotics, showed no evidence of cancer. Subsequent CAT scans have confirmed that she is completely cancer-free as of this writing.[8]

Mona's story is one of the remarkable cases presented in *Cancer Free: 30 Who Triumphed Over Cancer Naturally* (see Resources). Other people who healed themselves macrobiotically, as documented in the book, include a nine-year survivor of cancer of the pancreas with metastasis to the liver, an eleven-year survivor of metastatic prostate cancer, a twenty-year survivor of uterine cancer, a nine-year survivor of stomach cancer, and a twelve-year survivor of malignant melanoma. Additional case histories can be found in Michio Kushi's *The Macrobiotic Approach to Cancer* (see Resources).

Macrobiotic practitioners point to the need for further scientific studies to evaluate the therapeutic effectiveness of macrobiotics. In 1984 to 1985, researchers at the Tulane School of Public Health undertook a study to determine whether persons with pancreatic cancer who adopted a macrobiotic regimen survived longer than those who did not. The study tracked twenty-three pancreatic cancer patients who had practiced a macrobiotic diet for at least three months and a control group consisting of pancreatic cancer patients from the national tumor registry, diagnosed during the same period, who did not use the macrobiotic approach. A total of 55 percent of the macrobiotic patients survived at least one year, compared to 10 percent of the control group. These results were termed highly statistically significant, although not conclusive.

Researchers at Harvard Medical School and Ghent University in Belgium analyzed the blood of people who were eating macrobiotically. They were astonished at the results. The amount of blood fats, including cholesterol, was extremely low. The overwhelming majority of persons tested at Harvard had cholesterol levels below 150 milligrams per deciliter, and all were below 170. Several were below 100. The blood pressures of more than 200 macrobiotic people tested were found to be ideal.[9]

The researchers at Ghent University found similar results and began to eat macrobiotically themselves. Dr. J. P. Deslypere, a member of the Ghent research team, concluded, "In the field of cardiovascular and cancer risk factors this kind of blood is very favorable. It's ideal, we couldn't do better; that's what we're dreaming of. It's really fantastic, like children, whose blood vessels are still completely open and whole. This is a very important matter, deserving our full attention."[10] Even when compared to vegetarians, macrobiotic people were found to have the most favorable blood levels.

Japanese scientists in 1970 reported that polysaccharide preparations from the shiitake mushroom, commonly available in groceries, markedly inhibited the growth of induced sarcomas in mice, resulting in "almost complete regression of tumors with no sign of toxicity."[11] Several other studies conducted over the last decade have shown that other basic foods in the macrobiotic diet reduce the risk of many types of cancer and have antitumor properties.

Resources

Kushi Institute of the
  Berkshires
P.O. Box 7
Becket, MA 01223
Phone: 413-623-5742

For information on programs about macrobiotic health care, diet, cooking, and philosophy held in Becket and in cities throughout North America.

One Peaceful World
P.O. Box 10
Becket, MA 01223
Phone: 413-623-5742

For information on macrobiotics and the relationship between diet and degenerative disease, as well as for moral support.

Reading Material

The Macrobiotic Approach to Cancer, by Michio Kushi with Edward Esko, Avery Publishing Group (120 Old Broadway, Garden City Park, NY 11040; 800-548-5757), 1991.

Cancer Free: 30 Who Triumphed Over Cancer, compiled and edited by the East West Foundation with Ann Fawcett and Cynthia Smith, Japan Publications (distributed by Farrar, Straus and Giroux, 19 Union Square West, New York, NY 10003; 800-631-8571), 1991.

The Cancer Prevention Diet: Michio Kushi's Nutritional Blueprint for the Prevention and Relief of Disease, by Michio Kushi with Alex Jack, St. Martin's Press (175 Fifth Avenue, New York, NY 10010; 800-221-7945), 1983.

Doctors Look at Macrobiotics, edited by Edward Esko, Japan Publications (distributed by Farrar, Straus and Giroux, 19 Union Square West, New York, NY 10003; 800-631-8571), 1988.

Cancer and Heart Disease: The Macrobiotic Approach to Degenerative Disorders, by Michio Kushi et al., Japan Publications (distributed by Farrar, Straus and Giroux, 19 Union Square West, New York, NY 10003; 800-631-8571), revised edition, 1985.

Recalled by Life: The Story of My Recovery From Cancer, by Anthony Satillaro, M.D., with Tom Monte, Houghton Mifflin (One Beacon Street, Boston, MA 02108; 800-225-3362), 1982. A survivor story.

Recovery From Cancer, by Elaine Nussbaum, Avery Publishing Group (120 Old Broadway, Garden City Park, NY 11040; 800-548-5757), 1992. A survivor story.

Chapter 16

MOERMAN'S ANTI-CANCER DIET

For fifty years, Dutch physician Cornelis Moerman (1893–1988) fought Holland's medical authorities to have his anticancer dietary system recognized as an effective therapy. Despite hundreds of documented cases of complete remission, even in advanced cancer patients who had failed conventional treatment, the Dutch medical and pharmaceutical community labeled Dr. Moerman a quack and blocked a clinical investigation of his methods.

Yet Moerman ultimately triumphed. In January 1987, Netherlands' Ministry of Health—an agency roughly equivalent to the United States' Food and Drug Administration—finally granted official approval to his treatment. Dr. Moerman, still vigorous and active, died a year later of natural causes at the age of ninety-five with the satisfaction of having won his lifelong battle for recognition. Almost until the end of his life, Moerman worked eleven hours a day, never went to bed before midnight, and saw patients until seven in the evening. He clearly was a beneficiary of his own nutritional methods.

Today, the simple Moerman therapy, a drug-free diet and supplement program without side effects, is popular in the Netherlands. The group dedicated to Moerman's work, the Moerman Vereniging (Moerman Association), claims a membership of 10,000, including many cured patients. Patients who don't want to travel to Holland can read the book *Dr. Moerman's Anti-Cancer Diet: Holland's Revolutionary Nutritional Program for Combating Cancer*, by Ruth Jochems (see Resources). They can also check with the Moerman Vereniging to see whether any North American physicians currently prescribe the Moerman therapy for cancer patients. Another option for Americans is to seek out a nutritionally oriented physician who agrees with Moerman's approach and who would offer guidance in following the program.

In late 1989, the Dutch Ministry of Health issued a report on the results of various treatments for cancer. In a study group of 350 recovered cancer patients, 35 percent were certified in remission using the Moerman therapy alone. Of these patients, 10 were successfully treated by the Moerman therapy after having been sent home as terminal cases by their orthodox doctors.[1]

Dr. Moerman believed that cancer cannot develop in a body in optimum health. He maintained that every cell in the body contains a latent virus capable of developing cancer. Yet the disease can only occur, he insisted, as the result of a disturbed metabolism, "a sick condition of the tissues" arising from a long period of malnutrition. Put simply, faulty metabolism triggered by faulty eating is the fundamental cause of cancer.

The Moerman regimen uses sound nutrition in attempting to reverse the course of the disease. It aims to create a balanced, oxygen-rich bodily environment that is hostile to cancer cells and, at the same time, beneficial to all existing healthy cells. Through this process, tumors become encapsulated, reduce in size, and often disappear altogether. There is no one type of tumor that responds best, and not every form of cancer can be cured with the Moerman therapy. Yet all forms of solid-tumor cancer have reportedly responded to it, and the treatment has brought remissions or tumor regressions, as well as relief from pain and debilitation, in many patients. The Moerman regimen has been used both on its own and as an adjunct to immunotherapy and surgery. Not just for cancer patients, this immunity-enhancing approach could benefit anyone who wants to build up his or her natural defenses against illness.

The Moerman therapy consists of two principal components: a meatless, high-fiber diet rich in vitamins and minerals; and eight supplements found to be of vital importance to ideal health—citric acid, iodine, iron, sulfur, and vitamins A, B-complex, C, and E.

The basic diet includes fresh, preferably organic vegetables and fruits; fruit and vegetable juices, consumed in place of water and other beverages; whole cereals of all kinds; whole-grain breads; buttermilk; other dairy products in small amounts; and natural seasonings. Large amounts of fruit are eaten as excellent sources of vitamin C, citric acid, and other vitamins and minerals.

Dried green garden peas (not split peas) are eaten every day either in a vegetable soup or cooked. "Red beet juice with added vitamin C is also taken to detoxify the blood, especially during or after radiation or chemotherapy," says G. G. Strating-IJben of the Moerman Association.

Moerman's diet allows more fat than do other nutritional approaches. Egg yolks are included as a rich source of pyridoxine (vitamin B6), which facilitates the metabolism of protein and produces a substance called *properdin*, part of the body's natural immune system. A protein present in blood serum, properdin destroys bacteria and viruses in the blood. Egg yolks contain fifty times as much vitamin B6 as does skim milk of the same weight. Egg yolks are also rich in pantothenic acid (vitamin B5), important in the production of hemoglobin and the breakdown of cholesterol and believed to be essential for cell growth. Egg yolks should be eaten raw, the rationale being that cholesterol in cooked eggs does not break down as easily in the body.

The Moerman diet also allows small amounts of milk, butter, and cheeses with low fat and salt contents. One teaspoon of honey per day is permitted. The theory is that B vitamins are also produced in the body by "good" intestinal bacteria, which require fat and milk sugar to reproduce.

The diet strictly forbids the consumption of foods believed to damage the body and prevent nutritious foods from being properly used. Forbidden foods include meat, fish, shellfish, animal fats, cheeses with high fat and salt contents, egg whites, alcoholic beverages, coffee, tea containing caffeine, cocoa, hydrogenated (heat-pressed) vegetable oils and vegetable shortenings, margarine, potatoes, most beans and peas, and all added salt. Also forbidden are refined white sugar, sugar substitutes, and all foods containing them, such as cakes, chocolates, sodas, and ketchup; white flour and all foods containing it, such as breads, pastas, cakes, cookies, and crackers; artificial colorings; and chemical preservatives.

It was the pigeon that led Moerman to a cure for cancer. After graduating from medical school in the early 1930s, Moerman decided to dedicate his life to cancer research. From his rural native town of Vlaardingen, he wrote to a scientific supply company in Germany to order equipment. A pigeon fancier, he mentioned in his letter that he was planning to experiment with that bird. The supply house wrote back that this kind of experiment would be a waste of time: "In healthy carrier pigeons one cannot generate cancer."

That one sentence set Moerman on his course. "As long as these birds are in perfect health," he reasoned, "there must be something in their metabolism that protects them from" cancer.[2] Observing wild pigeons in their natural environment, he meticulously recorded everything they ate. He noticed how they liked to nibble grains in the fields before harvest. He observed that they regularly flew to the seashore to nibble sand, not for food, he believed, but for the iodine and other trace minerals that washed up from seaweed and other life forms in the ocean. Through careful observation, he discovered that the pigeons' natural diet consisted of whole grains and tiny bits of garden vegetables and orchard fruits.

Moerman's next challenge was to isolate the nutritional elements that keep healthy pigeons cancer-free with a strong immune system. By testing numerous substances on his own carrier pigeons over a ten-year period, he concluded that there are eight nutrients of fundamental importance to ideal health. Some of the major benefits of these eight substances in humans are summarized below:

- *Vitamin A*, like vitamins C and E, is a potent anticancer agent that reduces the risk of cancer in animals. The rationale for its use in treating human cancer patients is that it nurtures and protects the epithelial (lining) cells of the body, helping these cells to differentiate or mature. Tests in Cambridge, England, in the 1930s showed that a majority of lung cancers occurred when epithelial cells in the bronchi of the lungs failed to mature. There is often a marked deficiency of vitamin A in the blood of cancer patients. Many studies have demonstrated the protective anticancer effects of beta-carotene, which is converted into vitamin A in the body.

  In a series of experiments at the Dutch Cancer Institute in 1983, Dutch biochemist L. den Engelse identified vitamin A and its derivatives as anticarcinogens, substances that work on the DNA of cancer cells by stopping the enzymatic activity of carcinogens and thereby halting the growth of cancer cells. Under the microscope, the Dutch researchers saw that vitamin A could not only slow the growth of a tumor but that in some cases, it could actually transform a malignant tumor into a benign tumor.[3]

- The *B-complex vitamins* offer protection against cancer through their detoxification of cancer-causing chemicals, stimulation of immune response, and maintenance of oxygen metabolism. The body utilizes the B vitamins as components of enzymes and coenzymes. Thus these vitamins are building blocks of the compounds that control the chemical reactions of life. *Thiamine* (vitamin B_1) is essential for the metabolism of carbohydrates, and *riboflavin* (vitamin B_2) helps the cells breathe properly. *Niacin* (vitamin B_3) forms part of the coenzyme NADH, which, together with enzymes called aryl hydrocarbon hydroxylases (AHH), detoxifies the body of cancer-causing pollutants.

Nobel Prize–winning German biochemist Otto Warburg in 1966 told a meeting of fellow Nobel winners that a plentiful supply of vitamins B_2 and B_3 and pantothenic acid (B_5) affords the best possible protection against cancer. In 1970, he demonstrated that a deficiency of Vitamin B_1 would start the cancerous process in cells.[4]

The role of pyridoxine (vitamin B_6) in combating bacteria and inactivating viruses has already been discussed (see page 175). A contrary view of vitamin B_6 is given by Kedar Prasad, Ph.D., a professor of radiology and director of the Center for Vitamins and Cancer Research at the University of Colorado Health Sciences Center in Denver. According to Prasad, supplemental vitamin B_6 should be avoided during the treatment of cancer. He points to several animal studies reporting that supplemental B_6 actually enhances the growth of cancer while the restriction of B_6 retards it. "The relevance of this observation for human cancer is not known at this time," he states, but he recommends limiting the intake of vitamin B_6 in the diet.[5]

- *Vitamin C* (ascorbic acid) has been shown to help cure a percentage of "terminal" cancer patients in controlled clinical studies. It also has a preventive action, strengthening the body's defenses against cancer by increasing the effectiveness of the immune system in destroying cancer cells. Vitamin C makes it more difficult for cancer cells to spread by strengthening the "cellular cement," or "ground substance," the intercellular material that holds tissue cells together. In addition, this vitamin helps the body dissolve cholesterol, directly detoxifies some cancer-causing substances, and protects us against the effects of other carcinogens, such as harmful nitrites in cheese and meat.

Linus Pauling, two-time Nobel laureate, believes that "a high intake of vitamin C is beneficial to all patients with cancer." Pauling and his associate, Scottish-born surgeon Dr. Ewan Cameron, showed that terminally ill cancer patients given ten grams of vitamin C per day lived more than four times longer than control patients in the same hospital who did not receive vitamin C. Furthermore, for 10 percent of the vitamin C-treated patients, survival time was increased by a factor of at least twenty. Some patients declared terminal in the early 1970s were still alive over five years later.[6]

Dr. Pauling endorses the Moerman therapy as a valid approach to treating cancer. He testified on Moerman's behalf some twenty years ago when the Dutch physician was under attack by Holland's medical authorities.

- *Vitamin E* causes cancer cells to revert to normal in laboratory experiments and inhibits the growth of other cancer cells. It stimulates the human immune response, which can destroy precancerous cells before they develop into a malignancy, and it has been shown to help prevent cancers caused by many chemicals in the environment. Vitamin E (like vitamins A and C and selenium) is an antioxidant, protecting body cells against unwanted reactions with oxygen. Antioxidants hold in check free radicals, extremely reactive atoms or groups of atoms routinely produced in the body that can damage DNA and cause it to make the abnormal cells that become cancer.

- *Citric acid* is found in the lemon, a prominent fruit in the Moerman diet. This nutrient lowers the viscosity of blood by taking water from the body tissues. In so doing, it prevents fermentation in the cells. According to Otto Warburg's controversial theory, all cancer cells live by fermenting sugar, unlike normal cells, which obtain their energy by taking in oxygen.

    The lemon, a rich source of vitamin C and citric acid, also contains citrin, which is known as vitamin P. Citrin helps the blood flow freely through even the tiniest capillaries.

- *Iodine* regulates the thyroid gland, producer of the hormone thyroxine, which governs the rate of metabolism. Thyroxine helps the cells absorb oxygen in order to burn glucose for energy. But this process is impaired if the mitochondria do not get enough iodine. (Mitochondria, tiny rodlike structures found in the cytoplasm of most cells, serve as centers of enzyme activity.) If the mitochondria do not get sufficient iodine, the cells do not get enough oxygen, and the cells begin to ferment sugar in an anaerobic (airless) reaction. Dr. Moerman, like Otto Warburg, believed that a fermented environment is a breeding ground for cancer cells.

    The average person can get adequate dietary iodine by using iodized salt. However, refined salt is prohibited on the Moerman diet, so supplemental iodine is taken.

- *Iron* is a component of hemoglobin, the oxygen-carrying pigment of red blood cells. Iron deficiency leads to anemia. According to Dr. Moerman, "Cancer patients nearly always show the symptoms of anemia in a greater or less degree. . . . A shortage of iron, also with people who do not suffer from cancer and apparently in good health, occurs more frequently than people generally think."[7]

- *Sulfur* helps the body get rid of poisonous materials and serves as a fuel for the cells' energy-producing mitochondria. Many studies have shown that the sulfur compounds found in broccoli, Brussels sprouts, cabbage, and cauliflower—vegetables featured in the Moerman diet—have antitumor and cancer-preventive actions in laboratory animals.[8]

Correct doses and timing for taking the supplements are considered essential to the success of the therapy.

After years of working with his carrier pigeons on a trial-and-error basis, Moerman felt he had devised a list of food substances that promoted ideal health in pigeons and prevented them from getting cancer, either spontaneously or through injection of cancer cells. He believed that the absence of these same nutrients in the human body leads to a "sick basic condition." So perhaps, he reasoned, these substances might also work therapeutically, causing a tumor to shrink and disappear.

In 1939, Moerman got a chance to test his theory on a patient. Leendert Brinkman was diagnosed as terminally ill with metastatic stomach cancer so widespread that the surgeon wrote to Dr. Moerman, "The tumour is . . . inoperable, so that I have closed the belly again without removing the tumour. As soon as the stitches have been removed and the wound has healed, he can go home to die."

Moerman put Brinkman on a rudimentary form of his standard therapy: the eight supplements, plus unrefined barley, millet, and whole-wheat bread; fresh vegetables and fruits grown locally; rice with butter and green vegetables; one-half to one liter of buttermilk a day; lemon and orange juices; currant juice; egg yolks; and brown rice. (Today, only brown rice—no white rice—is used.) Brinkman ate oranges and lemons "by the truckload," he later testified, until he was "up to his eyes in vitamin C."

A year after Brinkman started the diet, his surgeon pronounced him cancer-free. He lived for more than twenty years after his "terminally ill" diagnosis, in excellent health, and died at the age of ninety.

Soon hundreds of cancer patients treated by Moerman were reporting similar positive results. Over the next decade, Moerman performed many experiments in an attempt to determine the optimum proportions, quantities, and interactions of the vitamins and minerals he prescribed. In 1956, doctors at Rotterdam's South Hospital sent home to die an "incurable" man diagnosed with advanced lung cancer, with metastases to the liver and brain. The patient rapidly went downhill. Moerman began treating the man with his nutritional therapy and noticed a visible improvement in a few weeks. A year later, X-rays revealed that the cancer had completely disappeared, and although the man was seventy-one, he was able to work at his trade again.

Further support for Moerman's method came in the mid-1950s, when an analysis of wartime records revealed a strong correlation between diet and cancer. The Nazis' 1940-to-1945 occupation of the Netherlands in World War II forced a nation of 9 million people to switch to a different dietary regimen. White bread was replaced by whole-meal-corn and rye bread. Sugar, coffee, and tea were nonexistent. Honey was used, if available. The production of margarine was halted, and people consumed small amounts of butter. They also hoarded as much fruit and vegetables as possible, buying fresh produce from local farmers. Alcoholic drinks were a very scarce luxury; the Dutch drank fruit juices instead. Meat was extremely hard to obtain, and consumers ate small amounts of dairy products.

This wartime diet was remarkably similar to the Moerman diet. But in 1945, the Dutch nation's forced experiment in healthy eating suddenly ended, and people went back to an unwholesome diet of high animal protein, white bread, sugar, and only a few vegetables and little fruit.

The curve of cancer incidence reveals what happened. Before the dietary changes were widespread, the incidence of cancer continued its steady rise, from 160,000 cases in 1940 to a peak of 180,000 in 1942. Then, from 1942 to 1945, the curve fell sharply to a low point below 130,000. As soon as highly processed foods began flooding back into Holland after the war, the cancer rate rose again, reaching 160,000 by 1950. Despite these provocative findings, the medical profession all but ignored Moerman's claims and his clinical results.

A country doctor without any affiliation with a hospital, university, or big drug company, Dr. Moerman stubbornly continued his work, shunned by his fellow cancer researchers. The tide slowly turned as mainstream scientists were compelled to investigate the continuing stories of successful cures of "terminal" cancer patients. In 1983, an interdisciplinary research group named SIKON, formed by several Moerman doctors, found that the Moerman therapy brought long-term remission in roughly half of the treated cancer patients who had been labeled "incurable" by orthodox medicine.[9] Their conclusion was based on a study group of 150 patients.

A larger retrospective study of Moerman patients—an outgrowth of the SIKON project—was carried out by the Dutch Ministry of Health in cooperation with the Moerman Vereniging. This study, which will soon be published in book form, includes the case histories of 35 patients cured by the Moerman approach, selected from a group of 400 recovered patients who volunteered to share their experiences.

In an April 1991 lecture to members of the Moerman Vereniging, Dr. Joop Klinkhamer commented on these 35 cases:

> For 14 among the 35, you could still say: "Yes, the Moerman treatment helped, but traditional therapy may also have contributed." For the other 21 it is clear: this was indeed the result of Moerman's treatment. Among those 21, there are 11 patients who never underwent any treatment other than Moerman's!
>
> These 35 patients are almost all cases that had been "given up." Or they were all patients who were told, "If you do not have this operation or treatment, you will not live much longer." Or: "I cannot do anything more for you, it is finished." If this was the case for these 35, it is also much more likely that many among the 400 were cured by the Moerman treatment.[10]

Dr. Klinkhamer went on to speculate:

> If it is possible for the Moerman therapy to cure people who have been given up, how many more people could have been cured if they had started with the treatment in the first year cancer was discovered, rather than after years of traditional treatment? We do not know, because the percentage of people who immediately start with the Moerman therapy is still very small. Frequently patients grab "the last straw" after a number of operations. On the basis of these 35 well-documented cases then, you might wonder . . . how much misery many people could have been spared if they had started the Moerman therapy early, whether in combination with traditional treatment or not.

Dr. Klinkhamer's overall conclusion was that "the Moerman therapy is indeed capable of curing patients, of having the tumor disappear or creating a remarkable, favorable change that lasts a very long time." Yet, despite the large retrospective study, he expected continued resistance from the medical establishment: "You all know the story—when someone visits a physician stating that he started Moerman's therapy and is still alive two years after the physician had given up on him, the classical answer is, 'Well, then you never had cancer.' Hence the study must contain so much information from conventional medical reports that this can never be said again. It has not been easy to collect all that information. But we succeeded."

Klinkhamer's comments on the politics of medicine in his own country have striking parallels with the state of affairs in the United States. He described how two major negative reports on the Moerman therapy were allegedly riddled with false information and outright fabrications. One study, commissioned by the Dutch House of Commons, initially found favorable results, so the researcher was asked to rewrite it. The subsequent negative report implied that the therapy was of little or no value.

"The big pharmaceutical companies," says Dr. Klinkhamer, "have no interest whatsoever in researching the healthful effects of carrots and peas. They have a vested interest in their own products. That is where the money is and that is where the research is done. This situation finally is making us realize that traditional medicine cannot solve the cancer problem by itself."

Resources

Moerman Vereniging
Mrs. G. G. Strating-IJben
Postbus 14
6674 ZG Herveld
Netherlands
Phone: 011 31 8880 51221

For further information on the Moerman therapy and a list of North American physicians who prescribe it.

Reading Material

Dr. Moerman's Anti-Cancer Diet: Holland's Revolutionary Nutritional Program for Combating Cancer, by Ruth Jochems, Avery Publishing Group (120 Old Broadway, Garden City Park, NY 11040; 800-548-5757), 1990.

A Solution to the Cancer Problem, by Dr. Cornelis Moerman, International Association of Cancer Victors and Friends (see page xviii for address and phone number), no date ("Postscript" translated into English in 1962). Out of print; available through the Moerman Vereniging (see above for address and phone number).

Part Five

METABOLIC THERAPIES

Metabolic therapy is based on the principle that many factors are involved in cancer causation and, therefore, a multifaceted healing program is required to reverse cancer. Metabolic approaches use detoxification to flush out toxins and waste materials that interfere with metabolism. Detoxification methods include cleansing the colon, flushing the liver and gallbladder, and drinking large quantities of fruit juices and herbal teas. Anticancer diets rich in grains, raw vegetables, and fruits supply essential nutrients to cells and help detoxify the body and repair damaged tissues. These diets are based on whole foods free from additives. Sugar, white flour, processed foods, coffee, and alcohol are not allowed. As in the dietary therapies discussed in the previous section, metabolic nutrition emphasizes vitamins, minerals, and enzymes that stimulate immune function and are thought to have a direct antitumor effect.

Supplementation includes intensive doses of nutrients such as vitamins, minerals, enzymes, laetrile, and glandular extracts. Taking supplements is said to strengthen natural immunity, deactivate toxins created by tumors, and directly attack tumor masses.

High doses of proteolytic (protein-digesting) enzymes are often given. These enzymes are believed to break down the protein coating that shields the walls of tumor cells, thereby enabling white blood cells to kill the malignant cells. The ability of enzymes to dissolve cancer-cell walls was noted as early as 1888. The enzyme treatment of cancer is widely practiced in Europe and in many clinics around the world, though it is not accepted by the medical establishment in the United States.

Metabolic doctors may also utilize immune-enhancing vaccines, herbal salves, ozone therapy, chelation, live-cell therapy, hydrazine sulfate, dimethyl sulfoxide (DMSO), psychological counseling, and other methods. The multipronged metabolic approach attempts to apply the best possible combination of methods to improve the synergistic functioning of glands, organs, and systems—not just the functioning of the organ that is under direct attack. The goal is to restore the patient's physiology to metabolic balance and thus eliminate the conditions that allowed the tumor to develop in the first place.

Laetrile, also called vitamin B_{17}, is a basic component of metabolic therapy at many clinics. "Laetrile" is another name for amygdalin, a type of carbohydrate occurring naturally in 1,200 different plants including chick peas, lentils, lima beans, buckwheat, brown rice, cashews, wheatgrass, and mung-bean sprouts. Amygdalin is present in the seeds of all common fruits, most abundantly in apricot pits. Commercially sold laetrile is derived from kernels of apricots, peaches, or bitter almonds. The Chinese used fruit-kernel preparations against tumors some 2,000 years ago. Ancient Greek, Roman, and Arabic physicians also used amygdalin to treat tumors.

Laetrile has been the subject of heated controversy in the United States since the early 1950s, when it was introduced by San Francisco biochemist Ernst T. Krebs, Jr., whose father, Dr. Ernst Krebs, Sr., first administered it to a cancer patient in 1929. There are over thirty clinical studies in the world medical literature reporting the effectiveness and safety of laetrile. A ten-year trial in Europe involving 150 patients found that "50 percent of all cases in treatment showed objective improvement" and concluded that laetrile was "an extremely useful chemotherapeutic drug."[1]

Skeptics remain unconvinced, however. In *Cancer and Its Nutritional Therapies,* biochemist Richard Passwater says the data "still presents a confusing picture." Passwater interviewed many physicians who reported that laetrile therapy produces swift, noticeable improvement in most cancer patients and significant improvement or remission in some patients with solid tumors. But most of these doctors also administered megavitamin therapy simultaneously and couldn't say whether laetrile was a key factor in the patients' improvement. "I have not witnessed a groundswell of laetrile-cured cancer patients, despite the legalization of laetrile in many states," concludes Passwater.[2]

Laetrile dramatically inhibited the growth of tumors in mice in a series of experiments performed by Dr. Kanematsu Sugiura at Memorial Sloan-Kettering Cancer Center in New York between 1972 and 1976. A notorious clinical trial at the Mayo Clinic in 1982, sponsored by the National Cancer Institute, concluded that laetrile was ineffective as a treatment of cancer. However, Dr. James Cason of the University of California at Berkeley, using infrared spectrophotometry, determined that the compound used in the Mayo study did not contain amygdalin (laetrile). Critics also charged that the so-called laetrile was not given in conjunction with a proper diet and nutrients.

In an NCI best-case review of patients on laetrile, six out of twenty-two evaluable cases showed objective remission, including two complete remissions.[3]

Vitamin C, or ascorbic acid, is another key component of metabolic therapy. The American Cancer Society, which for many years stated that vitamin C was worthless in preventing or treating cancer, in 1991 reversed its position and now suggests an increased intake of vitamin C to help control this disease.[4] A multipurpose vitamin, ascorbic acid stimulates immune mechanisms that kill cancer cells. It also detoxifies carcinogens and reduces the ability of malignant cells to spread.

Vitamin C increases the production of lymphocytes, white blood corpuscles that destroy cancer cells. Studies from the National Cancer Institute have demonstrated a direct association: the more vitamin C taken, the more lymphocytes in the blood. Cancer-killing antibodies that circulate in the blood are also more plentiful in people with high levels of vitamin C. Another positive effect of this versatile vitamin is the stimulation of activity by interferon, the antitumor, antiviral substance produced by T-cells. Like vitamin E, vitamin C can prevent the conversion of nitrites in the stomach into cancer-causing nitrosamines. Nitrites are commonly used as preservatives in meat.

Well-known studies by Dr. Linus Pauling, the Nobel Prize–winning chemist, and his collaborator, Dr. Ewan Cameron, showed that large doses of vitamin C markedly improved cancer patients' survival times. Many patients on vitamin C therapy reportedly feel better, gain weight, and experience less pain. Cancer cells produce an enzyme, hyaluronidase, which breaks down the cellular cement, the intercellular material holding tissue cells together. Dr. Cameron showed that vitamin C strengthens this cement, or ground substance, making it less vulnerable to tumor growth.

Like vitamins A and E and selenium, multitalented vitamin C is a free-radical scavenger, mopping up free radicals (highly reactive compounds formed in the body) to prevent damage to the DNA.

Some metabolic doctors advise against the use of chemotherapy, radiation, and surgery. The immune-destroying effects of conventional treatments, and their bombardment of the body with toxins, interfere with metabolic healing. Many metabolic practitioners believe that prior treatment with chemotherapy or radiation limits a patient's chances for recovery on a metabolic program. On the other hand, invasive therapies sometimes save a patient's life, and there are many metabolic physicians who at times do recommend conventional treatment. In such cases, a metabolic program combined with surgery, chemotherapy, or radiation will lessen the side effects of invasive treatment, help prevent cellular damage, and bolster immunity.

Metabolic therapies are available through clinics and individual practitioners in the United States, Europe, and Canada, with a concentration of clinics in Mexico. Numerous metabolic clinics are clustered in Tijuana, Mexico, just across the United States border. Assessments of the clinics vary widely, even among sympathetic observers within the alternative cancer field. Supporters say that some of the Tijuana clinics get positive results and attain five-year survivals (the American orthodoxy's definition of "cure") in metastatic cancer at rates much higher than conventional medicine. They assert that the most advanced technologies in treating cancer are available at the better Tijuana clinics. But critics charge that some of these clinics purvey "the latest in high-tech quackery."

Persons interested in researching the practitioners in Mexico can take the bus tour of Tijuana cancer clinics sponsored about four times a year by the Cancer Control Society. For information on the bus tours, contact the Cancer Control Society at P.O. Box 4651, Modesto, CA 95352; 209-529-4697. Another source of information is Sally Wolper's survey *Tijuana Clinics: Where and How to Go,* which features a number of clinics not covered on the bus tour. To order this survey, contact Wolper Publications, 14134 Gladeside Drive, La Mirada, CA 90638; 213-921-8495.

One promising new therapy used by metabolic physicians involves shark cartilage. Unlike mammals, sharks have no bones. The shark's cartilaginous skeleton is the same today as it was when this fish evolved over 400 million years ago. Shark cartilage is gristle made of long strands of tough, elastic connective tissue. The cartilage gives the shark immunity against carcinogens, mutagens, and pollutants. Furthermore, a substance in shark cartilage strongly inhibits the growth of new blood vessels toward solid tumors *in humans*, thereby starving cancer cells and shutting down tumor growth, according to scientists at the Massachusetts Institute of Technology (MIT). In the respected journal *Science*, MIT researchers Robert Langer, Ph.D., and Anne Lee, Ph.D., suggest that the abundance of this antitumor substance in sharks explains why these creatures don't get cancer and also makes the shark an ideal source of this inhibitor for the treatment of human cancer.[5] Other studies with animals and people confirm that shark cartilage blocks angiogenesis, the creation of new capillary blood vessels required for tumor growth. Shark cartilage also reduces pain and joint inflammation in arthritis and osteoarthritic conditions.

In a preliminary report, eight terminal cancer patients with an expected survival time of three to six months were given thirty grams of nontoxic shark-cartilage material daily. After just six to seven weeks of treatment, six of the eight patients (75 percent) showed positive response and substantially reduced tumor size. A woman with inoperable advanced uterine cancer with invasion to the bladder experienced an almost 100 percent reduction of the tumor (only scar tissue can be palpated now). Another patient had an inoperable peritoneal carcinomatosis from colon cancer. After fifty-four days of treatment, most of the tumor was found to be transformed into a jellylike substance that was 80 percent removed. The shark cartilage was given to the eight patients as a retention enema or an aqueous suspension vaginally administered. For further information, contact I. William Lane, Ph.D. (Cartilage Consultants, 206 Main Street, Milburn, NJ 07041; 201-467-1108), or Ernesto Contreras, Jr., M.D. (P.O. Box 3793, San Ysidro, CA 92173; 800-523-8795). Another source of information is the book *Sharks Don't Get Cancer: How Shark Cartilage Could Save Your Life*, by Dr. I. William Lane and Linda Comac (Avery Publishing Group, 120 Old Broadway, Garden City Park, NY 11040; 800-548-5757).

Part V of *Options* focuses on three popular metabolic approaches: the Gerson therapy, the Kelley method, and the practice of Dr. Hans Nieper in Germany. Another program frequently called metabolic—the immune therapy developed by Dr. Josef Issels—is discussed in Chapter 8. For a listing of other metabolic practitioners, see John Fink's directory *Third Opinion: An International Directory to Alternative Therapy Centers for the Treatment and Prevention of Cancer and Other Degenerative Diseases* (see Appendix A).

Chapter 17

GERSON THERAPY

"There is no cancer in normal metabolism," wrote Max Gerson, M.D. (1881–1959). A pioneer of what is today known as nutritional metabolic therapy, the German-born physician, who lived in the United States for twenty-three years, believed that cancer cannot occur unless the functions of the liver, the pancreas, and the immune system as well as other body functions have degenerated. Cancer, in his theory, results from faulty metabolism due to poor nutrition and long-term exposure to pesticides, chemical fertilizers, air and water pollution, and other irritants that increasingly saturate the environment.

The Gerson therapy combines vigorous detoxification with nutrition aimed at restoring the body's natural immunity and healing power. Believing cancer to be a systemic rather than a localized disease, Gerson emphasized the rebalancing of the cancer patient's entire physiology. The therapy is thought to reverse the conditions necessary to sustain the growth of malignant cells. To rebuild the patient's healing mechanism, a twofold attack is mounted: a detoxification program helps the body eliminate toxins and waste materials that interfere with healing and metabolism; and a low-fat, salt-free diet floods the body's cells with easily assimilated nutrients that strengthen the natural immune defenses.

The diet, the core of the therapy, includes organically grown fresh fruits and vegetables and thirteen glasses of freshly squeezed juices daily, taken at hourly intervals. The emphasis on fresh fruits and vegetables means the patient receives high levels of vitamin C, beta-carotene, and other antioxidants that scavenge free radicals. Patients also receive supplements such as thyroid extract, potassium iodide, liver extract, pancreatic enzyme, and niacin. No meat is allowed. Animal protein is omitted for the first six to twelve weeks, then kept to a minimum. The diet is largely fat-free but includes some yogurt, pot cheese, cottage cheese, and churned buttermilk as well as linseed oil, a rich source of omega-3 fatty acids. Research shows that these fatty acids kill human cancer cells in tissue cultures without destroying normal cells in the same culture.

The key detoxification method is the coffee enema, which patients are taught to self-administer several times daily. Through his work with cancer patients, Gerson came to the conclusion that many patients on a radical detoxification program died not of the cancer itself, but rather from the liver's inability to absorb the toxic breakdown products of the rapidly dissolving tumor mass. Coffee enemas, long a part of more orthodox medicine, seemed to him a logical component of a detoxification program. Caffeine taken rectally is believed to stimulate the action of the liver, increase bile flow, and open the bile ducts so that the liver can excrete the toxic products of tumor breakdown more easily.

Although coffee enemas may sound bizarre, and are distasteful to some, many cancer patients taking them report increased energy, improved appetite, relief from nausea, and a marked decrease in pain. Coffee enemas have been used by a number of other metabolic and immunotherapeutic practitioners, notably William Kelley (Chapter 18).

As a further aid in detoxification, some patients take castor oil orally and by enema every other day.

Max Gerson, a refugee from Nazi Germany with impeccable scientific credentials, was an eminent if controversial figure in Europe because he successfully treated tuberculosis, migraines, arthritis, and cancer by means of his salt-free vegetarian diet. One of Gerson's patients was Albert Schweitzer, the Nobel Prize–winning doctor-missionary. Through a prescribed nutritional program, Gerson enabled Schweitzer, at the age of seventy-five, to control his diabetes so well that he stopped taking insulin. Gerson also cured Schweitzer's wife of apparently terminal tuberculosis. Schweitzer wrote of the nutritional healer: "I see in him one of the most eminent medical geniuses in the history of medicine."

But in the United States, where he emigrated in 1936, Gerson was persecuted and harassed by the medical establishment. Because of his unorthodox cancer therapy, Gerson was expelled from the New York Medical Society and deprived of his hospital affiliations. His therapy was prominently featured on the American Cancer Society's Unproven Methods blacklist, where it remains today, even though his anticancer diet is quite similar to the preventive diet now endorsed by the ACS, the NCI, and the American Heart Association.

Today, Gerson's legacy is kept alive by his daughter Charlotte, who runs the Gerson Institute in Bonita, California, and works closely with the Centro Hospitalario Internationale del Pacifico (CHIPSA) in Tijuana, Mexico. The hospital, which is an inpatient facility, employs the Gerson method in the treatment of cancer and other degenerative diseases. Over the years, the Gerson therapy has yielded an impressive number of long-term cancer survivors, all of whom had well-documented illnesses. A current brochure gives the mini-case histories of thirty-six cancer patients, reportedly termed "incurable" by their orthodox physicians, who achieved long-term remission using the Gerson regimen. The names, ages, and photographs of these "cured incurables" are given, along with the details of their illnesses and treatments. Several of these patients are featured in Max Gerson's 1958 book, *A Cancer Therapy: Results of Fifty Cases* (see Resources), and are still alive and well—and cancer-free—over thirty years later.

Among the thirty-six cases profiled are seven survivors of cancer metastasized to the lung, which usually kills patients quickly, and three survivors of "hopeless" spreading melanoma who have lived thirty-six to forty-four years free of cancer after diagnosis. Other recovered patients include two survivors of metastasized pancreatic cancer and a fifteen-year survivor of advanced liver cancer who was given three to five weeks to live by her conventional doctor. These two forms of the disease are incurable by chemotherapy, radiation, or surgery. Also profiled in the brochure are long-term survivors of inoperable brain cancer, uterine cancer spread into the pelvis, metastasized breast cancer, prostate cancer, recurring bone cancer, and colon cancer.

Dora Sherken, now in her late eighties, was brought unconscious by ambulance to Dr. Gerson at Gotham Hospital, New York City, in March 1944. Doctors at Mount Sinai Hospital had diagnosed her in June 1943 with an exceptionally large tumor of the pituitary gland that left her blind in the right eye, with the left optic nerve and surrounding bones partially destroyed. Dora, who lived in Brooklyn at the time, had noticed a progressive loss of vision in both eyes during 1941 and 1942. At Mount Sinai, she had been given X-ray treatments, which were ineffective. Told by many doctors that she had six months to live and would shortly go totally blind, Dora was advised to have surgery to remove the large tumor mass pressing on the optic nerve. She refused, having seen the adverse aftereffects in other hospitalized patients who underwent neurological operations.

Under Dr. Gerson's care, Dora remained unconscious during the first week of treatment, which began immediately. Teaspoon by teaspoon, day and night, she was induced to take fruit and vegetable juices. She was also given many enemas. After one week, she regained full consciousness. At the end of two months, she was feeling fine, was able to do housework, and had improved visual acuity. At the end of eight months, she resumed her part-time job as a secretary to her husband. Tests taken in 1945 indicated that her cancer was in remission. Dr. Gerson's treatment had saved her life and also saved the remaining vision in her left eye, allowing her to resume her active schedule.

Dora followed a strict Gerson regimen for seven years. Her husband assisted with the food preparation and gave Dora her liver-extract and vitamin injections as required. "My mother has a tremendous will to live, and once she decided to go on the Gerson diet, she never once cheated or went off it," recalls Diane Rosen, Dora's daughter. After seven years of strict adherence to the protocol, Dora gradually did go off it and has remained in good health. Two CAT scans in 1980 showed her brain, bones, and pituitary completely cancer-free.

Gregory Grover, at age fifty-six, was diagnosed by X-rays in October 1966 with an advanced, aggressive tumor in the bladder. The tumor, rated Stage III to IV, was removed, but doctors at Cedars-Sinai Medical Center in Los Angeles advised him to have his bladder removed also. They told him that even if the operation went well, he had only a 50 percent chance of survival, and that if the bladder was not removed, he had a 5 percent chance of survival.

Refusing further surgery, Grover started the Gerson therapy in January 1967. "I followed it 100 percent, by the book, with no deviations through the end of 1968." After he had been on the program one year, he had a cystoscopy performed at UCLA. According to Grover, the urologist was amazed to discover that his patient was completely cancer-free. "'How do we account for this?' the assisting physician whispered to the urologist as he did the cystoscopy," recalls Grover, who is now in his eighties, still in remission, and quite active.

Almost all types of cancer are said to respond to the treatment. The types that respond particularly well, according to personnel at the Gerson Institute, are melanoma and lymphoma. The Gerson therapy has not been effective in leukemia, in the opinion of various alternative therapists. Chemotherapy gives at least a 50 percent five-year survival rate with leukemia.

During his lifetime, Max Gerson claimed a 30 percent rate of remission in his terminal patients. The current patient literature states that "the Gerson Therapy is able to achieve almost routine recoveries in early to intermediate cancers. Even when the disease is advanced and incurable by conventional standards (i.e., involves the liver or pancreas or multiple internal sites) excellent results are possible." The patient literature also claims that for cancer patients with additional afflictions (for example, arthritis, heart disease, or diabetes), the treatment "usually heals the body of all diseases simultaneously." Norman Fritz, vice president of the Gerson Institute, stated in *Cancer? Think Curable! The Gerson Therapy*, by S. J. Haught (see Resources), that the Gerson treatment "can save about 50 percent or more of advanced 'hopeless' cancer patients" and that "the percentage who recover can exceed 90 percent for early cancers and some 'early terminal' cancers."

These claims should be taken with great skepticism, as should all such claims in the alternative cancer field. (A figure of 80 percent or greater for five-year survival seems to be a favorite among alternative practitioners.) The reality appears to be that remission remains the exception rather than the rule with Gerson patients, according to Michael Lerner in his study *Varieties of Integral Cancer Therapy*.[1] Lerner cites a resident of a Gerson halfway house in the San Diego area who reported that during her stay of several months, she observed one of the approximately twenty patients in residence make a significant recovery. This story, of course, is anecdotal, but even if roughly accurate, the 5 percent recovery rate is a far cry from the claims made by the Gerson clinic.

Another evaluation of the Gerson treatment's efficacy comes from Steve Austin, a naturopathic physician who recently completed a survey tracking twenty-one Gerson cancer patients over a five-year period.[2] Austin, who teaches nutrition at Western States Chiropractic College in Portland, Oregon, visited the Gerson clinic in Mexico in 1983 and, at random, asked approximately thirty cancer patients for permission to follow their progress. He was able to track twenty-one of these patients over a five-year period, or until death, from 1983 to 1988, through annual letters or phone calls. At the end of the five years, only one of the twenty-one patients was still alive. All the rest had succumbed to their cancers. This also suggests a recovery rate of around 5 percent.

Austin, who plans to publish his study, comments, "The patients tracked had a wide variety of cancers. Many appeared to do well when they were at the Gerson clinic, but when they went home they died 'on schedule.' I was favorably predisposed, even prejudicially so, toward the Gerson therapy, because you hear so many remarkable stories about recovered Gerson patients in alternative cancer circles.

But the reality turned out to be different. The Gerson staff may be out of touch with the ultimate results of the therapy. They see patients doing well while they're at the clinic, something I observed myself. When these people go back home, however, most of them go downhill. The data admittedly are based on a very small sample, but they suggest that the therapy does not work as well as its advocates claim."

Interestingly, Austin also tracked eighteen late-stage cancer patients at Hospital Del Mar in Tijuana, a clinic run by Drs. Francisco Contreras and Ernesto Contreras, which combines metabolic therapy with detoxification, laetrile, enzyme supplements, megadoses of vitamins, and special vaccines. All eighteen patients died within three years of their stay at the Contreras clinic, according to Austin. "On the basis of these results, I recommend that all cancer patients avoid the laetrile clinics, despite the fact that I've run across occasional anecdotes suggesting efficacy. Even if a rare patient is helped, zero out of eighteen is a terrible indicator," says Austin.

More positive evaluations of the Gerson therapy, and scientific research supporting the validity of key components in the Gerson protocol, will be discussed later in this chapter.

The Gerson clinic lacks the staff to monitor patients' conditions once they return home. Gerson Institute members tend to explain the therapy's failures by saying those patients either did not follow the regimen strictly enough or went off the therapy. This is often true, but sometimes patients discontinue the therapy because they are no longer seeing results: tumors continue to grow or the patient becomes too weak to adhere to the program.

What is beyond dispute is that the therapy is not easy to follow. It's a rigorously demanding approach and should not be undertaken without the intention to persevere. Sticking to the regimen may sometimes seem like a full-time job. In his book, Max Gerson cautions, "It is advisable not to start the treatment, if for any reason strict adherence to it is not possible." Each element in the therapy is important, and all are interrelated in their workings. The diet is restrictive. Milk, most cheeses, and butter are forbidden, as are tobacco, salt, coffee, tea, cocoa, chocolate, alcohol, sharp spices, refined sugar and flour, candies, ice cream, cakes, nuts, mushrooms, soybeans, pickles, cucumbers, and all berries with the exception of red currants. Also taboo are canned, frozen, processed, smoked, salted, dehydrated, powdered, or bottled foods.

Juices must be freshly squeezed every hour so that the oxidizing enzymes will not be destroyed by light or air. Even the type of juice extractor and grinder are specially selected. Standard home juicers are not recommended because the electric charge produced by their centrifugal actions destroys enzymes and their preparation process mixes oxygen into the juices, hastening their decomposition. Gerson patients are encouraged to buy a more expensive, stainless-steel grinder and press.

After treatment at the Gerson hospital, patients are advised to continue the regimen at home for one and a half years or more, until the liver, pancreas, and oxidation, immune, and other systems have been restored sufficiently to prevent a recurrence of cancer. The support of family and close friends—both emotionally and on a practical level—is believed to play a vital role in the therapy's success.

For those who do persevere, the benefits can be dramatic. "It's a lot of work," says Charlotte Gerson, "but those people who want to be well, and remain well, with their bodies rebuilt, with their organs rebuilt, and normal and functioning, they go through it, and they do the job, and they regain health in all areas, whether we are talking about cancer, multiple sclerosis, rheumatoid arthritis, glaucoma, kidney disease, or even diabetes."

The therapy is multifaceted. Dr. Gerson placed great emphasis on the liver, which he believed to be the body's most important organ in defeating malignancy. He maintained that nearly all cancers were allowed to develop because of poor liver function. Support for this view comes from Dr. Jesse Greenstein, former chief of the National Cancer Institute's biochemistry laboratory. In his 1954 book, *Biochemistry of Cancer*, Greenstein wrote, "There seems to be little doubt that hepatic insufficiency is a concomitant phenomenon with cancer." According to Dr. Raymond Brown, former investigator at Sloan-Kettering Institute for Cancer Research, Gerson's "thesis that a damaged liver is a primary precursor of degenerative disease is consistent with current concepts that liver status reflects the functional capacity of the reticuloendothelial system."[3] The reticuloendothelial system defends against infection and disposes of the products of cell breakdown. It is composed of macrophages, liver cells, and cells of the lungs, bone marrow, spleen, and lymph nodes.

The liver, the body's largest organ, weighs seven to ten pounds and performs a multitude of tasks. Among its vital functions are metabolizing essential fats (and thus preventing their accumulation in the bloodstream), synthesizing necessary blood proteins, breaking down and eliminating toxic substances, and secreting bile, which is stored in the gallbladder and the enlarged bile duct. Bile, which empties into the small intestine, acts as a carrier for all liver wastes. One reason animal proteins are drastically reduced on the Gerson diet is that they have been found to interfere with liver-boosting medications and to impede the detoxification process. Keeping animal protein at a minimum frees the protein-dissolving enzymes to "digest" cancer tissue rather than food, according to Max Gerson.

Gerson also found that both animal and vegetable fats have the effect of promoting tumor growth. Whenever he eliminated fats from his cancer patients' diets, the results improved substantially. Recent research supports his finding. Studies show that the higher the level of cholesterol and fats in the blood of cancer patients, the less chance the patients have of surviving. Cancer patients receiving Gerson therapy therefore avoid both animal and vegetable fats. An exception is linseed oil, which helps the body transport vitamin A. Linseed oil has been shown to have antitumor action, and it is rich in an essential fatty acid that reduces blood viscosity. Low blood viscosity correlates with a decreased tendency to spreading (metastases) of cancer.

Eliminating animal protein is only one aspect of Gerson's liver therapy. Patients are also given injections composed of liver extract, administered daily for four to six months, sometimes longer. These liver injections provide vitamins, minerals, and enzymes believed to help restore the liver to its proper functioning. Intramuscular injections of liver extract are combined with vitamin B_{12} injections, which Dr. Gerson held to be important for proper protein synthesis. Full restoration of the liver may take from six to eighteen months, during which time patients should have their blood monitored by a physician so that the supplements and diet can be adjusted.

Nobel Prize–winning biochemist Dr. Albert Szent-Gyorgyi believed that the liver may hold the secret of cancer prevention and cure. In 1972, he reported that extracts of mouse liver "strongly inhibited" the growth of inoculated cancer in mice. He and his associate, Dr. Laszlo Egyud, isolated from liver extract a potent anticancer substance, which they dubbed retine. This liver derivative proved so effective in the laboratory, Dr. Szent-Gyorgyi was moved to predict, "We are on the verge of finding the key to curing cancer. . . . Retine stops the growth of cancer cells without poisoning other cells."[4]

Another major feature of the Gerson therapy is restoring the balance of potassium and sodium in the body. Dr. Gerson maintained that cancer alters the body's normal sodium-to-potassium balance, already disturbed by the modern oversalted diet. Liver, brain, and muscle cells normally have much higher levels of potassium than of sodium, but in cancer patients, observed Gerson, the ratio is reversed. The Gerson therapy aims to remove as much sodium from the cancer patient's body as possible, replacing it with potassium. The diet stresses foods rich in potassium and low in sodium, with no salt added.

In addition, patients receive a potassium solution, added to juices ten times daily. Edema, or fluid retention, caused by an excess of sodium, reportedly disappears with great frequency when patients ingest high amounts of potassium in juices. Restoring potassium levels to normal in the major organs of severely ill patients can take a year or two.

Gerson's emphasis on restoring the potassium balance in cancer patients finds considerable support in modern research. Several studies outline rationales to explain Gerson's theory that elevating the potassium level while restricting sodium in the diet acts against tumor formation.[5] Freeman Cope, M.D., wrote in *Physiological Chemistry and Physics* in 1978, "The high potassium, low sodium diet of the Gerson therapy has been observed experimentally to cure many cases of advanced cancer in man, but the reason was not clear. Recent studies from the laboratory of Ling indicate that high potassium, low sodium environments can partially return damaged cell proteins to their normal undamaged configuration. Therefore, the damage in other tissues, induced by toxins and breakdown products from the cancer, is probably partly repaired by the Gerson therapy through this mechanism."

Supplying oxygen to the cells is another central feature of the Gerson therapy. Dr. Gerson believed that cancer cells thrive by fermenting sugar in an oxygen-depleted cellular environment. This still-controversial theory, put forward by the great biochemist Otto Warburg in 1930, has some support in modern research. To enhance the patient's oxidation function, Dr. Gerson gave patients oxidizing enzymes through vegetable, fruit, and raw-calves'-liver juices. The Gerson clinic discontinued the use of raw-liver juice in 1989, but the present diet is still a rich source of oxidation enzymes. These enzymes are also produced naturally by a healthy, restored liver. Through the Gerson treatment, "oxidation is usually more than doubled," says the patient brochure, which adds that "most 'incurable' diseases are oxygen deficiency diseases also (heart attack, strokes, cancer, etc.)."

Tumor breakdown begins, according to Max Gerson, when the detoxification process is active, the repaired liver is producing oxidative enzymes, and the potassium-to-sodium balance has been restored. Once the body starts breaking down and eliminating the tumor, detoxification is critical so that the liver is not overloaded with toxins. Here is where the coffee enema becomes especially important. Some recent scientific research gives credence to the coffee enema as a detoxification measure. In 1981, for example, Dr. Lee Wattenberg and colleagues demonstrated that substances found in coffee promote the activity of a key enzyme system that detoxifies a vast array of electrophiles from the bloodstream. According to Gar Hildenbrand of the Gerson Institute, this "must be regarded as an important mechanism for carcinogen detoxification." This enzyme group is responsible for neutralizing free radicals.

Dr. Peter Lechner, who is investigating the Gerson program in Graz, Austria, has reported that "coffee enemas have a definite effect on the colon which can be observed with an endoscope." Two chemicals in coffee, theophylline and theobromine, dilate blood vessels and counteract inflammation of the gut. Palmitates, a group of substances also found in coffee, enhance the enzyme system responsible for the removal of toxic free radicals from the serum. (*Note:* While coffee enemas are part of the Gerson program, drinking coffee is forbidden.)

For a full review of the scientific research supporting the use of coffee enemas, see Ralph Moss's two-part article "Coffee: The Royal Flush," in *The Cancer Chronicles*, Autumn 1990 and December 1990.

The Gerson diet features three organic vegetarian meals daily. Along with a potassium supplement, six of the thirteen daily juices contain three drops of half-strength Lugol solution, an iodine-potassium compound, plus a small amount of thyroid extract. Dr. Gerson theorized that these substances are absorbed by the cancer mass along with the oxidizing enzymes. The combination makes it impossible for the cancer cells to ferment, and they die, he held. Iodine appeared to him to be a decisive factor in the normal differentiation of cells. He believed that iodine also counteracted the cancer-stimulating effect of certain hormones. Several studies validating Gerson's hunches have shown that thyroid extract boosts natural resistance to infection by increasing antibody formation and augmenting the power of reticuloendothelial cells.

Most cancer patients have a deficiency of digestive enzymes. To aid digestion, patients on the Gerson therapy take tablets of pancreatic enzyme (pancreatin), which helps restore stomach acid to normal levels. They also take tablets of niacin, which, according to Gerson, helps to check cancerous growth, restores cell energies, and raises depleted liver stores of glycogen and potassium.

Through carrot juice, liver supplements, and other foods, the

Gerson diet supplies an enormous amount of beta-carotene, vitamin A's precursor, which the body converts to vitamin A. Recent research suggests that vitamin A inhibits the cancer-causing action of tumor promoters and tumor initiators. Furthermore, in laboratory experiments, vitamin A has been shown to transform cancer cells to cells that resemble normal cells. This effect has been noted with tumors such as lung cancer, prostate cancer, colon cancer, and neuroblastoma (a tumor of embryonic nerve cells).[6] In a 1960 German study in *Nutritional Abstracts and Reviews,* 218 cancer patients received large amounts of vitamin A along with vitamin C for approximately three to seven months. Tumor growth generally stopped or regressed with no side effects.

Since 1983, the Gerson clinic has offered ozone therapy as an adjunct to its basic protocol. Available in many countries for cancer treatment but officially barred in the United States, ozone therapy has been shown to shrink tumors. (For a further discussion, see page 229.)

Max Gerson's nutritional treatment for cancer might never have come into being if not for his migraines. A brilliant medical graduate of the University of Freiburg (Germany) in 1909, Dr. Gerson was disabled by recurrent migraines for which his own doctors had no cure. By the early 1920s, Gerson had cured himself by devising a diet very high in fresh fruits and vegetables and very low in fats. He then prescribed his diet for migraine sufferers who came to him as patients. Their headaches disappeared. Next, using a slightly modified version of his diet, he cured patients with lupus vulgaris, a form of skin tuberculosis then considered incurable.

Gerson's success brought an invitation in 1924 from eminent German surgeon Ferdinand Sauerbruch, M.D., to test Gerson's diet in a lupus clinic at the University of Munich. Over a three-year period, the two doctors treated 450 lupus patients with the diet; 446 of them recovered, according to Sauerbruch in his autobiography *Master Surgeon.* Gerson extended his therapeutic system to other forms of tuberculosis. In 1928, he reluctantly accepted his first cancer patient, at the insistence of the patient—a woman who had undergone unsuccessful surgery for cancer of the bile duct that had spread to the liver. Within six months, the woman seemed fully recovered. Gerson's next two patients, both with inoperable stomach cancer, had the same good results.

After the rise of Hitler forced him to leave Germany, Gerson lived in Vienna and Paris, moving to the United States in 1936. He got his New York medical license in 1938 and was soon attracting more and more cancer patients, obtaining remissions even in far-advanced cases.

In 1946, Gerson testified before a Senate subcommittee along with five of his patients, all of whom had recovered from advanced cancer. One of the five was fourteen-year-old Alice Hirsch, whose orthodox doctors had predicted would be paralyzed by the end of 1945 due to an inoperable spinal cord tumor that would quickly kill her. Also testifying was George Miley, M.D., professor of medicine and medical director of Gotham Hospital, where Gerson was treating patients. Dr. Miley called the Gerson therapy "a highly encouraging approach." He presented the committee with signed statements from five other doctors who said that they had observed advanced cancer reversed by the Gerson regime.

After Gerson's congressional appearance, his anticancer diet surged in credibility and prestige. But it was just at this time that chemotherapy was seeking public acceptance, soon to become a gigantic money-making operation for the medical-pharmaceutical industry. Within five months of Gerson's Senate hearing, the American Medical Association launched a vehement campaign intended to discredit his therapy. Gerson was attacked in the pages of *JAMA*, the association's prestigious journal, for treating cancer patients with diet and for warning against cigarettes. In the same issues, *JAMA* ran ad copy in praise of cigarettes: "Many leading nose and throat specialists suggest, 'Change to Philip Morris,'" read a typical ad. Cigarette maker Philip Morris was the main source of advertising dollars for *JAMA* during the years of its assault on Max Gerson. The marriage of medicine and the tobacco industry, which helped addict hundreds of thousands to cancer-causing cigarettes, was "one of the most outrageous alliances in the history of medicine," says Gar Hildenbrand of the Gerson Institute.

Dr. Gerson's medical privileges at Gotham Hospital were revoked, and he was unable to secure an affiliation with any other hospital. In 1953, he was denied malpractice insurance because his therapy was not "accepted practice." Refusing to give up, he opened a sanatorium of his own. However, laboratories used by Dr. Gerson were threatened with economic ruin if they continued to provide services to him. In 1958, the New York Medical Society suspended him for "advertising." He died a year later.

A modified version of the Gerson therapy was tested, beginning in 1984, by Dr. Peter Lechner at the Krankenhaus in Graz, Austria. Lechner's program excluded niacin and liver juice and used thyroid supplements only in hypothyroid patients. In addition, it limited coffee enemas to two per day because the four enemas per day originally recommended by Gerson led to colitis (inflammation of the large intestine) in three patients at the very beginning of the project.

Lechner's study involved sixty post-operative cancer patients using this modified Gerson regimen as an adjunct, often with chemotherapy or radiation, over a four-year period. In several forms of cancer, the Gerson-derived therapy made an impressive difference in comparison to a control group of sixty cancer patients who chose not to try it. For example, breast cancer patients with liver metastases who received the Gerson-based treatment tolerated chemotherapy better, and one of three was reported in a steady state for more than a year. (The remaining five patients died.) Patients with brain metastases on the modified Gerson treatment experienced decreased edema and lived four months longer than their counterparts in the control group.[7]

In a highly suggestive 1988 study of cancer patients who underwent so-called spontaneous regressions, Harold Foster, Ph.D., of the University of Victoria, British Columbia, presented data on 200 recovered patients who had used various alternative treatments, including the Gerson therapy, Hoxsey's herbs, Kelley dietary approach, macrobiotics, Moerman diet, and Jason Winters Herbal Tea.[8] Over half of the group had used some form of detoxification, such as coffee enemas, castor-oil enemas, saunas, colonics, or fasting. In addition, 88 percent of the patients had made major dietary changes, usually switching to a strictly vegetarian diet. A total of 65 percent of the patients had taken mineral supplements, potassium and iodine being by far the most frequently used. Niacin, digestive enzymes, bioflavonoids, red clover, and vitamins A, B_{12}, and C were also taken frequently.

Foster noted that the "spontaneous" cancer regressions "tended to occur most frequently in vegetarian non-smokers, who did not use table salt, white flour, or sugar and who avoided canned, smoked, or frozen foods. Typically such individuals eschewed alcoholic beverages, tea, coffee, and cocoa, but instead drank freshly pressed fruit and/or vegetable juices. Many took vitamin and mineral supplements together with various herbs. The time spent by patients eating such special diets varied from one month to 15 years, the median time period being 41 months."

Foster pointed out that "there is really no such process as spontaneous regression" since there must always be a cause for the regression. The data, in his judgment, support the view that many dramatic remissions occurred "in association with major dietary changes, which must inevitably have resulted in alterations in the availability of bulk and trace elements to both the immune system and to tumors."

The Gerson therapy is heavily represented in the summary of cancer patients "who exceeded their anticipated lengths of survival by at least a factor of ten." In this group were persons who followed the Gerson protocol and recovered from brain tumors, lymphosarcoma, basal cell carcinoma, kidney sarcoma, spreading melanosarcoma, breast cancer, spinal cord tumor, metastasized testicular cancer, and cancer of the pituitary gland. Recovered Gerson patients were represented in nearly every category of cancer mentioned in the study. In summary, Foster concluded that "the potential role of diet in the treatment of cancer appears to merit far greater attention than it is currently receiving."

Resources

Gerson Institute
P.O. Box 430
Bonita, CA 91908
Phone: 619-472-7450

For further information on Gerson therapy, details on treatment, and books, audiocassettes, and videotapes.

Centro Hospitalario Internationale del Pacifico, S.A.
Playas, Tijuana
Mexico

For further information on Gerson therapy and details on treatment.

Reading Material

A Cancer Therapy: Results of Fifty Cases, by Max Gerson, M.D., Gerson Institute (see above for address and phone number), fifth edition, 1990.

Cancer? Think Curable! The Gerson Therapy, by S. J. Haught, Gerson Institute (see above for address and phone number), 1983.

Cancer: A Healing Crisis, by Jack Tropp, Exposition Press (New York), 1980. Out of print; check your local library.

My Triumph Over Cancer, by Beata Bishop, Keats Publishing (27 Pine Street, New Canaan, CT 06840; 203-966-8721), 1986.

Gary Null's Complete Guide to Healing Your Body Naturally, by Gary Null (see Appendix A for description).

The Cancer Survivors and How They Did It, by Judith Glassman (see Appendix A for description).

Special Gerson therapy issue, *Cancer Control Journal,* vol. 3, no. 1–2, 1975.

Healing Newsletter, published by the Gerson Institute (see page 202 for address and phone number). Semi-monthly magazine.

Chapter 18

KELLEY'S NUTRITIONAL-METABOLIC THERAPY

Over a twenty-five year period, Dr. William Donald Kelley, a dentist by training, developed a complex approach to treating many chronic and degenerative diseases, including cancer. The three main elements of his metabolic program are nutrition, detoxification, and supplements of pancreatic enzymes. Although the controversial Kansas-born practitioner was condemned as a charlatan by the orthodox medical establishment, thousands of severely ill patients sought his advice and followed his program, many with reported good results. Today, a number of practitioners claim to be using the Kelley regimen, though whether they actually are is open to question.

Interest in Kelley's therapy has increased dramatically in recent years, largely due to the work of Nicholas Gonzalez, a New York City physician who treats cancer patients in advanced or terminal stages using a modified version of the Kelley program. A graduate of Cornell University Medical School, Dr. Gonzalez undertook a five-year case study of Kelley's own cancer patients who had done well on the program.[1] Gonzalez's 500-page study was prepared under the sponsorship of Robert Good, M.D., Ph.D., then president of Memorial Sloan-Kettering Cancer Center. It is "widely regarded as the finest case review ever conducted concerning an alternative cancer therapy," according to *Misinformation From OTA on Unconventional Cancer Treatments,* by Robert G. Houston.[2]

"Gonzalez has given us convincing evidence that diet and nutrition produce long-term remission in cancer patients almost all of whom were beyond conventional help," wrote the late Harold Ladas, Ph.D., a biologist and former professor at Hunter College. "Because the cases [in Gonzalez's study] represent a wide variety of cancers, the implication is that the paradigm has wide applicability to cancer treatment. . . . What should happen is that ACS or NCI should immediately follow up with a half million dollar study to evaluate the rest of Kelley's cancer patients. But don't hold your breath," added Ladas, who concluded, "The evidence is in, and it is stunning. Kelley is vindicated."[3] Dr. Gonzalez's findings on Kelley's patients are discussed later in this chapter.

William Kelley held that a root cause of cancer is the body's inability to metabolize (digest and utilize) protein. "The person gets cancer because he's not properly metabolizing the protein in his diet," said Dr. Kelley. "Then, to make matters worse, the tumor has such a high metabolism that it uses up much of the food which is eaten." If a person's disordered protein metabolism is not corrected, Kelley continued, "it will give rise to more tumors in the future, even if the first one is successfully removed. This, by the way, is the unfortunate reason why so many seemingly successful cancer operations end up in recurrences a year or two later. The tumor was removed, but the cause—improper protein metabolism—remained."[4]

Dr. Kelley linked faulty metabolism to a deficiency of pancreatic enzymes, which he regarded as a fundamental cause of cancer. He believed that certain pancreatic enzymes, especially those that are proteolytic (protein-digesting) enzymes, are the body's first line of defense against malignancy. This theory stands in marked contrast to conventional medicine, which holds that the immune system, with its natural killer cells, protects people against cancer.

As every biology student learns, the pancreas releases enzymes directly into the small intestine to aid digestion. But Kelley maintained that the pancreas also secretes enzymes into the bloodstream, where they circulate, reaching all body tissues and killing cancer cells by digesting them. Studies in the clinical literature lend support to this theory, first proposed by Dr. John Beard, a Scottish embryologist working at the turn of the century.[5]

Imbalance of mineral metabolism is another condition that allows malignancy to occur, according to Dr. Kelley. He identified mineral imbalance as a root cause of the breakdown of the immune system. Additionally, he said, cancer cells produce immune-blocking factors and seem to generate an electromagnetic force field that inhibits the proper response of the immune system.

The Kelley anticancer program combines therapeutic nutrition, supplements intended to destroy cancer cells, and vigorous detoxification of the body. Kelley divided people into what he called ten metabolic types, with slow-oxidizing vegetarians at one extreme and fast-oxidizing carnivores at the other. Each person is different, he asserted, not only in nutritional needs but also in food utilization.

For each of the ten different metabolic types, a different nutritional program was recommended. An individualized diet was tailored to match the metabolic character of each patient, taking into account his or her physiology, neurological and physical make-up, basic metabolic rate, and personality. Some common threads ran through the diets, however. The consumption of raw, organic fruits and vegetables was emphasized, while protein intake was reduced considerably in order to preserve the enzymes needed to digest the fruits and vegetables.

In addition to following a diet, Kelley's patients also took up to 150 supplement pills per day, including pancreatic enzymes, vitamins and minerals, and concentrates of raw beef or organs and glands believed by Kelley to contain tissue-specific growth factors, hormones, natural stimulants, and "protective" molecules.

A direct antitumor effect has been observed repeatedly in patients on various metabolic therapies who receive enzymes either orally or by injection. As the enzyme "digests" the tumor, large amounts of cellular debris are released into the bloodstream and surrounding tissues, according to Kelley. These breakdown products from cancer cells are foreign to the normal body and can be very toxic, he maintained. Even though the liver and kidney can filter these substances out of the bloodstream, the wastes from tumor destruction form so quickly during enzyme therapy that the body's normal detoxification processes may become overloaded.

To assist their bodies in detoxification, Kelley's patients periodically discontinued their enzymes and other supplements for several days. This rest period, Kelley believed, allows the liver and kidneys to catch up with the body's load of tumor by-products. As a second aid in detoxification, Kelley advised all his patients to take at least one coffee enema daily. His reasoning was that coffee enemas clean out the liver and gallbladder and help the body get rid of the toxins produced during tumor breakdown.

During a coffee enema, claimed Kelley, the caffeine that is rapidly absorbed in the large intestine flows quickly into the liver. He held that in high enough concentrations, caffeine causes the liver and gallbladder to contract vigorously, releasing large amounts of stored wastes into the intestinal tract and greatly aiding elimination. Kelley also believed that enemas are important in stimulating the immune system, since most waste products eliminated by detoxification are enzyme inhibitors. Frequent enemas prevent the suppression of protein-digesting enzymes. These enzymes can break down the cancer cells' fibrin (protein) coats, making the cancer cells more vulnerable to the immune system.

Nonorthodox doctors other than Kelley, among them Dr. Max Gerson (Chapter 17), have recommended coffee enemas.

The original Kelley program also included purges to cleanse the liver, gallbladder, intestines, kidneys, and lungs. Like many other metabolic therapists, Kelley believed that the functioning of these organs is severely impaired in the cancer patient. Colonic irrigations, liver and gallbladder flushes, and controlled sweating accomplished the cleansing tasks. Kelley also often recommended some form of manipulative therapy, such as chiropractic adjustment or osteopathic manipulation, to stimulate enervated nerves.

A frequently overlooked aspect of the Kelley system is its spiritual component. Kelley called his approach metabolic ecology, taking into account the cancer patient's total environment—physical, mental, emotional, and spiritual. He urged the patient to "accept the fact that you are afflicted with a symptom (malignant cancer) and that recovery is possible. Establish a faith in a power greater than yourself and know that with His help you can regain health and harmony."[6] Patients were encouraged to conduct a searching self-analysis and to eliminate negative behavioral patterns and emotions.

The rigorous Kelley regimen is not easy. It requires self-discipline and a strong will to alter established dietary and other habits. Some patients experience fear and anxiety during "healing crises" involving lymph-system swelling, pain, and fever, all normal responses as the body detoxifies and heals. Critics of the system are deeply troubled by the enormous number of pills the patient is required to consume. Orthodox medicine holds that megadoses of vitamins and minerals are unnecessary and can be harmful. Excessive amounts of the fat-soluble vitamins (A, D, E, and K) are stored in the body and can be toxic, according to mainstream physicians.

But Kelley proponents counter that the nutritional program supplies various aids to the digestive system enabling the large doses of supplements to be absorbed and fully utilized. These digestive aids include hydrochloric acid, said to be abnormally low in many people, lessening their ability to digest proteins. Kelley also prescribed a combination of the herb comfrey and the digestive enzyme pepsin. These supplements dissolve the mucous coatings that cover the villi (the fingerlike projections) of the small intestine and block the absorption of nutrients.

Kelley's theory that people are genetically carnivorous, vegetarian, or somewhere in-between is rejected by many vegetarians and by others.

Some prospective patients were put off by the idea of frequent enemas, although Kelley claimed that most of his patients quickly adapted to this procedure. In fact, many patients on metabolic-therapy programs have reported a dramatic increase in energy and improved outlook after a coffee enema, presumably because of the elimination of toxins from the bloodstream, cells, and liver. The procedure appears to calm and soothe the nervous system, dispelling nausea, irritability, lethargy, lack of appetite, and sometimes even severe pain.

Pat Judson, a woman from Dearborn, Michigan, became Dr. Kelley's patient in 1972, having been operated on for cancer of the colon two years earlier. She is now in excellent health and completely cancer-free after her original diagnosis of "incurable" cancer. As she told a Michigan State Legislature committee investigating alternative cancer treatments in 1977, "I speak as . . . a cancer patient who seven years ago was sent home to die by a doctor who told me there was nothing more traditional medicine could do for me. . . . One of the doctors that performed my surgery told me that I had the fastest-growing type known to man and cobalt or chemotherapy would not help me. Expressing surprise that I even survived the surgery, he told me I had six months to a year to live. However, I was given diethyl-stilbestrol [DES] for hormone balance since they had also removed my ovaries. I have wondered many times why a medical doctor would prescribe a cancer-producing drug to a cancer patient."[7]

In January 1972, almost two years after the original surgery, Pat had a recurrence of the blockage of her colon, and the cancer had metastasized to the lymph glands. Reluctant to go through the ordeal of surgery a second time, she turned to a different doctor, who advised her that she might survive "possibly three months" with surgery. At that point, she heard of the nutritional therapy of Dr. Kelley and went to visit him in Texas.

After taking a blood sample and conducting diagnostic tests that were subjected to computer analysis, Kelley determined that Pat had a cancer index of 600. This scale was devised by Kelley to gauge the body's ability to defend itself; it runs from an optimal 1 (normal) to 1,000 (terminal, beyond help). Following these tests, Kelley prescribed a combination of diet, rest, exercise, and detoxification.

When Pat Judson returned to Kelley's office five months later for a checkup, her index rating had dropped to 300 and her cancer was under control. Eleven months after the initial visit, a shrivelled mass of excreted material was found to be necrotic, or dead, tissue from the colon tumor. Pat's next cancer-index reading with Kelley was 50, which is within the normal range. Standard diagnostic tests subsequently confirmed her to be in remission.

During Pat's first operation in 1970, her surgeon had noticed a lump in her throat that she had had since girlhood. He said it might have been a "leader" for the cancer. As Pat continued on a Kelley maintenance protocol after being diagnosed in remission, she also took Essiac (Chapter 10), the Canadian herbal tea that has helped many cancer patients. By 1978, the lump in Pat's throat was completely gone, and it has never returned. (*Note:* Some practitioners strongly advise against combining the Kelley program with Essiac or any other herbal remedy. They contend that the herbs work against the enzyme supplements.)

Pat Judson served as president of the Metro-Detroit chapter of the Foundation for Advancement in Cancer Therapy (FACT), in which capacity she told a Michigan State Legislature committee, "If I had accepted the advice of my doctor, if I had not been directed to Dr. Kelley, I would be another cancer statistic." In her speech, she also rebuked the medical establishment for its constant harassment of Dr. Kelley.

Kelley's problems with the medical orthodoxy intensified in 1969, when he self-published his book *One Answer to Cancer*, which became a best-seller in the "nutritional underground." The dietary program presented in the book was a distillation of his personal battle against illness. In 1964, according to Kelley, he was told by a doctor that he had metastasized pancreatic cancer, one of the deadliest forms of the disease, and that he had only weeks to live. There is no biopsy verification for his cancer. His internist recommended surgery, but the surgeon felt Kelley wouldn't survive the operation.

With nothing to lose, Kelley, who holds a Doctorate of Dental Surgery (D.D.S.) from Baylor University in Dallas and has an extensive background in nutrition, began his own impromptu course of nutritional therapy and lifestyle changes. As he gradually recovered, he felt he had stumbled across a scientific discovery and undertook further research to refine his program.

As *One Answer to Cancer* soared in popularity, Texas medical and legal officials launched an investigation of its author in 1969. Undercover officials posed as patients. A restraining order prohibited Kelley from treating nondental disease, and a local district court made it illegal for him to distribute *One Answer to Cancer* or any other publication discussing his approach to degenerative illness. Dr. Kelley appealed the decision to the United States Supreme Court, arguing that the restraining order was a flagrant violation of his First Amendment rights. But the Supreme Court upheld the ruling. "To my knowledge, Dr. Kelley remains the only scientist in this country's history ever forbidden by court decree from publishing," notes Dr. Gonzalez.

In 1971, the American Cancer Society put Kelley's therapy on its Unproven Methods blacklist, where it remains. To this day, no ACS scientist has ever attempted a direct, objective evaluation of Kelley's methods and results.

After the Texas dental board suspended his license for five years in 1976, Kelley moved to Winthrop, Washington, where he continued his nutritional practice. He later moved to Pennsylvania.

Kelley's most highly publicized encounter with the medical establishment began in 1980, when he agreed to treat actor Steve McQueen, suffering from advanced mesothelioma, a rare, nearly always fatal form of lung cancer. McQueen's malignancy was too extensive for surgery, and his terminal condition was completely hopeless. Nevertheless, on Kelley's advice, McQueen entered a small Mexican hospital where doctors claimed to use the Kelley program. McQueen never followed the full Kelley protocol; he smoked and smuggled junk food into his room. Even so, after eight weeks on a partial Kelley regimen, his tumor had stopped growing, he no longer felt a need for painkillers, and he had put on weight. His doctors expressed some cause for optimism. However, McQueen eventually discontinued the program. He died in November 1980, just hours after undergoing surgery to remove an apparently dead tumor mass in his abdomen.

The ensuing publicity triggered a media assault on Kelley organized by the American medical community. Spokesmen for the ACS, NCI, and leading medical schools condemned Kelley and his methods vociferously, without ever bothering to examine the details of McQueen's treatment.

Kelley claimed a high success rate with patients on his therapy. For those with a predicted life expectancy of about three months, he said that a well-designed nutritional program would yield "slightly better than a 50–50 chance of survival." For those with a very advanced disease, given less than three months to live, he claimed a success rate between 25 and 35 percent. These figures have not been verified and should be treated with caution. Yet according to Ruth Sackman, executive director of FACT, an educational organization that leans toward a nutritional-metabolic approach, "Enough of Kelley's patients lived ten years or more to suggest a pattern of survival and to indicate that he was using a basically sound system."

In Kelley's elaborate system of diagnosis and treatment, patients answered a detailed questionnaire, a nutritional survey consisting of up to 3,200 questions. The results were assessed by computer, and each patient was then fitted into Kelley's classification system of metabolic typing, which he used in treating a wide variety of diseases.

To understand Kelley's metabolic typing system, let us quickly review the ABCs of metabolism. The human body has two nervous systems. The *central nervous system* regulates conscious movement, and the *autonomic nervous system* (*ANS*) governs unconscious actions such as digestion, the secretion of enzymes and hormones, breathing, blood circulation, and heartbeat. The ANS plays a key role in the way cells transform food into energy.

There are two branches of the ANS—the *sympathetic system,* which tends to speed up body metabolism, and the *parasympathetic system,* which slows down metabolism. Kelley's thesis is that people can be divided into three genetically based categories that evolved in distinctive environments under evolutionary pressure. Each metabolic type reflects an inborn balance in the activities of these two subsystems.

According to Kelley, people who are slow-oxidizing "sympathetic dominant" types thrive on high-carbohydrate, low-protein foods and are meant to eat a largely vegetarian diet. Fast-oxidizing "parasympathetic dominants" grow hungry and weak between meals, so Kelley suggested that they follow a diet providing at least half of their total calories from fatty meat. "Balanced types," having both branches of the autonomic nervous system equally developed, were said to thrive on a wide variety of foods.

If a person follows the "wrong" diet, in Kelley's theory, disease is more likely to develop. For each of the three basic types (broken down into ten metabolic subtypes), he recommended a diet that would push the autonomic nervous system toward metabolic equilibrium. Furthermore, he linked specific syndromes and illnesses with each of the three types. "Hard tumors"—malignancies of the internal organs such as lung or colon cancer—were held to be more likely to afflict severely imbalanced "sympathetic dominants." "Soft tumors"—cancers of the white blood cells and lymph system—were linked with "parasympathetic dominants."

Dr. Nicholas Gonzalez, the New York City physician mentioned at the beginning of this chapter who uses a modified Kelley program, visited Dr. Kelley in Texas in 1981 and was given access to all of Kelley's records. Gonzalez was amazed to discover case after case of patients with advanced metastatic cancer who were healthy and active five, ten, and fifteen years after diagnosis.

Gonzalez interviewed 455 Kelley patients in depth, then narrowed down the group to 160 after eliminating the patients whom he considered inadequately diagnosed, others who had received intensive orthodox therapy, others who had been apparently "cured of their disease before they consulted Dr. Kelley," and still others who did not meet the selection criteria. Eventually, Gonzalez selected 50 patients whom he considered representative cases rather than Kelley's best cases.

These 50 patients represented a broad spectrum of cancer types, including long-term survivors of cancer of the breast, colon, ovaries, pancreas, and prostate. According to Gonzalez's findings:

> . . . 22 of the patients . . . experienced *documented* regression of cancer while pursuing the Kelley program. None in this group received orthodox therapy during this period of improvement. . . . Another 5 patients described regression of superficial, biopsy-proven malignancies, such as breast tumors or cancerous lymph nodes . . . [but] never returned to their orthodox physicians for follow-up studies.
>
> . . . six patients were found at surgery to have extensive inoperable abdominal or pelvic disease, such as metastatic pancreatic or prostate carcinoma. All these patients were given terminal prognoses. None have ever returned to their orthodox physicians, so strictly speaking I have no proof of tumor regression . . . [although] each of these people has survived for years with cancer that usually kills within months.[8]

Pancreatic cancer is one of the deadliest forms of the disease; the five-year survival rate in orthodox medicine is essentially 0 percent. Dr. Gonzalez reviewed the records of all 22 patients whom Kelley had diagnosed with pancreatic cancer between 1974 and 1982. Five of these 22 patients followed the Kelley program completely. Their median survival (at the time of Gonzalez's study in 1987) was nine years, and 4 of the 5 are alive today; one died of Alzheimer's disease. This is a 100 percent remission rate for those who adhered to the full Kelley regimen. (The 10 patients with pancreatic cancer who never followed the treatment had a median survival time of 67 days. Seven who partially followed the program had a median survival time of 233 days.)

These reported results are virtually unheard-of in conventional treatment. Orthodox medicine gives a median survival time of two to six months for pancreatic cancer.

One of Kelley's patients whom Gonzalez investigated was Robert Dunn, a sixty-two-year-old man from Missouri diagnosed with inoperable pancreatic cancer in June 1977. The formal diagnosis, as it appears in the medical records, reads, "Carcinoma of the pancreas—unresectable, incurable." Although his traditional physician recommended both chemotherapy and radiation, Dunn was told he would probably not live a year even with aggressive treatment. Refusing both options, he took a brief course of laetrile in Mexico, then consulted Dr. Kelley and, in August 1977, began the full Kelley protocol.

Within a year, Dunn said, he felt better than at any other time in his life. A follow-up CAT scan indicated that the once-large pancreatic tumor had completely regressed. Exploratory surgery in 1983 to remove a small bowel obstruction further confirmed that the tumor was gone. When last contacted by Dr. Gonzalez more then ten years after his original diagnosis, Dunn was following a maintenance protocol and was in excellent health.

Dr. Gonzalez treats advanced cancer patients with a Kelley-derived program. He keeps careful records of his own patients and also monitors many of Kelley's patients who have survived ten years or more. He claims that approximately 80 percent of his patients are doing well on his therapy. Most of his patients have already been heavily treated with surgery, radiation, or chemotherapy and, having failed these modalities, come to him with a prognosis of two to three months to live.

In May 1985, doctors removed roughly ten pounds of tumor from Bonnie Randolph, a clinical psychologist from Bala Cynwyd, Pennsylvania. They also performed a total hysterectomy. Bonnie's ovarian cancer had grown silently for eight years, according to the doctors, and had spread to her abdominal organs. The survival rates in such cases are less than 20 percent.

Over the next year, Bonnie underwent eight courses of chemotherapy and two more major operations, all of which failed to eradicate the cancer. By the fourth chemotherapy treatment, her bone marrow was suppressed to such an extent that her white blood count had plunged from a normal of 4,000 to less than 100. After the second major surgery, in March 1986, her doctor injected a massive dose of radioactive phosphorus into her abdomen, "which he said would be my quota of radiation for the rest of my life," according to Bonnie. Six ovarian cancer specialists then told her that despite the radiation treatment, she had a year to live at the most.

Bonnie, who tells her remarkable, moving story in the November

1991 issue of *East West*, began investigating alternative therapies through a cancer referral service. "I had known there were cancer survivors who had beaten the odds by using nontraditional forms of treatment. What I did not know was that there were so many of them—and that they were doing so well." She became a patient of William Kelley, and her CA 125—a standard medical test for ovarian cancer—dropped from 29 to 11. (A reading above 35 indicates tumor growth.) Her pelvic exams were negative. But Dr. Kelley abruptly moved away into semiretirement. A few months later, the ovarian cancer returned.

Her conventional doctor insisted that Bonnie undergo radiation once more, even though it would not save her life. When Bonnie refused to submit her body to more damage from radiation therapy, her doctor became incensed. "'You'll be dead in two months,' he yelled at me over the phone."

For two months, Bonnie followed a strict nutritional program, which she believes kept her alive, while searching for a responsible alternative practitioner. In January 1988, she began the Kelley-derived program with Dr. Gonzalez in New York. "He warned me that it could be years before I became completely well again because of all the damage the chemo and radiation had done to my immune system," she says. Under Dr. Gonzalez's supervision, Bonnie followed an organic vegetarian diet (one of the ten diets prescribed) and took massive doses of pancreatic enzymes, nutritional supplements, and coffee enemas.

Today, more than six years after her initial diagnosis, Bonnie is alive, free of pain, and writing a book about her experience. Her last three Pap smears were normal. Although she still has evidence of cancer and works hard to maintain good health, she keeps the cancer under control with a maintenance protocol of pancreatic enzymes, supplements, and sound nutrition and hopes to achieve complete remission. "The Gonzalez regimen requires discipline," Bonnie reflects, "but this is a small price to pay for having the chance to live out my life. And implementing the program is in my hands, so I feel that I am in command of my health care."

In a review of the Gonzalez study published in a leading insurance-industry journal, Robert Maver, vice president and research director of Mutual Benefit Life, stated, "The Research Division has been evaluating Dr. Gonzalez' results over the last four months, including numerous site visits. . . . The results are indeed extraordinary." He added, "This is a prime example of an innovative therapy that merits evaluation, but is being ignored. As costly as cancer is to our industry, and in light of such promising and cost-effective preliminary results, our industry should consider funding such a trial."[9]

Resources

Nicholas Gonzalez, M.D.
737 Park Avenue
New York, NY 10021
Phone: 212-535-3993

For further information on the modified Kelley therapy and details on treatment.

Reading Material

Dr. Kelley's Answer to Cancer (combining *One Answer to Cancer*, by Donald Kelley, and *Metabolic Ecology*, by Fred Rohe), Wedgestone Press (Winthrop, Washington), 1986. Out of print; check your local library.

The New Approach to Cancer, by Cameron Stauth, English Brothers Press (New York), 1982. Out of print; available from the Cancer Control Society (see page xv for address and phone number). Contains a good deal of information on metabolic therapies and the case histories of twenty cancer survivors who followed a Kelley-type program.

One Man Alone: An Investigation of Nutrition, Cancer, and William Donald Kelley, written and distributed by Nicholas James Gonzalez, M.D. (see above for address and phone number), 1987. Unpublished manuscript. Includes a biographical profile of Kelley, a detailed explanation of his system, and an analysis of fifty case histories documented with hospital and patient records.

Cancer Forum. Back issues of this magazine have numerous articles and case histories.

Chapter 19

HANS NIEPER, M.D.

One of the most prominent practitioners of unconventional cancer therapy in Europe, Hans Nieper, M.D., of Hanover, Germany, has developed a complex metabolic-nutritional therapy. Its multifaceted components include correction of mineral imbalances in the body, use of "deshielding" enzymes to dissolve the mucous layer that often surrounds tumor cells, and "gene-repair therapy" with natural substances, said to reprogram incorrect genetic information in the cancer cell.

Dr. Nieper calls his approach *eumetabolic therapy,* a term he coined to refer to the use of a variety of substances that work as a natural partner with the human metabolism in healing the body and keeping it healthy. He prescribes varying combinations of vitamins, minerals, laetrile, animal and plant extracts, pharmaceutical drugs, and vaccines such as BCG (bacillus Calmette-Guérin), a weakened strain of tuberculin bacillus that stimulates natural immune defense mechanisms and slows tumor growth. Patients may receive low-dose chemotherapy and radiation, in combination with other methods, to kill or impair tumor cells directly. Dr. Nieper's program includes an essentially vegetarian diet emphasizing whole-grain cereals, vegetables and fruits, skim milk, and juices, especially carrot juice. Meat, sausage, and shellfish are strictly avoided; refined sugar, white bread, cheese, and alcohol are drastically limited.

Nieper, who received his Doctorate of Medicine from the University of Hamburg, specializes in the treatment of cancer, multiple sclerosis, and heart disease, and treats many other conditions as well. He practices in a modern facility, the Silbersee Hospital in Hanover, and also maintains an outpatient practice. His wide-ranging interests extend from the causation of cancer to theoretical physics. A hobbyist in gravity theories, he is active in the emerging field of free-energy physics, which attempts to harness the energy-rich gravitational field of space by converting it directly into electrical current.

Dr. Nieper claims that 45 to 48 percent of his outpatients, mobile but diagnosed as incurable by orthodox medicine, have their cancer brought under control within eighteen months on his program. For "incurables" who are so ill that they require hospitalization when they see him, he says the disease is brought under control within eighteen months in roughly 20 percent of cases. Once people have survived about eighteen months on eumetabolic therapy, he maintains, their life expectancy tends to become normal. He calls this eighteen-month survival pattern a quasi-cure rate. In cancer patients who are in very early stages of the disease but still at risk, Dr. Nieper reports that long-term eumetabolic therapy achieves a quasi-cure in 75 to 80 percent of patients. But, he cautions, these figures should be regarded "only as pointers."

Opinions differ sharply about Nieper's program and its alleged effectiveness. Some critics from within the alternative cancer field charge that he uses toxic chemotherapy routinely or indiscriminately. They contend that he spends precious little time with patients and does no systematic follow-up. Detractors portray him as a charismatic, often abrupt doctor whose methods are improvisational and whose ideas change so rapidly that it is difficult to keep abreast of his current mode of practice.

But to his admirers, Dr. Nieper is a brilliant clinician, a medical genius who speaks five languages and assimilates the latest research on cancer from around the world, applying the knowledge in his own innovative practice. They describe him as a caring, insightful physician, the most advanced practitioner of an integrated metabolic-nutritional cancer therapy in the world today. Persons who are contemplating a trip to Germany to see Dr. Nieper might do well to talk to his patients, both current and former; names and phone numbers can be found in the Cancer Control Society's listing of patients treated with various alternative therapies. They should also contact the patient referral and information services discussed in "Guidelines for Choosing a Therapy," page xi, for help in forming a balanced opinion.

In 1985, Katherine Mayer of Sherman Oaks, California, was diagnosed with advanced multiple myeloma, a rapidly spreading bone cancer characterized by extensive bone destruction and multiple fractures. Katherine, then age sixty-five and down to seventy-nine pounds in weight, was told that orthodox medicine held out no hope for her after doctors in Switzerland performed the standard diagnostic tests, including electrophoresis, bone marrow aspiration for biopsy, and a myelogram, in which dye is injected into the fluid around the spinal cord and followed by an X-ray. The survival time for patients with multiple myeloma is roughly two years from the time of diagnosis.

Katherine returned to California with her husband, Lou, and consulted a physician who urged her to undergo palliative chemotherapy. She refused, saying, "If I'm going to die, let me do it the right way." She had already purchased a crypt when she attended the Cancer Control Society's annual convention in Los Angeles in 1986 at the insistence of her husband, who hoped they might learn of some alternative therapy that might help. There she heard about Dr. Nieper.

In August 1986, the Mayers flew to Germany, and Katherine, barely able to walk, went to the Silbersee Hospital without an appointment. Dr. Nieper put her on a program combining a strict diet and medication, including calcium and magnesium *mineral transporters*, laetrile, liver extract, and various minerals and enzymes. "Nieper takes a blood sample and X-rays," she recalls, "then he takes home the tests and studies them at night. The next day when you come in, he tells you what to do and prescribes medicine. During the two weeks that I was in Germany on my first visit, I felt that he had figured out exactly what was wrong with me. He is not really abrupt or rude, he's just hard-pressed for time. I would rather be treated by a brilliant doctor like him than to go to an American doctor with a pleasant bedside manner whose mind is closed to new ideas or discoveries in medicine that could save a patient's life."

One of the medications Katherine received was calcium orotate, a substance developed by Dr. Nieper between 1958 and 1960 while he was a research fellow at the Paul Ehrlich Institute in Frankfurt. Used routinely on patients since 1964, calcium orotate helps to recalcify bone metastases in persons with cancer. It is one of a class of substances known as *mineral transporters,* which carry minerals to specific sites within a cell by means of active transport. Calcium orotate contains calcium and orotic acid, which forms a complex salt with any mineral. Calcium orotate penetrates the cell's outer membrane and is metabolized only at the site of the mitochondria and at structures found in the cell plasma. Only here is the calcium released. Different mineral transporters go to different structures inside the cell.

Virtually unknown in the mainstream American medical community, calcium orotate is legally available in Germany. It is widely utilized in the treatment of lupus, multiple sclerosis, and amyotrophic lateral sclerosis (Lou Gehrig's disease). The use of this mineral transporter in combination with other substances brings success in about 40 percent of all cases of metastatic disease of the bones, with recalcification of lesions and no side effects, reports Dr. Nieper.

Another mineral transporter that Dr. Nieper prescribed for Katherine, calcium–2-AEP, was also developed by him between 1958 and 1960. The transporting half of this compound is the 2-AEP, colamine phosphate (2-aminoethanol phosphate), one of the body's natural substances. Dr. Nieper believes that 2-AEP is a cell-membrane protector, perhaps the prime mechanism our bodies have to prevent our immune-system defenses from turning against some element of our bodies. This self-destructive warfare occurs in autoimmune disorders, leading to chronic degenerative disease, the body's cell-by-cell destruction of itself.

The compound 2-AEP is a basic component of the cell membrane, as proven in the 1950s by the eminent American biochemist Erwin Chargaff. According to Dr. Nieper, in people with autoimmune disorders, especially multiple sclerosis, the body does not produce enough 2-AEP, as shown by its deficiency in the blood and urine. When calcium, magnesium, or potassium are attached to colamine phosphate (2-AEP), this mineral transporter goes to the outer layer of the cell membrane, where it releases the mineral and, at the same time, protects the cell.

When Dr. Nieper prescribed shark-liver oil for Katherine, she was taken aback. The doctor explained that sharks almost never get cancer, very much in contrast with other fish, which develop tumors when they swim in polluted waters. Investigations by researchers at the Smithsonian Institution in Washington, D.C., revealed that only 1 malignant tumor was found in about 25,000 sharks. Nieper believes the shark's remarkable cancer-prevention mechanisms include squalene, an oily substance that constitutes 70 percent of shark-liver oil and also 2 percent of olive oil.

According to Nieper, squalene intensifies the "docking" of immune-defensive cells onto cancer cells and may activate the formation of "surveillance steroids," free-floating substances that circulate in the blood and monitor for cancer. He theorizes that squalene exerts these effects due to its ability to "convert space energy into photoelectric energy." In Nieper's controversial and untested theory, a shark obtains a large share of its energy by tapping the "free energy" locked into the space-time flux of the universe, and only a small part from food. Insects likewise get 90 percent of their energy from this "universal energy" rather than from food, he asserts. He claims that many cancer patients have shown marked improvement on squalene. Squalene is only effective with high doses of vitamin C, according to both Nieper and American chemist Linus Pauling, who researched vitamin C. The dosage Nieper generally uses is 1 gram of squalene with 1 gram of vitamin C.

Deep-sea fish, especially sharks, recycle the ocean water's salt back into the sea thanks to taurine and isaethionic acid, agents produced by their livers. Nieper contends that this helps make sharks extremely resistant to cancer formation by eliminating sodium from their cells. Persons suffering from cancer nearly always have an excess of sodium in their blood. Eliminating superfluous sodium from the cancer patient is a primary goal of Nieper's therapy. Nieper believes the substances in shark-liver oil, when ingested by humans, facilitate the process of sodium elimination in cancer cells. For this purpose, he also prescribes substances such as lithium orotate. Toxic side effects are practically nil using dosages of 150 to 450 milligrams per day, he reports. In addition, he says, there is no need for a blood test because lithium orotate is absorbed into cells.

Katherine Mayer was given injections of thymus extract several times a day. The purpose of these shots was to boost her thymus gland's build-up of tumosterone, a steroid occurring in the thymus and in all of the body's lymph cells. "According to the investigations by the biochemist Matter at Hoffman-LaRoche, tumosterone apparently migrates directly into the nucleus of the cancer cell," writes Dr. Nieper.[1] Nieper posits tumosterone as a natural gene-repairing factor that erases the erroneous genetic programming in the cancer cell; this either kills the cancer cell or causes it to revert back to normal. According to Nieper, tumosterone repairs—and prevents—gene defects and also seems to block the tumor cell's ability to fatten itself on cholesterol and other lipids.

Magnesium supplements were also given as part of Katherine's regimen. Magnesium improves the activity of white, granulocytic blood cells and increases the production of immune-defensive substances such as antibodies and complements (factors that activate specific antibodies). Studies have shown that the higher the magnesium intake is—for example, through drinking water—the lower is the cancer incidence.

Katherine also took laetrile, or amygdalin, which Dr. Nieper recommends for many patients and nearly always for those undergoing calcium therapy. "This does not work on all patients having bone lesions for various reasons, but it is an important way to treat these lesions," he observes. Laetrile is found naturally in bitter almonds, apricot pits, and hundreds of other fruit seeds, berries, grains, and vegetables. Nieper says laetrile only works when the body's natural defense mechanisms are operating. He calls the banning of laetrile in the United States "the greatest and most depressing tragic comedy of modern medicine."

After two weeks in Germany, Katherine went home and continued on the Nieper protocol. Soon she could walk again and felt relief from the severe bone pain that accompanies multiple myeloma. "I noticed a definite improvement after six months," she recollects. "When I went back to Germany at the end of the six months, Dr. Nieper did another blood analysis, and tailored my program accordingly. He constantly tailors the program with each visit, and I was able to reduce my pill intake." Gradually, all the lesions along her spine and bones disappeared, followed by the two lesions on her tongue and one on her neck. Her weight bounced back to her normal 108 pounds.

During her recovery, Katherine accidentally fell down and was also in a car accident. "I have very fragile bones to begin with, but there were no fractures at all, only whiplash from the car accident." This is noteworthy since multiple myeloma itself causes bone damage and frequently produces broken ribs, vertebrae, or pelvic bones.

In August 1990, Katherine had a series of diagnostic tests, including blood and urine analyses, performed by a conventional doctor in California. The doctor said that Katherine was completely cancer-free and expressed amazement that she had only five years earlier been at death's door, a hopeless "incurable." Katherine goes back to Nieper for periodic "tune-ups," still follows her largely vegetarian diet (with some fish), and takes twenty different pills per day. Her husband continues to give her thymus-extract injections as a preventive.

To stimulate thymus function, Dr. Nieper often uses zinc and dry beta-carotene. Zinc plays a key role in helping the lymphocytes (white blood cells) attack and destroy cancer cells. Zinc ions act as a "spark plug" to activate the enzymes within lymphocytes that digest cancer cells. "Cancer patients nearly always show a deficit of zinc in their total blood," according to Nieper. Nieper therefore often gives his patients zinc orotate, a mineral carrier that transports zinc across cell membranes and deposits it. This increases the activity and number of T-lymphocytes, especially when a large amount of dry beta-carotene is given at the same time, he says. He maintains that without zinc and beta-carotene, the thymus gland will not "inform" the lymphocytes to fight the cancer cells.

Patients drink carrot juice, rich in beta-carotene, mixed with cream, butter, or margarine. Dr. Nieper feels that beta-carotene is only absorbed from the intestine in the presence of a fatty emulsion. If people take beta-carotene supplements, Nieper believes, the supplements must be in a dry form (capsule or powder) to maintain the beta-carotene's electrical properties. He administers beta-carotene with minute doses of selenium, which, he says, enhances the electrical charges necessary to trigger the thymus gland to produce T-cells for immune defense.

In 1974, Nieper told the second annual convention of the Cancer Control Society, "We run whole blood analyses by the thousands. What is most interesting is that all patients who have malignancies, even in beginning stages and even in small children, have a very much deteriorated mineral picture." Some of these mineral imbalances have already been described.

Another important factor is energy-rich phosphates, which are actually the donor of the energy needed to ensure optimal functioning of the host's defense against disease. The energy extracted from the food we eat is transported to a kind of "battery system," a phosphate system including ATP (adenosine triphosphate). "This battery always has to be charged," says Nieper. To achieve this, he administers substances like potassium and magnesium aspartate, which activate the formation of ATP.

Also a major component of Nieper's cancer therapy is the use of the enzyme bromelain, found in pineapple root, to help remove the protective shield surrounding cancer cells. "The cancer cell itself develops many pretty mean methods to elude the body's defenses," Nieper notes. One such method is a mucous substance that coats the surface of the cancer cell, thus shielding the cell from identification and docking by lymphocytes. To dissolve the mucous sheath, he recommends 600 to 1,200 milligrams of bromelain daily, taken thirty minutes before meals. Beta-carotene from carrots also deshields cancer cells, according to Nieper. "In my opinion, this is the most simple and efficacious therapy in the frame of immune therapy. However, in patients with bone lesions one should be cautious because the resorbed enzyme may inhibit the formation of new bone."

Wong Hon Sun, a naturopathic physician, once contracted cancer but fully recovered with the help of a raw foods diet and bromelain. His return to health is detailed in the book *How I Overcame Inoperable Cancer*.[2] Since bromelain was introduced as a therapeutic agent in 1957, over 200 scientific papers have dealt with its application in enhancing antibiotic absorption, reducing inflammation, preventing ulcers, and other positive effects.

So-called gene-repair mechanisms are central to Dr. Nieper's therapy. Scientists have linked the formation of some cancers to a host of viruses and a virus-like genetic material called an *oncogene*. In 1982, a group of researchers headed by Dr. Francis Dautry of the Massachusetts Institute of Technology reported that abnormalities in a minute portion of just one gene out of thousands—the oncogene—transformed cells grown in the laboratory into a cancerlike state. Oncogenes are found in the cells of cancer patients and promote the cancer process. No one is sure how they get there. Some scientists speculate that oncogenes are pieces of the genetic material of viruses that originally entered the body as an infection. Others think that oncogene pieces may have been inherited from a parent or some other ancestor who first became infected with a virus. Certain factors like geopathogenic stress zones, radiation, carcinogenic chemicals, strong electromagnetic fields, and viruses (for example, HIV, Epstein-Barr, and hepatitis B) are thought to cause oncogenes to become active.

Dr. Nieper employs natural and artificial substances that in his words "seal up" cancer-related genes or "extinguish the information they release." One such substance is the steroid tumosterone, mentioned earlier. In Germany, there are two commercially available preparations for cancer treatment—Resistocell and Ney-Tumorine—which incorporate substances from cell plasma allegedly capable of gene repair. Resistocell, when administered to women after surgery for breast cancer, doubled their survival rate in a study done at the Hanover Medical School.[3]

Valerian plants grown in the Himalaya Mountains contain a substance called didrovaltrate, an organic compound that according to Nieper has a marked gene-repairing effect on cancer cells. In Germany, didrovaltrate is available under the trade name Valmane. "You have to take a lot of this, but this is the first substance which is highly effective in metastasizing kidney cancer which so far was almost untreatable," says Dr. Nieper. By "a lot" he means about twenty 1,000-milligram tablets daily. "To prevent side effects, which are minimal, the patient must increase his intake of table salt."[4]

Insects, much like sharks, are extremely old phylogenetically and highly resistant to viral infections. Cockroaches, beetles, and ants may carry all kinds of viruses and infect humans with them, yet the insects themselves do not get sick from the viruses. "The insects have no immune system at all. . . . Now, how do they do this?" asks Nieper.

The answer is *iridodials,* substances found especially in ants that, he says, repair insects' body systems and may destroy virus genomes (chromosomes). Nieper claims that iridodial preparations obtained from insects "are extremely effective against cancer and viruses, also herpes virus . . . possibly also against AIDS. . . ."[5] Squalene, the oily substance found in shark-liver oil, is a chemical precursor of iridodials, "which very likely serve as gene repair substances," states Nieper.[6]

The Venus flytrap, a swamp plant whose hinged leaves snap shut to trap insects, is another source of a substance used to treat cancer. The pressed juices of this carnivorous plant yield a pharmaceutical agent called Carnivora, available commercially in Germany. It was developed by Helmut Keller, M.D., who in 1990 opened a treatment center for chronic and malignant diseases in Bad Steben, Germany. Since 1981, over 2,000 patients have been treated with Carnivora. Besides slowing the growth of tumor tissue, its reported effects include stimulation of the patient's T-helper cells, which mobilize immune-system defenses, and increased activity of macrophages, white blood cells that ingest and destroy invading microbes and other foreign matter.

Carnivora is used to treat cancer and other immunosuppressive diseases. It has been found to reduce the viability of the HIV virus implicated in AIDS. Persons diagnosed as HIV-positive have been restored to HIV-negative status through Carnivora treatment.[7] Former United States President Ronald Reagan took Carnivora drops for their healing and preventive powers against cancer after his operation for the excision of malignant polyps of the colon. Betty Williams, a retired school teacher from Ames, Iowa, recently was successfully treated with Carnivora by Dr. Keller for inflammatory carcinoma of the breast. She then followed a maintenance protocol of Carnivora intramuscular injections, administered by her husband.[8]

Dr. Nieper, who uses Carnivora in his practice, states that it contains at least six different chinoids that seem to inactivate the information released by unstable or erratic genes, especially oncogenes. Nieper also uses mistletoe extract (Chapter 11) and pau d'arco (Chapter 12) in treating cancer patients.

As for diet, Nieper gives explicit recommendations to cancer patients. Meat and dairy products are to be avoided since they increase the production of mucus in the body—the same shielding, or blocking, mucus that coats tumors, according to him. Meat and dairy products are also harmful because they usually come from animals that received synthetic hormones through injections or chemicalized feed; the residue from these contaminants is present in meat, eggs, and milk. One common synthetic growth hormone, DES, has caused cancer in laboratory animals and humans. It is still used illegally by numerous mechanized factory farms in the United States, even though the Food and Drug Administration finally banned it in animal feed after it was proven to cause cancer in even the smallest doses imaginable. As FDA biochemist Jacqueline Verrett reported, "Researchers from the National Cancer Institute assured Congressmen that it might be possible for only one molecule of DES in the 340 trillion present in a quarter pound of beef liver to trigger human cancer, as far as they know."[9] Those mechanized farms that stopped using DES simply switched to other synthetic growth hormones, which contain many of the same substances as DES and have similar effects.

Shellfish, lobsters, and crabs are avoided on the Nieper diet because their high concentration of nucleic acids is thought to be potentially cancer-activating. Foods that "zoom up" the blood-sugar level such as cakes, chocolate, candy, and ice cream must be avoided as well. Apple juice is shunned because it is "too rich in glucose." The Nieper dietary regimen emphasizes whole grains, fruits and fibrous vegetables, carrot juice, fish in limited quantities, and skim milk.

Nieper advises patients to avoid *geopathogenic zones*, locations in which harmful electromagnetic radiation is said to emanate naturally from the planet's geophysiology. Such regions may contain fault lines, underground water, mineral veins, or subterranean caverns that allegedly emit harmful electromagnetic vibrations. Nieper estimates that "at least 92 percent of all the cancer patients I examined have remained for long periods—especially with respect to their sleeping place—in geopathogenic zones." He urges patients to have a dowser come to their house to check for these zones. A dowser uses a diving rod, or forked stick, to search for water, minerals, or other phenomena beneath the Earth's surface. There are also electronics firms and electronic gadgets that test for geopathogenic stresses. Nieper tells cancer patients never to use electrically heated cushions or blankets "since the irradiating alternating-current fields may knock off cell membrane charges."

Geopathology is a young science dealing with the relationship between human health and geologic factors such as underground water veins and radiational currents. Still virtually unknown in the United States, geopathology is being vigorously pursued in Germany, where it has spawned a natural-home movement called *Baubiology*, for "biological architecture." Baubiologists suggest that a "sick-building syndrome" may result from an inappropriate combination of geo-pathogenic zone, unhealthy building materials (for example, paints, plywood, and artificial carpets), and indoor electromagnetic pollution.

Resources

Hans A. Nieper, M.D.
21, Sedanstrasse
3000 Hannover 1
Germany
Phone: 011 49 511 348-0808
Fax: 011 49 511 318417

For further information on eumetabolic therapy and details on treatment.

A. Keith Brewer International
  Science Library
325 North Central Avenue
Richland Center, WI 53581
Phone: 608-647-6513

For books and articles by and about Dr. Nieper and his therapy as well as literature on other alternative therapies and advances in health and biophysics.

Reading Material

Revolution in Technology, Medicine, and Society, by Hans Nieper, MIT Verlag (Oldenburg, Germany), 1985. Available from A. Keith Brewer International Science Library (see above for address and phone number).

Hope for Us! written and published by Claire V. Morrissette (Augusta, Maine), 1985. Available from A. Keith Brewer International Science Library (see above for address and phone number). A survivor story by a Nieper patient with multiple sclerosis. Covers many aspects of Nieper's therapy that may be of interest to cancer patients.

Part Six

ADJUNCTIVE TREATMENTS

The treatments discussed in Part Six of *Options* are oxygen therapies, hyperthermia, DMSO (dimethyl sulfoxide), chelation, and live-cell therapy. While they are most often used as adjuncts to alternative or conventional treatment, this in no way diminishes their potential value to the cancer patient. In fact, some of these approaches do serve as powerful primary therapies for some patients. A number of other treatments described in this book are frequently or usually adjunctive, for example, hydrazine sulfate (Chapter 5), Iscador (Chapter 11), and mind-body activities like meditation, guided imagery, and psychotherapy (Chapter 29). Other alternative approaches such as nutrition, exercise, and herbs can also be used adjunctively as components in a custom-tailored anticancer program.

Chapter 20

OXYGEN THERAPIES

Without oxygen, we would die very quickly. Oxygen therapies supply life-giving oxygen to the body. This chapter will focus on two such therapies, ozone therapy and hydrogen peroxide, both used in alternative cancer treatment.

German biochemist Otto Warburg, a two-time Nobel Prize winner, stated in his 1930 book, *The Metabolism of Tumors,*[1] that the primary cause of cancer is the replacement of the process of oxygenation in normal cells by the fermentation of sugar. The growth of cancer cells, he maintained, can be initiated only in the relative absence of oxygen. In the mid-1950s, Warburg showed that cancer cells die in the presence of a high oxygen concentration.[2]

More recent efforts to explain the effects of oxygen therapies in various diseases focus on free radicals, unstable, highly reactive molecules that form continuously in the body and can severely damage cells. Oxidative treatments are thought to create "good" free radicals that counteract the dangerous ones. Other mechanisms of action will also be discussed in this chapter.

The first oxygen therapy to be discussed, ozone therapy, combining ozone and oxygen, has been extensively used in Europe for over fifty years to treat infections of all kinds, cancer, circulatory disturbances like arteriosclerosis and diabetes, wounds, gangrene, asthma, and many other conditions. In the clinical experience of many doctors in Europe and Mexico, ozone has shrunk tumors. It has also proven effective in helping AIDS patients. It increases the oxygen supply to the cells and destroys viruses and bacteria in the bloodstream.

Despite ozone therapy's wide and routine acceptance abroad, the medical orthodoxy in the United States considers it unproven, unimportant, and potentially hazardous. The FDA has put manacles on the clinical use of ozone. Cancer patients who want to be treated with ozone must go to Europe, Mexico, the Bahamas, or elsewhere, or get their own machines. Like other oxidative therapies, ozone has been "literally overlooked or 'left on the shelf' primarily because it is not a creature of the petrochemically based synthetic drug industry whose influence over (and often outright control of) Western medicine is, to many, obvious," according to Michael Culbert, editor of *The Choice,* a magazine devoted to restoring medical freedom of choice in the United States.[3]

Ozone (O_3), the most chemically active form of oxygen, is a powerful germicide that kills or inactivates bacteria, fungi, and viruses. Because ozone zaps germs and destroys toxic industrial impurities so effectively, over 3,000 cities in Europe use ozone to purify their drinking water. The tap water you drink in Paris, Florence, Zurich, Brussels, Singapore, and Moscow is ozonated, not chlorinated. In Germany, 90 percent of all swimming pools are ozonated.

Los Angeles, with one of the highest rates of throat cancer in the United States, recently switched to an ozonation system for the purification of its drinking water. After a five-year study, the City of Los Angeles found that ozone was the only means that could effectively remove carcinogens from its water supply. In contrast, chlorination of drinking water creates cancer-causing trihalomethanes (THMs), extremely toxic by-products formed when the chlorine added to water interacts with organic waste materials like dry-cleaning fluids. The widespread practice of chlorinating public drinking water increases the risk of gastrointestinal cancer over a person's lifetime by 50 to 100 percent, according to the United States Council on Environmental Quality. Ozone is a safe, nontoxic alternative, yet it is rarely used in the United States because of petrochemical-industry pressure.

Most people associate ozone with one of two things—the ozone layer or smog. A natural product formed in the stratosphere, ozone gas makes our lives possible by shielding us from the Sun's harmful ultraviolet rays. The presence of ozone in smog has led some people to the erroneous notion that ozone is always toxic. Ground-level ozone is produced when the Sun's ultraviolet light strikes the "toxic soup" of auto exhaust, industrial gases, and oxygen. This ozone can irritate the eyes and mucous membranes and inflame the upper respiratory tract. There is evidence that ozone synergistically interacts with these chemical pollutants to hamper breathing temporarily. The root problem here is the pollutants, however, not the ozone. Even so, this ozone is totally different from that administered in a clinical setting, where an ozone generator delivers pure, medical-grade ozone-oxygen mixtures in precise dosages.

"Ozone is Nature's natural disinfectant," observes Ed McCabe, author of *Oxygen Therapies* (see Resources). "You breathe it yourself on clear, sunny days outdoors, and after lightning storms." Through the action of lightning flashes, Nature produces ozone, which purifies the upper atmosphere. "When man dumps pollutants into the air, Nature tries to clean it up by, in effect, sending ozone into the affected area, to oxidize and clean up the pollution," states McCabe. "Ozone is one of the most beneficial substances on this planet. It is strictly, always, only O_3—pure oxygen, and never anything else. The bad science that people hear on the news, referring to 'ozone smog,' is a gross misrepresentation that causes people to be subconsciously afraid of Nature, and of life itself."

Compared to the most common form of oxygen (O_2), ozone (O_3) has much greater germicidal, antiseptic, and oxidizing power. The ozone molecule contains a large excess of energy and is highly unstable, reverting back to O_2 quickly. These properties increase ozone's interaction with tissues and blood. Ozone is toxic to infecting germs but appears to be harmless to patients when given at low, prescribed doses.

In the treatment of cancer, ozone is usually an adjunctive therapy, at times prescribed on a daily basis for several weeks; sometimes it is used as a primary therapy. It can be administered in a variety of ways. The most common method is *major autohemotherapy*, or blood infusion, in which 50 to 100 milliliters of blood are drawn from the patient, mixed with a dose of ozone-oxygen, then returned via the same intravenous catheter. The ozonated blood is rapidly distributed throughout the patient's body to all tissues. Some patients receiving this treatment report feelings of well-being lasting from a few minutes to several hours.

Another method, *minor autohemotherapy*, involves drawing 10 milliliters of blood, mixing the blood with ozone-oxygen, then injecting it into a muscle. Alternately, up to 10 milliliters of pure ozone-oxygen mixture can simply be injected into the gluteus maximus muscle or the deltoid. *Ozonated water*, used routinely in dental surgery, is sometimes swallowed by patients with gastric carcinoma or gastritis.

"Ozone therapy used in combination with other anti-cancer agents shows great promise," says Gerard Sunnen, M.D., associate clinical professor at New York University, who published the first full review of scientific papers about ozone therapy in the world medical literature.[4] A number of studies suggest that when ozone is used in combination with radiation or chemotherapy, lower dosages of the conventional agents will achieve either the same effect or an even better effect.[5] In this way, ozone could play an important role in combination therapy somewhat analogous to hyperthermia (Chapter 21). This may be another reason why the profit-oriented medical-pharmaceutical industry ignores or opposes ozone therapy.

Ozone treatment infuses high amounts of oxygen into the bloodstream. Although Otto Warburg's theory that cancer cells exist in an anaerobic (oxygenless) state has been amended considerably by subsequent research, ozone therapy is thought to capitalize on the disturbed metabolism of cancer cells and on the biochemical differences between normal and malignant cells. Some researchers report that tumor cells possess an intolerance for peroxide radicals but lack sufficient enzymes to inactivate them. Exposing malignant cells to ozone may induce metabolic inhibition, shutting down cancer cells.[6]

Dr. Sunnen proposes a plausible mechanism that might at least partially account for ozone's anticancer action. According to his ingenious theory, the blood taken from a patient presumably contains some of the patient's cancer cells, the fragile "seedling" cells that migrate from the original tumor site and enable the cancer to metastasize to other parts of the body. When the patient's extracted blood is mixed with ozone-oxygen, these "seedling" cancer cells are destroyed. They are then reintroduced into the patient's body with the blood, and the immune system produces antibodies in response to this necrotic (dead) cancerous material. These antibodies then work to destroy the primary tumor. In effect, the ozonated blood re-entering the body functions as a vaccine.

Another key anticancer property of ozone proposed by Dr. Sunnen hinges on the fact that certain cancers have been linked to viruses. For example, the Epstein-Barr virus is associated with nasopharyngeal cancer and Burkitt's lymphoma. Thus far, about 30 percent of all cancers have viruses implicated as causal factors, and the total percentage of viral-related cancers may be much higher. In ozone therapy, any viruses present in the blood drawn from the patient will presumably be killed or inactivated by the ozone-oxygen mixture. The virus, in fact, will be split apart into fragments upon exposure to ozone-oxygen. Now, when these viral fragments are reinjected into the patient, the immune system springs into action, producing antibodies to fight the dead viral fragments. These antibodies will also help destroy the *live* cancer-related viruses lurking in the patient's body, according to Dr. Sunnen.

In a remarkable 1980 study reported in *Science,* cultured human tumor cells of different cancer types were exposed to ozonated air for eight days. The growth of the cancer cells was inhibited *by 90 percent* upon exposure to 0.8 parts per million of ozone in cancers of the lung, breast, and uterus, and endometrial carcinoma.[7]

In October 1991, the prestigious journal *Blood* published a study reporting that ozone inactivates HIV, the AIDS virus, in factor VIII, a component of blood serum essential to hemophiliacs. This means hemophiliacs can now have a safe, HIV-free blood supply thanks to ozone.[8] Dr. Alexander Preuss, a German physician from Stuttgart, has reported dramatic success in treating AIDS patients with a combination therapy involving ozone, the drug suramin, immuno-modulation, minerals, and vitamins.[9]

Ozone destroys viruses, bacteria, and fungi by any one of a variety of mechanisms, according to Dr. Sunnen. Since ozone is highly reactive and disappears from the patient's body within five to fifteen seconds, it is ozone's by-products—mainly lipid compounds—that are believed to interact with viruses' nucleic acid and inactivate them. In one scenario, ozone combines with blood lipids (fats), which results in the creation of beneficial free-radical scavengers called *hydroxyperoxides*. Introduced into the bloodstream with ozonated blood, these scavengers go only to the diseased cells while ignoring normal cells. The scavengers see the virus-infected cells' lowered enzyme activity as an enemy "flag"and attack it. The diseased cells and scavengers "join together in their eventual mutual destruction and elimination, benefiting the patient," says Sunnen.[10] Normal, healthy cells with balanced enzyme activity are said to be invisible to the scavenging hydroxyperoxide agents.

Dr. Sunnen traveled to Europe in 1987 to investigate how ozone therapy is used at various clinics there to treat cancer and other conditions. One of his stopovers was Dr. Renate Viebahn's clinic in Iffezheim, Germany, where intramuscular injections of ozone are given daily to cancer patients. Viebahn's book *The Use of Ozone in Medicine* lists twenty-two scientific papers that show the effects of ozone against cancer. Sunnen found that ozone seems to have a "therapeutic window," in the experience of German practitioners. Patients receive ozone dosages in a range of a few to 100 micrograms per milliliter. Anything less is ineffective; anything more is considered potentially damaging to the normal cells.

Sunnen also found that Europeans prefer to start slowly, with low ozone dosages, then gradually increase the concentrations because they feel that too much ozone inhibits the immune system. Other doctors tend to advocate higher doses and to give them more frequently.

Critics of ozone therapy state that it is potentially toxic and may even be carcinogenic. They contend that ozone reactions produce free radicals that may attack DNA, proteins, and other biological molecules in uncontrolled ways. At least two studies present evidence that ozone acts in certain cell systems[11] and in animal models[12] as a carcinogen and/or cocarcinogen. Active oxygen introduced into the bloodstream promotes the growth of malignant cells in a variety of ways, according to the critics.[13]

Nonsense, reply the advocates of ozone therapy, who point out that *any* substance given in excessive amounts becomes toxic. They add that dosage and exposure time are crucial in administering any therapeutic agent. Many hundreds of thousands of patients, they say, have benefited from ozone therapy with no apparent side effects except a shortness of breath in extremely rare instances. "Metabolic processes take place in a milieu where there is a dynamic balance between oxidation and reduction," says Dr. Sunnen. "For certain pathological conditions, it may be highly advantageous to temporarily encourage oxidative processes in order to re-establish a healthy equilibrium."

According to Ed McCabe, "The reason ozone in very rare instances might seem to aggravate some conditions temporarily is explained by the deficient diets most people have. Their bodies do not have enough antioxidant enzymes to use the oxygen correctly." In the negative studies, contends McCabe, radiation damaged the cells, and the body sent oxygen to the site to repair the damaged cells while the ozone oxidized them. McCabe has visited scores of clinics around the world, interviewing hundreds of doctors and ozone-therapy patients whose positive experiences he distills in *Oxygen Therapies: Solutions for You, Your Animals, Your Plants, and Your Planet* (see Resources). "Thousands of people continue to use ozone air purifiers at home," he says, "and instead of getting lung cancer, they reduce or get off their medications as their diseases are oxidized by the body using the new-found source of atomic oxygen."

McCabe observes that medical ozone is used in clinics worldwide on a daily basis. In Germany, he points out, 644 therapists recently reported that among 384,775 patients who received 5.5 million ozone treatments, the rate of negative side effects was a very low 0.0007 percent. "This is far, far lower than side-effect rates from U.S. drug therapy, which each year kills approximately 140,000 people from prescription drug use," he says.

The other oxygen therapy to be discussed in this chapter is hydrogen peroxide. Administered by intravenous injection, hydrogen peroxide is considered an experimental and rather controversial therapy, even within alternative medical circles. Proponents say that this oxidative agent kills bacteria and viruses, oxidizes toxins, and stimulates the immune system. They also point to research indicating that it has demonstrated noticeable antitumor effects *in vivo* (within live organisms).[14] In a 1986 study, stomach cancer seemed to improve after hydrogen peroxide was administered.[15] But critics maintain that the therapeutic use of this substance is extremely dangerous and damages the body. They also point out that its long-term effects are unknown.

Dr. Kurt Donsbach of Hospital Santa Monica in Rosarito Beach, Mexico, has administered diluted solutions of hydrogen peroxide to patients with cancer and other diseases. "I have given more than 10,000 infusions to seriously ill patients, with a high percentage of miraculous results," he claims. "All my patients continue to use the substance orally after they leave the hospital. Four years of use and evaluation certainly should count for something."[16]

Intravenous hydrogen peroxide is also given in conjunction with radiation therapy. Dr. Vincent Speckhart of Virginia Beach, Virginia, reported on his work with this type of combination therapy at a conference on oxidative medicine in 1989. The results, he said, were particularly encouraging. It appeared that hydrogen peroxide prevented the radiation from causing damage to some healthy tissue and allowed the sick tissue around the cancer to recover more rapidly. The radiation was possibly also more effective than when used alone to treat the same type of cancer. "There was an excellent response of tumor metastatic to bone and brain," noted Dr. Speckhart. He and others additionally reported some positive results when intravenous hydrogen peroxide was used alone.[17]

Most people know hydrogen peroxide (H_2O_2) as a solution in the medicine chest used to cleanse minor cuts and abrasions. The white bubbling foam you see when you dab hydrogen peroxide on a wound is oxygen being released by the action of a specific enzyme, catalase, found in the blood and other body fluids. In addition, there are also oxidation enzymes in the body that produce hydrogen peroxide directly. Leukocytes (white blood cells) also produce natural hydrogen peroxide using an organelle, a special part of their anatomy that functions like an organ. Leukocytes emit hydrogen peroxide to surround and destroy harmful microbes. The hydrogen peroxide (H_2O_2) breaks down into water (H_2O) and oxygen (O_1). This form of oxygen (O_1), an unstable free radical, attaches itself to a virus or bacteria and disrupts it electrically, thus killing or inactivating it.

Hydrogen peroxide is "a naturally produced, purposeful molecule," observes Charles Farr, M.D., Ph.D., an Oklahoma physician and research chemist who supports the therapeutic use of intravenous hydrogen peroxide. Produced by almost every cell in the body, natural hydrogen-peroxide molecules aid membrane transport, act as hormonal messengers, regulate heat production, stimulate immune function, and perform many other important metabolic activities according to Dr. Farr. Farr reports good results from giving hydrogen-peroxide infusions to patients with chronic obstructive pulmonary disease, influenza, emphysema, and asthma.

Intravenous H_2O_2 was used as early as 1918 to markedly lower the death rate in the influenza epidemic. Its first recorded use, by Dr. T. H. Oliver, was reported in *The Lancet* in 1920; patients with influenzal pneumonia treated with hydrogen-peroxide infusions had a much better chance for survival. Researchers at many medical centers and universities have investigated the use of hydrogen-peroxide injections.

Critics assert that hydrogen-peroxide therapy is a major contributor to cellular damage caused by free radicals produced in the body. "The fact is excessive use of hydrogen peroxide is linked to a variety of conditions and disorders involving—but not limited to—inhibition of enzyme systems, inhibition of immune systems, cellular damage, chromosomal and genetic damage, and damage to specific organs," contend Robert Bradford and Michael Culbert, coauthors of a fifty-page monograph, *Hydrogen Peroxide: The Misunderstood Oxidant*[18] (see Resources). They claim that the concentrations of hydrogen peroxide commonly used in intravenous infusions (300 to 2,500 parts per million, or 0.03 to 0.25 percent) greatly exceed the levels of safe administration of this substance. To their way of thinking:

> Proponents do not seem to realize that hydrogen peroxide is generated by the body under certain conditions and for highly specific purposes. These purposes include the fighting of infections, the killing of invading microorganisms and defense of the body. . . .
>
> But as with antibiotics, hydrogen peroxide not only kills or inhibits the growth of microorganisms but it damages the host as well. For this reason the production of peroxide by the body's white cells is activated only when necessary. It simply does not follow that because a tiny amount of hydrogen peroxide may be beneficial in highly specific circumstances, that gigantic amounts will be better. Indeed, they may be highly damaging.

The body goes to great lengths, through an elaborate series of biochemical steps, to protect itself against the effects of the very hydrogen peroxide it has elicited to deal with specific problems, as in wound healing. The body produces the enzyme glutathione peroxidase. The function of this enzyme is to guard the body against the damaging effects of hydrogen peroxide.[19]

Bradford and Culbert are not proponents of orthodox medicine. Their Committee for Freedom of Choice in Medicine promotes patient empowerment so that people have greater access to alternative therapies. "One of the most alarming aspects of hydrogen peroxide," they write, "is its ability to peroxidize unsaturated fatty acids as found in lipids. The activity of membrane receptors and enzymes, as well as the active transport of cellular components across membranes are all dependent upon the compositions of the membranes in which these vital macromolecules—the lipids—are found."

Dr. Farr disputes the allegations of Bradford and Culbert. He believes that hydrogen peroxide's alleged role in free-radical damage has been completely misunderstood by scientists. Farr maintains, as do other researchers, that peroxidation of lipids may serve a useful purpose in the biochemical balance and may even need stimulating at times. He points out that nearly 5,000 articles in the medical literature describe beneficial effects of H_2O_2 treatment. Researchers in the 1960s treated several hundred patients with hydrogen peroxide infusions "with no reported serious side effects."[20]

The Bradford-Culbert critique is also disputed by McCabe. He states that many of the studies cited by Bradford and Culbert fail to indicate the concentrations of H_2O_2 used, which may have been excessive. Further, McCabe points out that American Biologics, the clinic in Mexico with which Culbert and Bradford are associated, sells Dioxychlor, a chlorinated product that produces singlet oxygen just like hydrogen peroxide. Finally, McCabe argues, theoretical scientists with little clinical experience in oxidative modalities do not understand how H_2O_2 given therapeutically works in the body. In his explanation, hydrogen peroxide selectively oxidizes dead, weak, diseased, and dying cells. "The theorists see this response and assume that normal cells are hurt," he says. "Not so. Hydrogen peroxide peroxidizes the *diseased* cells and their DNA, along with harmful free radicals, and after this cleansing reaction the body produces brand-new cells. The clinical experience of fully credentialed, blue-ribbon M.D.s who have spent years giving over 10,000 medical peroxide infusions has been overwhelmingly positive.

The criticisms are all theory that simply does not stand up to the test of real-world experience."

Dr. Gerard Sunnen maintains that higher organisms have enzymes that can restabilize disrupted DNA and RNA, whereas lower life forms do not. This could help explain why bacteria and viruses die from oxidative therapies while human cells are supposedly unaffected.

Where does all of this leave the cancer patient? Probably more bewildered than before. Anyone contemplating intravenous hydrogen peroxide as an adjunctive therapy should read up on the literature and get a diversity of viewpoints—pro and con—before making a decision.

Some people take diluted H_2O_2 orally as a self-help remedy. Hydrogen peroxide is called oxygen water in many countries around the world and is used as an all-purpose elixir. However, according to Dr. Farr, when hydrogen peroxide is taken orally, it can react with iron and fatty acids in the body to form the highly toxic, unstable hydroxyl radical, a powerfully destructive free radical that can erode the lining of the stomach and duodenum (the first part of the small intestine) and, in rats, cause cancer.

McCabe recommends that people taking any form of H_2O_2 or any other oxygen therapy should also consider taking wheat-sprout-derived superoxide dismutase (SOD), an antioxidant enzyme. The SOD will neutralize excess or harmful free radicals that might be formed by the hydrogen peroxide. The fifth most plentiful protein in the body, SOD is present in all cells. It converts free radicals into stable oxygen and hydrogen peroxide, which are then broken down into water and oxygen.

Resources

International Bio-Oxidative Medicine Foundation
P.O. Box 610767
Dallas/Fort Worth, TX 75261
Phone: 817-481-9772

For further information on intravenous hydrogen peroxide and a physicians' referral list.

Reading Material

Oxygen Therapies: A New Way of Approaching Disease, by Ed McCabe, Energy Publications (99-RD1, Morrisville, NY 13408; 315-684-9284 or 800-284-6263), 1988.

Oxygen Therapies: Solutions for You, Your Animals, Your Plants, and Your Planet, by Ed McCabe, Energy Publications (99-RD1, Morrisville, NY 13408; 315-684-9284 or 800-284-6263), 1991.

Health Consciousness, February 1989. Contains articles on the pros and cons of hydrogen peroxide.

Hydrogen Peroxide: The Misunderstood Oxidant, by Robert Bradford and Michael Culbert, Bradford Research Institute (1180 Walnut Avenue, Chula Vista, CA 92011; 619-429-8200), 1989.

Chapter 21

HYPERTHERMIA

Hyperthermia is the application of therapeutic heat to destroy or reduce cancer tumors. The rationale behind hyperthermia is that cancer cells are more heat-sensitive than normal cells. In fact, cancer cells break down when heat is in excess of around 107°F. The use of high heat to kill tumors dates back to ancient Egypt.

Modern hyperthermia takes many forms. In *local hyperthermia,* the tumor is heated from 107°F to 113°F using highly focused ultrasound, microwaves, or radio-frequency waves, which break down the tumor mass without harming the surrounding tissues. The intensity and placement of the heat are controlled with sensors and computer-guided applicators.

In *whole-body hyperthermia,* the patient is anesthetized and either placed in a heat suit or wrapped in thick rubber blankets through which hot water flows. The temperature is then slowly raised to 108°F and maintained for two or more hours. Another whole-body approach involves perfusion with heated blood that circulates through the body. This procedure can take up to thirty hours, during which time patients are lightly anesthetized.

Dosages of radiation and chemotherapy can be sharply reduced without lessening their effectiveness when used in conjunction with hyperthermia. This means that damage to healthy cells and to the immune system is diminished. Some radiation therapists claim to have seen cancerous tumors disappear twice as often with a combination of radiation and hyperthermia as with radiation alone.

Remissions of cancer have been reported with hyperthermia, usually when it is used as an adjunct to radiation or chemotherapy. Beneficial results have been noted not just with superficial external tumors but even with deeper cancers such as brain tumors, lung cancer, and bone cancer. Another application of hyperthermia is to shrink tumors to make them operable or more susceptible to chemotherapy.

Hyperthermia can also be used as a stand-alone modality. However, the results with heat therapy utilized alone in treating superficial tumors are "relatively poor, with response rates of less than 40 percent, and most of these are partial responses," says Haim Bicher, M.D., director of the Valley Cancer Institute in Los Angeles, the largest American nonprofit center specializing in the hyperthermic treatment of cancer. But according to Dr. Hye Koo Yun, Ph.D., head of the Eastwest Wellness Center in San Ysidro, California, "Hyperthermia by itself is often more preferable than in conjunction with radiation. This is because the job still gets done without further poisoning the body with cobalt radiation."

The American Cancer Society removed hyperthermia from its Unproven Methods list in 1977, and in 1984, the technique was approved by the United States Food and Drug Administration as a medical procedure to treat cancer. Yet most cancer patients in the United States have never heard of hyperthermia, even though it is currently being used on an estimated 10,000 patients per year. Advocates of hyperthermia call it the fourth modality, after surgery, chemotherapy, and radiation. However, while there has been a recent upsurge of interest in the approach, it is still available mostly at university medical centers. In Dr. Bicher's estimate, "Progress has been frustratingly slow. Hyperthermia needs to be more commonly utilized in community oncology practice. The use of combination treatment should be strongly considered before giving radiotherapy without hyperthermia." Many advocates of hyperthermia feel that the medical establishment's continued resistance to it can be explained partly by the huge monetary profits the supporters of chemotherapy and radiation might lose if use of hyperthermia became widespread.

Proponents say that heat therapy is nontoxic, noninvasive, and virtually without side effects. They cite studies that suggest it boosts the efficacy of radiation, yielding a response rate two to three times greater than with radiation alone. Radio-resistant tumors such as malignant melanoma and sarcomas have been treated with some success when radiation is administered in tandem with hyperthermia. "It therefore seems especially appropriate to use hyperthermia initially in the treatment of radio-resistant tumors," states Jack Tropp, a long-time student of alternative therapies.[1]

Heat therapy enhances the body's natural immune response, as numerous experiments have demonstrated. For example, physicians at Indiana University Medical Center used microwaves to raise the body-core temperature of advanced cancer patients above normal and maintain it for thirty to sixty minutes. The heat affected the patients' immune cells, causing their lymphocytes to divide faster. After heating, the immune cells were stimulated to divide by producing more interferon and interleukin, biologic response modifiers that activate the body's own defenses and increase the production of white blood cells. The number of monocytes (large white blood cells) and natural killer cells increased after the heat application, and their activity remained elevated for several days. "We have clearly demonstrated enhanced killing by natural killer cells and enhanced production of interleukin-2 and interferon," said Mahin Park, M.D., in a report presented at the annual meeting of the Federation of American Societies for Experimental Biology in Las Vegas in 1988.

Hyperthermia does have its critics, including those who say it is mostly a palliative measure, delaying the growth of tumors much more often than completely regressing them or bringing them under permanent control. Patients have seen their tumors recur within months or years of treatment. The critics add that the toxic and carcinogenic side effects of chemotherapy and radiation are still present with combination hyperthermia, though to a lesser degree.

Elmeria Teffeteller, an oncology clinical nurse specialist in the hyperthermia department of the Thompson Cancer Survival Center, Knoxville, Tennessee, is critical of heat-therapy practitioners who overstate the treatment's potential benefits. "The claim that heat treatment is noninvasive, by which they mean it is without pain, is totally misleading. It can be invasive and sometimes painful because probes are inserted into the body to monitor temperature levels. Hyperthermia is not a panacea. For patients with advanced disease or distant metastasis, it will make little difference in long-term survival and is best used as a palliative measure. Hyperthermia is a localized treatment for an often systemic disease. Patients need to realistically weigh the possible advantages of palliative hyperthermia against the potential disadvantages."

Dr. Haim Bicher has reported a "38% complete response rate."[2] However, in nearly 90 percent of patients, permanent control is not possible, the goal of treatment being relief of symptoms, improvement in quality of life, and extension of life. "In the few patients I have had the opportunity to treat with hyperthermia combined with radiation for previously untreated local-regional cancer, eighty percent have had complete response and most of these have no evidence of disease in limited follow-up of less than 5 years," Dr. Bicher reports.

With local hyperthermia, no toxicity has been reported other than occasional skin blisters, which occur in less than 10 percent of patients, or about 0.5 percent of treatment sessions. Otherwise, there appears to be no adverse effect from heat on normal tissue. The blood flow in normal tissue increases tenfold in response to heat application, while tumors retain heat due to their abnormal blood supply.

Reported side effects of whole-body hyperthermia include fever, transient arrhythmia, respiratory distress, and drowsiness. Many people feel sleepy and worn out for a day or two. More significant dangers associated with the whole-body approach stem from the fact that heat causes veins to dilate and increases the body's demand for oxygen; cardiac output therefore becomes twice the norm. Cardiovascular or renal complications may occur in some patients due to absorption of the dead tumor material into the bloodstream. Within twenty-four hours of total body immersion, tumor cells rapidly break down, and the waste products can place undue stress on the liver and kidneys.

There is no agreement as to the optimal number of hyperthermia sessions; contradictory reports abound. Most clinics give heat therapy twice a week. Practitioners and researchers are still trying to determine the optimal doses and treatment schedules and the best combinations of hyperthermia with chemotherapy and radiation.

Another problem is the variation in equipment. Pain or systemic stress occurs in 45 percent of patients with deep tumors treated with the most commonly used equipment.[3] Deep treatment utilizing magnetic induction has also been associated with poor patient tolerance and compliance.[4] However, a treatment using external microwave applicators developed by Dr. Bicher seems to be better tolerated by patients. It is said to treat deep tumors more easily, with patients experiencing no side effects other than perspiration, the body's mechanism for avoiding overheating.[5]

Even though hyperthermia is still in its developmental stages as an auxiliary or primary treatment for deep tumors, hyperthermia for superficial tumors has been considered a standard treatment since 1984. Several studies over more than a decade have had encouraging results, for example:

- A Public Health Service study found that for certain cancers producing tumors close to the skin, 75 percent of the tumors disappeared after combination therapy with hyperthermia and radiation, compared to 44 percent after radiation only.[6]

- Dr. Ned Hornback of Indiana University treated seventy-two patients with advanced cancer. Complete remission was achieved in 92 percent of those given hyperthermia following radiation.[7] Dr. Hornback compared the results obtained in the treatment of advanced cervical cancer using radiation alone and using radiation combined with hyperthermia. Complete local control rates were 53 percent and 72 percent respectively.[8]

- Dr. Ronald Scott of Roswell Park Memorial Institute treated fifty-nine patients with superficial malignancies using radiation either alone or combined with hyperthermia. The complete tumor response at six months was 39 percent and 87 percent respectively. By one year, nearly half of the tumors eliminated with radiation alone had recurred, while all the tumors given the combination treatment remained controlled.[9]

- A tabulation of worldwide results obtained in 2,330 patients by hyperthermic oncologists revealed at least a partial response in 67 percent of the patients treated with combination hyperthermia and radiation, versus 33 percent of those treated with radiation alone.[10]

- Several patients with melanoma recurrent in a limb as well as metastatic showed complete regression of all lesions following heated chemotherapy perfusion of the limb, with disease-free survival at follow-up for up to fifteen years.[11]

In 1980, Harry LeVeen, M.D., then with the Veterans' Administration Hospital in Brooklyn, New York, reported tumor regression in eleven of thirty-two inoperable and "untreatable" lung cancer patients who had received hyperthermia with radio-frequency energies. Six of the patients became disease-free, with two still alive and well after three years. Dr. LeVeen also reported dramatic symptomatic relief—including weight gain, increased strength, and relief from pain—in twenty-seven of the thirty-two cases. Secondary metastasized growths had sometimes vanished after heat treatment of the primary site, indicating that localized heat had stimulated the whole immune system.

Egyptian papyri show that doctors in the Nile Valley apparently treated breast tumors with heat millennia ago. These doctors must have known that a fever is Nature's response to a threat to the body's integrity. Under heightened temperature, white blood cells immediately begin to reproduce more rapidly. A fever is simply the body's way of combating illness.

The ancient Greeks also recognized the value of heat in some medical treatments. The word *hyperthermia* comes from the Greek *hyper* ("over" or "above") and *therme* ("heat"). After the Renaissance, there were reports of "spontaneous" tumor regressions in patients with smallpox, influenza, tuberculosis, and malaria. The common factor was a fever of about 104°F.

Some fifty-five years ago in central Italy, a marshy area called the Pontine Swamps was a breeding ground for malaria. Nearly everyone who lived in that 300-square-mile region got malaria and the recurrent fevers associated with it. Yet, strikingly, cancer was virtually unknown to the natives living there.

In 1896, Dr. William B. Coley, a young New York surgeon fresh out of Harvard Medical School, shook the medical community with his "mixed bacterial vaccine," which he used to deliberately induce a fever in cancer patients for therapeutic purposes. Dr. Coley's daughter, Helen Coley Nauts, executive director of the Cancer Research Institute in New York City, has analyzed 896 of her father's cases. In a 1953 review, she reported complete regression and five-year survival in 46 percent of 523 inoperable cases and in 51 percent of 373 operable cases.

Despite the wide use of heat therapy through the centuries, research on this modality languished in the United States until the 1970s. In 1978, when an American Cancer Society assistant vice president was asked why hyperthermia had been officially condemned as an unproven method, he said that hyperthermia had undergone experimentation only in Europe, that it was reviewed only in European journals, and that American doctors have a tough enough time keeping up with American journals.[12]

Scientists now have a better understanding of how hyperthermia works. In normal tissue, blood vessels dilate when heat is applied; this dissipates the heat and cools down the cell environment. But a tumor is a tightly packed group of cells with restricted, sluggish circulation. Application of heat cuts off the nutrients and oxygen vital to the tumor cells by causing a collapse of the tumor's vascular system.

The great majority of cancer patients who seek out heat therapy either have tumors that failed to respond to other forms of treatment or have metastatic disease. In those few cases where a patient uses hyperthermia as the primary external treatment for a locally advanced cancer, favorable results are reported. In such cases, "complete local control" of the cancer in the 70 to 80 percent range has been claimed both for superficial lesions and for deep-seated cancers of the cervix[13] and lung.[14]

Thomas Terry of Placentia, California, had a tumor larger than a golf ball surgically removed from his neck in October 1988. Two months later, a new lump, about the size of a quarter, appeared above the area of excision. His doctor strongly recommended that Terry undergo a standard course of radiation and chemotherapy. Instead, Terry began a ten-week regimen with Dr. Bicher at the Valley Cancer Institute combining low doses of radiation with hyperthermia every day. The radiation was given within two hours after the heat therapy. "There were no feelings of pain or discomfort," says Terry. By about the eighth week, the lump was gone, and Terry has remained cancer-free.

In late 1986, Rita Engel, age fifty-nine, consulted her doctor about pain in her right shoulder and a cough. Her lung cancer was diagnosed as inoperable when a CAT scan showed it was "densely adherent to the chest wall" and impinged on the trachea. Her symptoms were relieved after a full course of radiation, but the tumor remained, and she consulted Dr. Bicher in June 1987. She received three weeks of hyperthermia alone and an additional three weeks of hyperthermia combined with very low doses of radiation. She was well, with no evidence of disease, in December 1991. During her struggle against cancer, Rita practiced relaxation and guided imagery with the help of a cassette tape by Carl Simonton, M.D. (Chapter 29). She says, "I was able to relax and gain a feeling of control over my illness. It was important for me to feel that I could participate in my treatment and cure rather than be a passive victim. I preferred to maintain a positive attitude. I also ate well, took vitamins, went for walks, and tried to lead as normal a life as possible."

Dick Evans of Anaheim, California, was diagnosed in early 1983 with a brain tumor that "came on very quickly." He had surgery to remove the benign meningioma, which affected the physical coordination on the left side of his body. Four years later, the tumor recurred, and after a wait-and-see period, the doctor recommended a second operation. Evans refused and began investigating alternative methods of healing. At the annual convention of the Cancer Control Society in Los Angeles, he came across a booth with information on hyperthermia. He then contacted the Valley Cancer Institute and decided to embark on a course of hyperthermia with low-dose radiation. "When I told the surgeon who had performed the original operation that I was planning to have hyperthermia, he said, 'It's a farce, it'll never work,' and he abruptly walked out of my hospital room."

Evans underwent a seven-week course of treatment with local hyperthermia at 112°F to 113°F for two hours a day, followed immediately by low-dose radiotherapy given at a different facility by an independent radiologist. "I would simply lie down, and the doctor would bring the heat applicator right down to my forehead," he recalls. "There were no side effects from the heat therapy, except for perspiration. The tumor got smaller and smaller as the weeks progressed." Evans' last CAT scan showed that the tumor seems to be encapsulated and is greatly reduced in size. He has no symptoms, has been able to go back to work, and, in his late sixties, is full of energy.

Resources

Valley Cancer Institute
12099 West Washington Boulevard
Suite 304
Los Angeles, CA 90066
Phone: 310-398-0013
        800-488-1379

For further information on hyperthermia and details on treatment.

For a partial listing of other treatment centers that offer hyperthermia, see *Third Opinion: An International Directory to Alternative Therapy Centers for the Treatment and Prevention of Cancer and Other Degenerative Diseases,* by John Fink (see Appendix A for description).

Reading Material

Consensus on Hyperthermia for the 1990s, edited by H. I. Bicher et al., Plenum Publishing (233 Spring Street, New York, NY 10013; 800-221-9369), 1990. A technical book for the medical professional.

The Cancer Survivors and How They Did It, by Judith Glassman (see Appendix A for description).

Cancer Victors Journal, Summer–Fall 1988, Summer 1989, and Winter–Spring 1991.

Chapter 22

DMSO THERAPY

DMSO (dimethyl sulfoxide) is an organic sulfur compound widely used in alternative cancer treatment, particularly in biologic and metabolic therapies. A clear, colorless, viscous, and essentially odorless liquid, it is administered to patients by intravenous infusion, intramuscular injection, topical application, or oral solution.

Proponents of the use of DMSO point to a body of research indicating its value as an antitumor agent. Laboratory studies with animals show that DMSO delays the development of breast cancer[1] and colon cancer[2] in rats and, also in rats, retards the growth of bladder cancer[3] and leukemia.[4] Several studies indicate that dimethyl sulfoxide induces the differentiation of leukemia cells, causing them to revert to normal or benign cells.[5] A 1983 study concluded that DMSO has therapeutic value in treating skin cancer.[6] The compound also increases the effectiveness of cytotoxic chemotherapy drugs, as demonstrated by clinical use with patients and tests on mice.[7]

Despite nearly 6,000 articles about DMSO in the scientific literature and several international symposia on its efficacy and safety, DMSO has been approved for use by the FDA only in the treatment of a rare bladder ailment. Veterinarian physicians, however, routinely use DMSO, so your dog may have an easier time receiving the substance than you will. Meanwhile, DMSO is used as a prescriptive drug in fifty-five countries, including Switzerland, Germany, Russia, Austria, Great Britain, Ireland, Canada, Mexico, and several South American nations.

In cancer patients, DMSO relieves pain and acts as a free-radical scavenger that is efficacious against the side effects of radiation. Free radicals are renegade molecules having an unpaired electron, an arrangement that makes them highly unstable. In the human body, free radicals hunt down vulnerable proteins, enzymes, and fats, seeking a spare electron with which to bond. By stealing an electron from a normal molecule, free radicals can destroy enzymes, proteins, and cell membranes, disrupting vital processes and creating mutant cells. Any cancer patient who has undergone chemotherapy or radiation is loaded with free radicals. According to Dr. Morton Walker, drinking a small amount of diluted DMSO tends to relieve the free-radical symptoms and signs caused by orthodox treatments, such as sores at the corners of lips, loss of head hair, nausea, metallic taste in the mouth, and dry mouth.[8]

How DMSO protects against radiation and the side effects of radiation therapy is not well understood. One theory holds that DMSO's radioprotective properties are based on its ability to scavenge free radicals. Other theories maintain that dimethyl sulfoxide probably protects against the lethal effects of whole-body radiation through a number of different mechanisms.

One of DMSO's unique properties is its ability to bind very strongly to water. In fact, the hydrogen bonds formed between water and DMSO are stronger than the hydrogen bonds that exist between two water molecules. The *preferential binding* of water to DMSO rather than to water reportedly accounts for DMSO's wide-ranging biological activities.

Another unusual property of DMSO is its ability to penetrate the skin very rapidly and in high concentrations with little or no known tissue damage. The organic compound's innocuous passage through protein barriers is believed to occur through reversible configurational changes of the proteins. This is due to the substitution of water by DMSO, which causes a loosening of the protein structure.[9] (*Caution:* Do *not* mix DMSO with any chemical or drug and apply it to the skin. The relative dosage would be uncertain and quite possibly harmful.)

DMSO is able to pass through most membranes of the body without destroying their integrity. On its journey, it can carry with it a number of other chemical agents, including antitumor agents. Its ability to enhance the activity of other compounds dissolved in it is thought to be related to its membrane-penetration abilities.

DMSO's unique chemistry accounts for its versatile therapeutic use in a broad spectrum of medical conditions, including cancer, arthritis, cerebral edema, urinary-tract disorders, osteomyelitis, burns, and musculoskeletal disorders such as sprain, strain injuries, and acute bursitis. It has the broadest pharmacological action of any known chemical agent. Dr. Stanley Jacob, who initiated DMSO therapy in humans around 1961 at the University of Oregon Medical

School, has suggested that DMSO should be reviewed as a "therapeutic principle" rather than merely a "drug."

The most common side effect of DMSO is the garlic-like taste and breath odor experienced by a majority of patients. A portion of DMSO is metabolized into dimethyl sulfide (DMS), which is exhaled by the patient and causes the characteristic bad breath. The odor is also present in oil and sweat glands. Sulfur from the compound may remain in the body for several days.

Other side effects include occasional headaches, nausea, and dizziness, especially when DMSO is taken in very high doses. If DMSO is applied directly to the skin, a localized skin rash sometimes develops. One study of 4,180 patients found localized dermatitis in 3.5 percent of the patients. Many patients experience a slight burning or tingling sensation of the skin upon topical application, followed by itching after the DMSO has begun to dry. The burning or tingling is caused by a local histamine-releasing action. These temporary sensations disappear within roughly thirty minutes. (Note: DMSO should be administered under professional care only. Persons with cancer should not attempt to self-administer this substance, which could be dangerous and harmful.)

The toxic and injurious effects of chemotherapy drugs on the immune system and the body as a whole may be reduced if these drugs are administered in low doses in combination with DMSO. In Chile, sixty-five cancer patients were given low doses of a chemo drug combined with DMSO and amino acids. Many of the patients had earlier received orthodox forms of treatment that had proved useless. The patients' tolerance for the toxic chemotherapy agent when combined with DMSO was exceptional. Most of the patients experienced significant relief of pain. Very few exhibited white-blood-cell suppression or malformation, which so often occurs with chemotherapy. Of the sixty-five patients, forty-four obtained remission. In twenty-six of the patients with metastasized breast cancer, twenty-three obtained remission and three showed no improvement.[10]

Another intriguing finding is that minute doses of DMSO inhibit or kill pleomorphic bacteria, or "dwarf bacteria," associated with cancer. The bacteria in tumors are usually assumed to be secondary invaders, but investigators such as Virginia Livingston-Wheeler, Royal Rife, and Florence Seibert held that these organisms are actually a primary cause of cancer. Their research, rejected by orthodox medicine, suggests that bacteria can change their size and shape, becoming smaller and smaller until they are transformed into filterable, invisible particles the size of a virus.

The disease-causing effect of bacteria in cancer was explored by Florence Seibert, Ph.D, and her associates at the University of Pennsylvania and later at the Veterans' Administration Center in Bay Pines, Florida. In laboratory studies, Seibert showed that organisms isolated from tumor and leukemia patients stopped growing when exposed to a DMSO solution. Furthermore, no damage or change was observed in the growth patterns of normal cells. As Patrick McGrady, Sr., reports in *The Persecuted Drug: The Story of DMSO* (see Resources), "When the Seibert group added 12.5 percent DMSO to cultures of organisms isolated from sixteen of eighteen cancer patients' tumors and blood, their growth was completely inhibited for thirty days; in control tubes there was marked growth. Seibert's discovery that the hardy, drug-defying dwarfs can be both weakened and killed by innocuous doses of DMSO encourages speculation not only that DMSO may find a place among anti-cancer drugs but also that it may lead to an anti-cancer vaccine."[11]

In 1970, a three-year-old diabetic boy, Clyde Robert Lindsey of Pasadena, Texas, was taken by his mother to see Houston physician Eli Jordan Tucker, an innovator of one form of DMSO cancer therapy. The boy had an especially deadly cancer, a type of metastatic endothelioma known as Letterer-Siwe disease. Solid, visible tumors were lodged behind his ears, and multiple cancer lesions spread across his scalp and over his body. Clyde's orthodox doctors diagnosed his condition as hopeless. A young patient with this type of cancer rarely, if ever, lives over six or seven years.

Mrs. Lindsey sought out Dr. Tucker's help, having heard of his successful experimental approach. A respected orthopedic surgeon who had spent years investigating cancer, Dr. Tucker treated the disease with a solution combining DMSO and hematoxylon, a dye used by biologists for over 100 years as a pathologic marker for animal cells. The DMSO-hematoxylon solution is said to have an affinity for tumors, carrying the hematoxylon directly into them. Hematoxylon oxidizes readily into a red substance known as hematein. The combination of DMSO and hematoxylon is believed to produce a hematein reaction of oxidation with the tumor cells; this inactivates the ground substance, or protoplasmic material, surrounding the cancer cells. With the ground substance inactivated, the cancer cells are starved to death.

Dr. Tucker gave Mrs. Lindsey a small dropper bottle of DMSO-hematoxylon solution, with instructions to give Clyde five drops in distilled water each morning before breakfast. The boy's condition gradually improved, and today, in his twenties, Clyde is in good health and continues to take his anticancer medicine every day.[12]

In his book *DMSO: Nature's Healer* (see Resources), Dr. Morton Walker claims that "the FDA knows very well about this treatment's success for certain forms of cancer." He points out that FDA officials met with Dr. Tucker (now deceased) to study the doctor's DMSO cancer therapy. Walker's book includes a number of case histories of cancer patients, as well as a detailed report on the effect of Tucker's DMSO-hematoxylon therapy on different types of cancer.

For administering this treatment, Dr. Tucker was expelled from the staffs of two hospitals, despite his reputation as "the grand old man of orthopedic surgery." Dr. Walker comments, "It is about time the medical community, especially oncologists, took hold of this treatment and explored it further."

Dimethyl sulfoxide, a wood-pulp derivative, was first synthesized in 1866 in Russia by chemist Alexander Saytzeff. In the early 1960s, two American scientists, Stanley Jacob, M.D., and Robert Herschler, began successfully experimenting with DMSO as a vehicle to promote the penetration of antibiotics into wounds, to speed healing, and to reduce infection.

In November 1965, the FDA abruptly halted the clinical testing of DMSO in the United States. In lab tests of the drug, refractory lens changes had occurred in dogs, rabbits, and pigs, three species of animals not closely related to humans. When the DMSO treatments were terminated, these toxic effects to the lenses of the animals' eyes reversed. No such effects have ever been noted in studies with humans.

Nevertheless, the FDA was determined to block further research on DMSO. Critics have suggested that one or more pharmaceutical companies sabotaged the research because DMSO threatened their profitable products. In any event, FDA agents reportedly launched punitive investigations of DMSO researchers, photocopied their personal correspondence and private patient records, bugged their offices, and committed forgery and blackmail in an attempt to destroy the DMSO research. One scientist told Pat McGrady, Sr., author of *The Persecuted Drug,* "I'm afraid for my family and myself. I'm afraid for doctors and scientists. And I'm more afraid for our country. I can't believe these things are happening in the United States."

Another eminent researcher maligned by the FDA observed, "The academic community and industry are so completely intimidated that one cannot look for any leadership to counteract some of the punitive actions of the FDA." He added, "I am very pessimistic concerning the future status of medical research unless a mood arises to combat overzealous bureaucratic authority."

In March 1966, the New York Academy of Sciences held an international symposium on DMSO despite efforts by the FDA and the drug industry to prevent the conference from getting off the ground. Chairing the meeting was "the dean of American pharmacologists," Dr. Chauncey Leake of the University of California Medical Center. Dr. Leake said, "Rarely has a new drug come so quickly to the judgment of the members of the health professions with so much verifiable data from so many parts of the world, both experimentally and clinically, as to safety and efficacy."

The FDA allowed a limited resumption of clinical testing of dimethyl sulfoxide in December 1966 while still banning the medical use of the substance. In 1978, the FDA approved the prescriptive use of DMSO for the treatment of a rare bladder disease, interstitial cystitis. Today, according to Jonathan Collin, M.D., editor of the *Townsend Letter for Doctors,* "Many other applications of DMSO are also observed, but have not been given ample opportunity for investigation because of the adamant stance by the FDA to suppress DMSO research."[13]

Resources

For a partial listing of treatment centers that offer DMSO therapy, see *Third Opinion: An International Directory to Alternative Therapy Centers for the Treatment and Prevention of Cancer and Other Degenerative Diseases,* by John Fink (see Appendix A for description).

Reading Material

The DMSO Handbook, by Bruce W. Halstead and Sylvia A. Youngberg, Golden Quill Publishers (P.O. Box 1278, Colton, CA 92324; 714-783-0119), 1981.

DMSO: Nature's Healer, by Morton Walker, Avery Publishing Group (120 Old Broadway, Garden City Park, NY 11040; 800-548-5757), revised edition, 1992.

DMSO, by Barry Tarshis, William Morrow and Company (105 Madison Avenue, New York, NY 10016; 800-843-9389), 1981.

The Persecuted Drug: The Story of DMSO, by Pat McGrady, Sr., Charter Books (390 Murray Parkway, East Rutherford, NJ 07073; 800-631-8571), 1973.

Chapter 23

CHELATION

Chelation (pronounced key-LAY-shun), a procedure used to remove toxic metals such as lead, cadmium, and mercury from the body, is a standard technique in some metabolic cancer programs. Many physicians use chelation therapy to restore circulation to arteries partially blocked by plaque, the accumulated yellowish material on arterial inner walls that is held together by calcium deposits. Chelation enhances the free flow of blood. It increases the oxygen to the body's cells and inhibits the production of free radicals.

Chelation takes its name from the Greek word *chele*, meaning "claw." This refers to the way the chelating agent, a synthetic chemical or body protein, grabs on to certain minerals and forms a compound with them. In chelation therapy, a synthetic amino acid called ethylene diamine tetraacetic acid (EDTA) is administered by means of a slow intravenous drip. Once in the bloodstream, this chelating agent claws, or grasps, free-floating ions of heavy toxic metals, forming a tight chemical bond with them. As the EDTA passes through the kidneys and is expelled from the body, it takes these toxic metals with it. Patients usually receive EDTA infusions one to three times per week, with each session lasting about three hours. Other intravenous chelating substances are also sometimes used.

Chelation is best known to the public as a therapy for cardiovascular disease. Practitioners say that chelation has an impressive track record in preventing or reversing atherosclerosis (hardening of the arteries). It reduces the risk of heart attack and stroke, lowers blood pressure, and relieves angina pain. Chelation is "substantially more effective and infinitely less dangerous than bypass surgery," according to well-known author Robert Atkins, M.D.[1] As an alternative to invasive artery-clearing procedures such as coronary bypass surgery and balloon angioplasty, chelation has met with increasing acceptance among health-oriented physicians and the public. Positive results have also been reported in the use of chelation as a treatment for Alzheimer's disease, diabetes, emphysema, arthritis, osteoporosis, Parkinson's disease, kidney diseases, and gangrene.

Yet, while chelation is a preferred therapy for cardiovascular disease in some countries, the American medical establishment spearheaded by the AMA has waged an intensive campaign to stamp out this procedure. In fact, the only officially approved use of chelation therapy in the United States is to remove toxic metals such as lead. Chelation is also being used to treat Vietnam war veterans poisoned by Agent Orange.

The medical orthodoxy claims that the evidence for chelation does not meet acceptable scientific standards with controlled double-blind studies. However, only 10 to 20 percent of current orthodox medical procedures meet such criteria, according to a 1978 report by the Office of Technology Assessment. "A more likely explanation for widespread opposition to chelation is that it competes with many aspects of conventional cardiology and eliminates much vascular surgery," notes Raymond Brown, M.D.[2] In pure economic terms, chelation poses a direct threat to coronary artery bypass surgery, a thriving $3.3 billion-a-year industry "providing a financial windfall to hospitals, drug and equipment manufacturers, and . . . highly paid surgical and postsurgical coronary care teams."[3]

What role does chelation have in cancer treatment? According to Morton Walker, D.P.M., chelation therapy may be "a partial answer" in the treatment of some malignancies. One possible benefit of chelation to cancer patients is that the improved circulation it induces makes oxygen more readily available to cells. Cancer grows better in tissues that do not have as much oxygen as do healthy tissues. Where chelation allows the bloodstream to carry its full complement of oxygen, cancer cells may wither.

Some chelating physicians believe that EDTA and other chelating substances strip away the protein coat surrounding tumor cells. This protective coating shields the tumor cells from T-lymphocytes, white blood cells that kill invaders. It is the tumor's protein shield that makes it impossible for T-lymphocytes to identify the tumor. Once the chelator has stripped cancer cells of their protective coats, the T-lymphocytes identify the tumor cells and release numerous chemical factors to kill them.

Chelation also removes cancer-causing and cancer-promoting substances from the body. Lead, a poisonous legacy of the automobile age, has been implicated in cancer formation. Lead, cadmium, mercury, and other toxic heavy metals in our highly polluted environment chronically depress the immune system and poison the body's enzyme systems. Lead also inactivates macrophages, specialized immune cells that act as scavengers and engulf invaders. Removal of these toxic metals enhances natural defense and metabolic functions.

Toxic minerals such as iron, copper, and lead, when accumulated in the body, interact with oxygen to form free radicals. Free radicals, if they proliferate out of control, are troublemakers that can damage the DNA in normal cells, inducing mutations that lead to cancer. EDTA has been shown to be a free-radical inhibitor that controls oxidative damage by removing copper and iron from the body.[4]

To boost immune functioning, doctors who use chelation with cancer patients often administer an intravenous infusion combining a chelating agent with supplemental nutrients such as vitamins B and C, zinc, and selenium. High doses of vitamin C (20 to 100 grams per intravenous bottle) are often given by metabolic practitioners. Vitamin C reacts with copper in the blood, generating hydrogen peroxide, which breaks down to destroy tumors through oxidative reactions.

Not everyone believes that chelation is appropriate for treating cancer patients. Not even all alternative practitioners are convinced. "There is little evidence in any form that chelation is helpful in treating cancer," says David Steenblock, a holistically oriented osteopathic physician from El Toro, California, who has an eclectic approach to cancer treatment. He explains:

> Free radicals are bad for a healthy body since they damage normal molecules, but the very fact that they damage tissues can be used against cancer once it has occurred. Metals such as copper have an oxidizing effect on the body, and increased oxygen or oxidation inhibits cancer growth. If you are attempting to treat cancer with oxidizing substances, then you will want to leave the metals intact in the body to facilitate free radical generation and stimulation of the immune system with its oxygen-dependent, cancer-destroying mechanisms. These effects will be nullified if a person is treated with chelation therapy. I have personally seen cancer develop in three people who were undergoing chelation therapy. In these cases, the cancer was present at the start of the chelation but unrecognized at the time.

Deficiencies of zinc impair the immune system. Chelation,

which removes zinc and other essential metals from the body, can contribute to immune deficiency. Another possible danger of chelation is that the breakdown products from dissolving tumors and the chelating compounds all are excreted through the kidneys. This may precipitate kidney failure. . . . There is some evidence that iron chelators are potentially useful in certain types of cancers, but much more research needs to be done. Vitamin C is, however, a mild chelating agent and works extremely well in helping a person recover from chemotherapy or from a viral infection.

Steenblock is an officer of the American College of Advancement in Medicine (ACAM), which provides training in chelation therapy and certifies physicians who qualify.

Nephrotoxicity, or kidney poisoning, due to a sudden overload of heavy metals being removed from the body is a potentially lethal hazard of EDTA chelation. Too rapid an infusion of EDTA could produce a kidney overload. However, the general ACAM position is that the serious toxic effects of EDTA can be eliminated if the treatment is administered correctly by a physician trained by ACAM. Besides nephrotoxicity, other urinary symptoms have been reported following EDTA chelation therapy, including urgency to urinate and difficult or painful urination. "There have been sparse reports also of kidney insufficiency, kidney failure, blood in the urine, and one report of acute tubercular necrosis," observes Dr. Morton Walker.[5]

Other reported side effects of EDTA infusion include low blood calcium, cardiac arrhythmia, insulin shock, hypotension, fever, headache, joint pain, and thrombophlebitis (inflammation of a vein, with a blood clot forming within the vein). "Most of these side effects are very rare and shouldn't stop a person from having chelation therapy," according to Dr. Steenblock. However, chelation may be contraindicated in persons with damaged kidneys, acute or chronic liver disease, tuberculosis, brain tumors, or pregnancy.

Not only does chelation eliminate toxic metals and arterial plaque, it also removes some essential, beneficial elements from the body such as zinc, magnesium, calcium, copper, manganese, and other trace minerals. To restore these essential metals, the chelation protocol includes nutritional supplements taken orally on a daily basis plus a prescribed diet.

There is compelling evidence that chelation helps *prevent* cancer. Walter Blumer, a Swiss oncologist who practices general medicine and chelation therapy, investigated the high rate of cancer deaths among 231 adults living along a highway in an atmosphere polluted with lead from automotive exhaust. Over an eighteen-year period (1959 to 1976), 31 of these people died of cancer. But only 1.7 percent of those treated with EDTA plus vitamins C and B1 died from cancer, whereas 17.4 percent of the untreated subjects died from cancer. In other words, cancer mortality in the untreated people was *ten times greater* than in the chelated patients.[6]

Chelation may also play a role as an adjunctive therapy in AIDS. Some research has found EDTA to be an inhibitor of retroviruses.[7] There are unofficial reports that chelation destroys pleomorphic organisms, the form-changing microbes that some scientists link to cancer and AIDS. According to these accounts, AIDS patients whose blood showed many pleomorphic microbes under dark-field microscopic examination were found to be clear of them immediately after chelation.[8]

Resources

American College of Advancement in Medicine
23121 Verdugo Drive
Suite 204
Laguna Hills, CA 92653
Phone: 714-583-7666
        800-532-3688

For further information on chelation, a physicians' referral list, and a consumer-information pamphlet.

Reading Material

What Your Doctor Won't Tell You, by Jane Heimlich, HarperCollins Publishers (10 East 53rd Street, New York, NY 10022; 800-242-7737), 1990.

The Chelation Answer, by Morton Walker and Garry Gordon, M. Evans and Company (216 East 49th Street, New York, NY 10017; 212-688-2810), 1982. Includes a five-page section on cancer.

The Chelation Way: The Complete Book of Chelation Therapy, by Morton Walker, Avery Publishing Group (120 Old Broadway, Garden City Park, NY 11040; 800-548-5757), 1990.

AIDS, Cancer and the Medical Establishment, by Raymond Keith Brown, Robert Speller and Sons, Publishers (Box 461, Times Square Station, New York, NY 10108-0461; 212-473-2295), 1986.

Bypassing Bypass: The New Technique of Chelation Therapy, by Elmer Cranton and Arline Brecher, Medex Publishers (P.O. Box 44, Trout Dale, VA 24378; 800-426-3551), second edition, 1990.

Chelation Therapy: Special Report, written and published by the People's Medical Society (462 Walnut Street, Lower Level, Allentown, PA 18102; 215-770-1670), 1991. Pamphlet. Presents a cautionary view of chelation therapy.

Chapter 24

LIVE-CELL THERAPY

Live-cell therapy involves the injection of animal fetal or embryonic cells into the body. It is used as an adjunct in cancer treatment, not as a stand-alone therapy. Most often, cells are taken from an unborn calf, but other donor animals can be used, including sheep, horses, monkeys, and sharks. Proponents of cellular therapy maintain that it stimulates the immune system, regenerates tissue, balances hormonal production, and helps rejuvenate "target" organs. The rationale for using fetal or embryonic animal cells rather than adult animal tissue is that such cellular material is held to be immunologically silent—that is, it will not trigger an immune response in the patient that would lead to rejection of the cells.

Widely known in Europe, live-cell therapy is unapproved by the FDA and unlicensed in the United States, even though research on using human fetal tissue to treat incurable diseases has sparked much scientific interest.[1] Developed by Swiss physician Paul Niehans in the early 1930s, cellular therapy is available at some European clinics. Several clinics in Tijuana, Mexico, offer it as a component of nutritional-metabolic anticancer programs. It has been used to treat a wide variety of complaints ranging from chronic skin disorders to arteriosclerosis, multiple sclerosis, Down's syndrome, liver cirrhosis, Alzheimer's disease, Parkinson's disease, epilepsy, lupus, muscular dystrophy, and infertility.

In treating cancer, live-cell therapy is more effective the earlier the patient is diagnosed and the less he or she has been exposed to chemotherapy or radiation, according to endocrinologist Wolfram Kuhnau, M.D., former head of the live-cell program at American Biologics–Mexico S.A. Medical Center in Tijuana. Dr. Kuhnau, who retired in 1991 at the age of eighty-one, is still a consultant to the clinic.

He worked with Paul Niehans in Switzerland and introduced live-cell therapy to Mexico.

Dr. Kuhnau points out that the full effects of a round of cellular treatment typically do not manifest for three to four months, a critical time in which the patient must be kept alive and strengthened. At American Biologics, cellular therapy is part of a metabolic program including detoxification, diet, and supplements of vitamins, minerals, enzymes, amino acids, and antioxidants. If the patient can be maintained, says Dr. Kuhnau, the cellular treatment has a chance of taking hold. With terminal cancer, he has written, live-cell therapy is usually not directly beneficial.[2]

Live-cell practitioners maintain that the material from the donor animal is transported in the patient's blood to its counterpart organ and tissues (for example, heart cells to the heart, lung cells to the lungs). This effect was demonstrated, at least in animal experiments, by Professor H. Lettré of the University of Heidelberg. Lettré tagged cellular material from rats with radioactive isotopes and injected it into other animals, tracing it with a Geiger counter. The injected live-cell material was brought through the host's macrophages to the corresponding tissues: the liver cells went to the liver, the kidney cells went to the kidneys, and so on.[3]

Patients at American Biologics are given injections of calf-thymus extract, along with fibrous tissue from a bovine umbilical cord. The human thymus, once thought to be the chief regulator of the immune system, is a primary target of cellular therapy. It produces T-cells and *B-cells*, key players in mobilizing the body's immune response. Well-developed in childhood, the thymus shrinks later in life as the production of T-cells begins to decline. In a clinical trial reported in the *New England Journal of Medicine* in 1981, ten of seventeen children with an immunosuppressive condition, histiocytosis-X, entered complete remission after being treated with daily intramuscular injections of thymus extract from five-day-old calves.[4] In September 1982, the *Journal of the American Medical Association* reported experiments indicating the value of thymosin, a thymus extract, in treating AIDS.

In treating cancer patients with animal fetal cells, American Biologics physicians generally begin by giving live-cell injections weekly for three weeks. Patients then return for shots at three months and six months. The shots consist of fresh cellular material suspended in an isotonic salt solution and are given intramuscularly or subcutaneously. At some clinics, the animal fetal preparations may be freeze-dried or frozen in liquid nitrogen before being injected. When frozen in liquid, the preserved cells can be tested for bacteria, viruses, or parasites before use, whereas fresh cells are used before testing can be performed. Other cellular therapies employ rehydrated concentrates in tablet or capsule form.

Dr. Kuhnau believes that freeze-drying and other techniques cause the animal cells to lose a good deal of efficacy. "Nobel Prize winner Dr. Rita Levi-Montalcini in Rome found in her work on chicken eggs and xenotransplants from murine brain tumors that freeze-dried cell preparations simply did not work," he says.

One innovation in live-cell therapy at American Biologics is the use of shark-embryo cells. According to Kuhnau, sharks never get cancer or contagious diseases and have a placenta resembling that of humans. Scientists think the mystery substance in shark cartilage responsible for the shark's seemingly perfect health can also inhibit tumor growth in mammals. In 1983, Dr. Robert Langer of the Massachusetts Institute of Technology reported, "Shark cartilage contains a substance that strongly inhibits the growth of new blood vessels toward solid tumors, thereby restricting tumor growth."[5]

Live-cell therapists contend that their modality has no serious toxic side effects, although it may cause transient-fatigue reactions. Dr. Kuhnau, who has treated over 20,000 patients with cellular therapy, states, "The responsible administration of live-cell preparations causes no side effects at all—and I say this from the vantage point of four decades of experience, during which time I have never experienced an allergic reaction. Neither is it possible for responsibly prepared live-cell suspensions to transmit infections."

In Europe, the overuse of live-cell products has led to tragic deaths. In 1987, West German health authorities suspended the use of the freeze-dried cellular products of several companies for one year after the death of an athlete who reportedly had received several hundred injections and had a fatal allergic-type reaction. But this fatality apparently does not reflect on regular live-cell practices—more than six injections are rarely given in any one treatment. However, a recent report in *The Lancet* noted a number of serious immunological reactions to cellular treatment in Germany, including encephalitis, immune vasculitis, polyradiculitis (inflammation of the nerve roots), and a delayed effect of chronic progressive neurological disease.[6] A 1957 survey of 179 West German hospitals revealed eighty cases of severe immunological reaction, thirty of them fatal, in patients who had received cellular treatment. According to Dr. Kuhnau, these deaths resulted from a gross overuse of cellular preparations. A 1984

FDA "talk paper" claims that live-cell therapy poses a risk of transmitting both bacterial and viral infections, such as brucellosis (a generalized bacterial infection characterized by fever, sweating, and pain in the joints) and encephalomyelitis (a viral infection characterized by inflammation of the brain and spinal cord).[7]

The precise mechanism of action of live-cell therapy is not fully understood. The implanted cellular material is believed to go to "earmarked" amino acids. The donor cells' RNA, DNA, mitochondria, and enzymes are held to play a part in the rejuvenation of the organ or bodily system at which the cellular therapy is aimed. Injection of cellular extracts from animals' embryonic endocrine organs is supposed to harmonize the hormones produced by the human endocrine system, which impacts on virtually all other bodily systems, including the immune system, as well as the emotions.

Live-cell therapy, a form of treatment condemned by animal-rights advocates, was early on embraced by movie stars, athletes, politicians, and others seeking physical rejuvenation. Since little documented evidence exists as to its reputed value in treating cancer, patients considering this adjunctive treatment should weigh the moral arguments and get as much hard information on the treatment as possible from the clinic or practitioner offering it.

Resources

For a partial listing of treatment centers that offer live-cell therapy, see *Third Opinion: An International Directory to Alternative Therapy Centers for the Treatment and Prevention of Cancer and Other Degenerative Diseases,* by John Fink (see Appendix A for description).

Reading Material

The Biochemical Basis of Live-Cell Therapy, by Robert W. Bradford, Henry W. Allen, and Michael L. Culbert, with a foreword by Rodrigo Rodriguez and Wolfram Kuhnau, Robert W. Bradford Foundation (Chula Vista, California), 1988. Available from the Cancer Control Society (see page xv for address and phone number). A discussion of live-cell therapy and its application in various diseases.

The Choice, Winter 1990 and Summer 1990.

Treatment of Cancer by Means of Cell Therapy, by Dr. Federico Ramos, Foundation for Advancement in Cancer Therapy (see page xvii for address and phone number), 1977. Booklet.

Part Seven

ENERGY MEDICINE

Energy medicine encompasses many ancient and some modern medical practices. In energy (or bioenergetic) medicine, the human organism is viewed as a complex of interacting energy fields that underlie and help regulate the physical body. If these energy fields become imbalanced, disease can result. Bioenergetic healers attempt to rebalance the energy fields and restore patients to well-being by applying the energetics of magnetism, electricity, light, herbs, acupuncture, or other methods. Instead of manipulating body cells and organs through drugs and surgery, the energy-medicine practitioner attempts to heal illness by manipulating and working with the patient's energy fields.

For thousands of years, proponents of the ancient medical systems of India, China, Tibet, Japan, and other cultures have insisted the human body is pervaded and surrounded by a basic energy field that is observable. Healers within these traditions have noted both normal and abnormal patterns in the field. Centuries ago, Eastern physicians used the forces of electricity and magnetism as well as light, color, minerals, and prayer to influence the internal energy systems of the body.

The concept of bioenergy—a "life force" that creates order from disorder, promotes healing, and directs the process of growth—is central to many of the planet's major medical systems, although it is rejected by practitioners of mechanistic Western medicine. The Chinese call this energy *chi* (pronounced chee), the yogis of India speak of *prana,* while homeopaths refer to the *vital force.* All these terms relate to a fundamental force that assists healing. While many energy-medicine practitioners say they work with "subtle energies" that at present cannot be measured, there are also physicians and scientists in this field who believe it is not necessary to invoke mystical forces to explain the workings of bioenergetic therapies.

The four major systems of energy medicine and their application to treating cancer are as follows:

1. *Electromedicine* uses electrical and magnetic fields to treat cancer by altering the electromagnetic energies within the body. Albert Szent-Gyorgyi, who won a Nobel Prize for discovering vitamin C, outlined a bioelectronic theory of cancer causation in his 1976 book, *Electronic Biology and Cancer.* He said that his theory complemented, but in no way contradicted, the virus theory of cancer. In the 1930s, Harold Burr, M.D., a prominent professor at Yale University, concluded that all living organisms are controlled by "electrodynamic fields," which he named life fields, or L-fields. Using a microvoltage meter capable of measuring infinitely small gradations in an energy field, Burr determined that L-fields act as blueprints for the development of all life forms. He maintained that through these bioelectric fields, we are connected to the entire universe.

2. *Homeopathy,* based on the ancient healing principle of "like cures like," uses microdoses of substances that with each successive dose are more and more diluted until no molecule of the original medicine exists. The subtle effects of homeopathy on cancer and other ailments are said to occur through energy realignment.

3. *Ayurveda,* the traditional medicine of India, developed bioenergy to a sophisticated science long before the birth of Western technologic science. Ayurveda holds that weakened life force, or low energy, lies behind most diseases, including cancer, and that wrong diet, wrong breathing, stress, and most modern Western methods of treating disease reduce vitality.

4. *Chinese medicine,* rooted in a conception of the body as a unified energy system, treats cancer and other illnesses through the energetics of herbs, diet, acupuncture, massage, manipulation, exercise, and meditation.

Part Seven of *Options* examines in full each one of these four major systems of energy medicine.

Chapter 25

BIOELECTRIC THERAPIES

If the body is a bioelectric system, then healing consists of correcting disturbed electrical fields and related energy flows. Electromedicine exploits the impact of different regions of the electromagnetic spectrum on health and healing. Electromagnetic and magnetic fields are force fields that carry energy and can convey information. Scientific evidence strongly suggests that electromagnetic energy systems within the body control growth and healing. The science of the body electric is still in its infancy. Electromedicine seems to have the greatest potential of any healing discipline; yet, for the cancer patient, it may hold the greatest number of potential hazards.

A wide array of bioelectronic equipment for diagnosis and treatment is currently being employed in medicine for diverse purposes. The use of electrical stimulation for the relief of pain has recently gained acceptance in hospitals and clinics. Dr. Robert Becker, an orthopedic surgeon in New York, twice nominated for the Nobel Prize, pioneered the application of electrotherapy to stimulate the body's innate capacity for tissue repair and regeneration. Electromagnetic devices have found widespread application in accelerating the healing of fractured bones.

However, Dr. Becker says, "My advice to any cancer patient contemplating any sort of electromagnetic or biomagnetic therapy is *don't*." He explains, "All of the work is seriously flawed. It is not backed up by any thorough research, and there is a real possibility for serious harm." That judgment may seem overly negative to some people, including those who may have benefited from these approaches. But it does point to the lack of comprehensive clinical studies or long-term follow-up to support most bioelectric therapies.

Readers who wish to explore any of these treatments should exercise caution and healthy skepticism in making their own evaluations.

One of the most important cancer cures, the Rife generator, was a device that destroyed cancer-causing microbes using specific electromagnetic frequencies. It was developed by Royal Raymond Rife (1888–1971), a San Diego scientist-inventor born in Nebraska. Rife successfully treated many cancer patients in the 1930s, but he aroused the wrath of the American Medical Association, which worked to destroy his therapy and his technology. Millions of lives might have been saved if this medical breakthrough had been accepted and properly developed.

Today, there is a plethora of purported Rife generators (also called Rife boxes) on the market, especially in California. Critics contend that virtually all of these devices are fraudulent and potentially hazardous because they do not faithfully reproduce the authentic technology used by Rife in his instrument.

Roy Rife built an extraordinary, powerful light microscope with a resolution of 31,000 and a magnification of 60,000X, which made it possible to study live bacteria and viruses. This was a stunning advance over the electron microscope, which kills its specimens. Using his Universal Microscope with its special "light-staining" technique, Rife discovered, observed, and photographed bacteria that could change their form, in effect becoming cancer-causing viruses. He identified four forms of the cancer microbe, ranging from a bacillus to a fungus and virus. One of these four forms, the monococcoid, was found in the blood of 90 percent of cancer patients. When properly stained, the monococcoid could be readily seen with a standard microscope. For experimental purposes, any of the four forms could be changed back within thirty-six hours into the "BX form," capable of producing cancer tumors in laboratory animals; the BX germ could then be isolated from those tumors.

Rife's detailed observations led him to conclude that bacteria are pleomorphic, or form-changing. He found that harmless bacteria could metamorphize into disease-causing virus forms and go through different stages of a life cycle. His pleomorphic cancer microbe was clearly visible in human cancer specimens at a microscopic magnification of 30,000X. This finding completely contradicted orthodox microbiology, which held that bacteria are eternally *monomorphic* and could never assume other or smaller forms. (See pages 35 and 78 for discussions of this controversy.)

At the same time he developed his microscope, Rife also invented a special frequency emitter on the theory that radiations beamed at particular frequencies would devitalize or kill specific germs. Under the microscope, he saw targeted germs that were subjected to specific electromagnetic energies actually explode and die. By 1932, Rife was reportedly using his Frequency Instrument to destroy the cancer microbe, the typhus bacteria, the polio virus, the herpes virus, and other viruses in culture and in experimental animals.

In 1934, the Rife instrument was used to successfully treat fourteen of sixteen terminal cancer cases at a University of Southern California clinic sponsored by the school's Special Medical Research Committee. This work was done under the supervision of committee chairman Milbank Johnson, M.D. According to Rife's report, "16 cases were treated at the clinic for many types of malignancy. After 3 months, 14 of these so-called hopeless cases were signed off as clinically cured by the staff of five medical doctors and Dr. Alvin G. Foord, M.D., pathologist for the group. The treatments consisted of 3 minutes duration using the frequency instrument which was set on the mortal oscillatory rate for 'BX' or cancer (at 3 day intervals). It was found that the elapsed time between treatments attains better results than the cases treated daily. This gives the lymphatic system an opportunity to absorb and cast off the toxic condition which is produced by the devitalized dead particles of the 'BX' virus."[1]

Follow-up clinics conducted in 1935 through 1938 achieved similar remissions of cancer using a painless, noninvasive, three-minute treatment administered every third day. Rife collaborated with some of the most respected physicians and researchers in the United States, including Dr. Edward Rosenow, a bacteriologist from the Mayo Clinic, and Dr. Arthur Kendall, a bacteriologist who worked at the Rockefeller Institute and Harvard Medical School and was dean of Northwestern University Medical School. Independent physicians utilizing the Rife Frequency Instrument successfully treated as many as forty people per day, reversing cancer, tuberculosis, and other deadly diseases and painlessly removing cataracts. Rife's breakthrough work was described in *Science* magazine and various medical journals, discussed at medical conferences, and explained in depth in the Smithsonian Institution's annual report.

In 1940, Arthur Yale, M.D., told a convention of the California State Homeopathic Medical Society about the astonishing results he had achieved with cancer patients using Rife's instrument:

> Having used this apparatus for almost two years, the writer has had the satisfaction of witnessing the disappearance of

every malignant growth, where the patient has remained under treatment, these included epitheliomas, carcinomas and some of undetermined origin. . . .

For purposes of elucidating, a few of the more remarkable cases are given in detail.

Mrs. L., age 49 years, came to me on June 5, 1939. . . . X-ray pictures showed a mass the size of a cantaloupe at pyloric end of the stomach. . . . Treatments were commenced immediately. . . . Pain rapidly disappeared and on October 20, 1939, a picture was made showing the entire mass had disappeared.

Mrs. A., age 59 years, came to me on January 7, 1939. . . . X-ray pictures showed irregular mass at pyloric end of the stomach the size of an orange with almost completed occlusion, the lymphatic involvement extending both upwards and downwards. . . . Rife-ray . . . were given three times a week . . . pain disappeared. . . . At the end of five months the mass entirely disappeared.

Mr. C., age 53 . . . three of our leading surgeons had diagnosed the case as inoperable carcinoma of the rectum. There was a large irregular shaped mass in the rectum the size of a grapefruit which had to be pushed out of the way before he could have a stool. . . . Treatments were instituted, pain disappeared before the completion of the first week's treatment. . . . The entire mass disappeared at the end of sixty days. . . .

Mrs. J., age 58. . . . The patient had lost sight in her left eye and the case was referred to Dr. Sherman, who diagnosed carcinoma of the retina. He advised immediate enucleation to save the right eye. In October 1938 I installed the Rife ray machine and discontinued all treatments except the Rife ray three times a week in this case. In December the vision returned to the eye and Dr. Sherman said the growth had entirely disappeared, leaving a scar on the retina. In January 1939, Dr. Sherman reported that all the growth had disappeared and also the scar on the retina, and the vision was the same in both eyes.

I have quoted in detail the four cases which were far advanced, each one of which would probably have proved fatal within 90 days. . . . The effect of the Rife ray on all malignant growth is so remarkable and so universally satisfactory that I felt this society should have the first report and the credit for advancing what evidently promises to be the first positive treatment for the ever-increasing curse of cancer and its resultant fatalities.[2]

But Rife's lifesaving medical technology never reached the American people. His work threatened powerful doctors and financial interests. As an inexpensive treatment for cancer and many other illnesses, the Rife generator was seen as a direct competitive threat to the big drug companies, surgeons, doctors, health bureaucracies, and other vested interests. As Barry Lynes shows in his dramatic, well-documented book *The Cancer Cure That Worked* (see Resources), the American Medical Association, with the California State Board of Public Health, launched a systematic campaign to destroy Rife and his therapy. By 1939, the AMA virtually stopped the Rife treatment by harassing physicians and threatening them with loss of license and jail terms and by forcing Rife into court. All scientific reports on Rife's work were censored by the head of the AMA; no major medical journal was permitted to report on Rife's medical discoveries and cures.

Doctors who used the Rife instrument were visited by officials and harassed. Any doctor who made use of Rife's methods was stripped of his privileges as a member of the local medical society. The author of the Smithsonian article was shot at while driving his car and never wrote about the subject again. A leading New Jersey laboratory that was independently verifying Rife's discoveries was "mysteriously" burned to the ground at 3 A.M. in March 1939 while the lab's director was visiting Rife in California.

John Crane, an engineer-inventor who was Rife's partner for a while, spent three years in jail following a 1961 trial. No medical or scientific reports documenting the Rife generator's effectiveness were allowed to be introduced at the trial. The foreman of the jury was an AMA doctor. The medical establishment succeeded in smashing Rife's therapy. His records were destroyed, and his microscope and life's work were tabooed by the American medical profession.

The Food and Drug Administration still bans Rife-like treatments for human medical use. The devices on the market that are called Rife generators are authorized only for "experimental/technical/educational/veterinary use." Critics say that *none* of these devices is the real thing and that a number of them are potentially very hazardous. If you are considering exposing yourself to the energies from a purported Rife generator, you should first talk to other patients who have done so. Ask the clinic or device vendor to show you documented case histories of recovered patients, with names and phone numbers. If they cannot produce such case histories or contacts, you should be highly suspicious.

One clinic purportedly using Rife technology is the American Metabolic Institute (AMI) in La Mesa, Mexico, just south of San Diego. The AMI device was developed by Bud Curtis, a former business associate of John Crane. Curtis claims his device is identical to the frequency instrument that Crane and Royal Rife developed in 1967 and that Crane copyrighted in 1978. The AMI's unit, still in the experimental stage, has been used in Mexican hospitals and clinics to treat many diseases. At AMI and nearby Rosarita Hospital, the Rife therapy is part of a metabolic anticancer program that includes chelation therapy, acupuncture, oxygen therapies, herbs, laetrile, immunotherapy, magnetic therapy, colon detoxification, nutritional counseling, and other modalities. American Metabolics claims "great success" with its Rife device and recommends that patients purchase a machine and take it home with them to self-administer treatment.

To demonstrate the reputed effectiveness of its modified Rife design, AMI uses live-blood-cell analysis. Critics, however, dispute the legitimacy of this test. For an evaluation of ten different models of Rife-like devices, see *Consumer Guide to Rife Generators,* a four-page pamphlet by Lyks Sieger, N.D., and Dieter Reisdorf, H.M.D (Uncommon Books, 2936 Lincoln Avenue, San Diego, CA 92104; or S.R.C.E., P.O. Box 1772, Santa Rosa, CA 95402).

According to the November–December 1991 issue of the *Journal of Borderland Research,* "John Crane devised the square wave pulse generator approach from his understanding of Rife's work. . . . Positive and negative results have been recorded from this approach, but it is definitely not what Rife was doing. However, Crane still has some of the original Beam Tube equipment and it is in use in a clinic in Mexico." People interested in the "original" equipment can contact Crane at 4246 Pepper Drive, San Diego, CA 92105; 619-281-0278. The same magazine cites a new book, *The Rife Way III,* which "is over 200 pages with photos, charts and other supporting documentation providing specific technical information on what Rife's work is really all about." The book can be ordered from Mark Simpson, Box 710088, Dallas, TX 75371.

A device somewhat similar to the Rife generator was the Lakhovsky multiwave oscillator, developed in Paris in the 1920s by Dr. Georges Lakhovsky. This French scientist used selective radio-frequency radiation to successfully treat cancer in plants and in humans, as well as other diseases in humans. Lakhovsky was granted a United States patent in 1934, but his instrument was suppressed by medical authorities. Modern Lakhovsky devices, still built by individual engineers, are banned by the FDA as quackery. The current crop of devices all carry the statement, "For experimental use only."

Antoine Priore, an Italian-born electrical genius working in France in the 1960s, developed a machine that uses a combination of magnetic and electromagnetic forces to eliminate tumors. The French government has poured millions of dollars into its development, but a proposal to build a Priore machine at the Massachusetts Institute of Technology was blocked.

A host of oscillating-wave generators and other types of bioelectronic devices has surfaced in the United States, with underground claims of having cured everything from cancer to AIDS. Since the manufacturers of these devices are trying to avoid interference or seizure by the FDA, getting reliable information about how the machines operate and whether they have any therapeutic benefit is especially difficult. A general rule of thumb: Let the buyer beware.

In the 1880s, a French surgeon, Professor Apostoli, treated cervical and uterine cancers by inserting a positive electrode into the tumor and passing electricity through the tumor to a negative electrode on the abdomen. Tumors shrank in size, but no long-term remissions were reported. A young American surgeon, Dr. Franklin Martin, later replicated Apostoli's results.[3]

Since 1978, Dr. Björn Nordenström, a Swedish radiologist, has been using a similar technique to treat otherwise inoperable cancers, chiefly of the lung and breast. Inserting a positive needle electrode directly into the tumor, with a negative electrode applied to the skin, Nordenström has prompted tumor regression and occasional remission in cases considered untreatable by conventional cancer therapies. His electrical therapy works only on isolated tumors; the largest have been four centimeters across, and most have been smaller. The treatment takes one to three hours and can be done under local anesthesia. Usually, a single treatment suffices for each tumor, and regression takes place over several months or years.

Nordenström, born in 1920, is the former head of Sweden's prestigious Karolinska Institute in Stockholm. He pioneered the needle biopsy, a diagnostic technique used in every major hospital in the world. In his 1983 book, *Biologically Closed Electric Circuits,* he postulates bioelectric circuits as part of a major, previously unrecognized "electrical circulatory system" in the body. These bioelectric circuits, he says, can be switched on by an injury, an infection, a tumor, or even the normal activity of the body's organs. This electrical system, says Nordenström, represents the very foundation of the healing process. In his view, cancer may result from a disturbance in this complex electrical network.

Nordenström has proposed a number of mechanisms to explain how his electrotherapy destroys tumors. He determined that white blood cells carry a negative electrical charge, so he reasoned that a positive electrode placed in the tumor would lure the tumor-fighting white cells to the site of the cancer. He also found that the electrical field generated between the two electrodes induces ionic tissue change and acid build-up, altering the local environment of the tumor in ways that destroy cancer cells. In his scenario, the acidic reaction around the tumor kills some red blood cells or damages their hemoglobin, preventing delivery of oxygen to the tumor. He held these and other reactions responsible for the tumor destruction.

Robert Becker rejects Nordenström's explanation. "Nordenström is not doing anything new. He is simply producing electrolysis and killing the tumor by a strictly physical technique," contends Dr. Becker. "Electrolysis and gas formation occurring within the tumor results in a highly acidic area where cancer cells will be destroyed. The destruction of the tumor is *not* the result of electrical factors acting alone."

Dr. Becker claims that Nordenström's technique poses "a very real hazard" of stimulating new cancer growth through the use of electricity. As the current spreads out and flows along a return path to the negative electrode, its electrical strength drops below the level of electrolysis. Through this, states Becker, a large volume of tissue is exposed to electrical currents that *stimulate* rather than *retard* tumor growth. If there are several cancer nodules present in one area, the zapping of one nodule may increase the growth of adjacent tumors, according to Becker. This unwanted effect did in fact occur in a number of Nordenström's cases, Becker alleges.[4] He sweepingly asserts that although electromagnetic therapy has a promising future, all the present techniques are based upon a simplistic view of the relationship between electromagnetic energy and cell growth.

Professor Nordenström denies that any of the negative effects described by Becker have ever occurred. He writes:

> I have not seen one instance of induction of cancer by my treatments. If Dr. Becker had known enough about physiologic flow of current in tissue, he would not come to that conclusion. Ions are transported in many closed circuits in the body, e.g., driven by metabolic or injury potential differ-

ences. These small current densities do not induce cancer growth. An acute exposure of tissue to electricity or chemicals will not lead to neoplastic formation. However, a *chronic* flow of even small currents in tissue will change the ionic micro-environment over a long time. The tissue then attempts to adjust its living conditions to the new *chronically* changed environment which may lead to neoplastic (benign or malignant) growth. This is the reason why all factors changing the environment can lead to formation of cancer. Chronic exposure to chemicals (tar, tobacco), mechanical repeated trauma, heat, and infection are therefore dangerous when they expose the tissue over weeks or years.

Nordenström adds: "I have introduced my method in several countries. Chinese doctors have performed over 1,000 treatments of cancer patients with the method with good results."

At American Biologics hospital in Tijuana, a bioelectric therapy called *accelerated-charge neutralization (ACN)* is used as part of a metabolic approach to treating cancer. The rationale behind ACN is that cancer cells carry a negative electrical charge that enables them to avoid immune surveillance. By replacing the negative charge with a positive one, ACN is said to draw the immune system's tumor-destroying cells to the area to attack the cancer. In ACN treatment, a positive electrode— an electrically insulated platinum wire—is placed directly into the tumor. The negative return is an inserted platinum probe or a saline soaked conductive sponge in contact with the leg or other nonrelated body part. ACN machines have been used to destroy tumors and to reduce their size. American Biologics considers ACN a way to attack tumors without surgery, not a cure for the tissue.

Magnetic-field therapy to treat various disorders including cancer has been practiced with reported successes in Europe, India, and the United States. The devices range from tiny magnets taped directly on the skin to magnetic pads to pulsed magnetic-field generators. The use of magnetic fields to treat cancer has "a long and shady history" involving outright fraud and very few serious scientific or clinical studies, observes Dr. Robert Becker. He warns that the application of pulsed electromagnetic fields (PEMF) to treat cancer could *promote* the growth of cancer cells instead of inhibiting them. In the past few years, PEMF treatment has reportedly slowed the growth of animal tumors and prolonged survival time, but Becker believes these experiments are deceptive because the immune response is only temporarily boosted and may be followed by enhanced tumor growth.[5]

"More harm than good is presently being done in applying biomagnetic fields," says Jesse Partridge, who gives lectures and workshops on magnetic therapy around the country. "These methods can be disastrous if improperly used." Partridge, a retired laboratory supervisor from Torrance, California, suggests that anyone contemplating magnetic therapy in any form should be extremely careful. "It's important to learn from someone who knows what happens, why it happens, and how it happens. Anyone of less knowledge is very apt to mislead you."

In *The Body Magnetic* (see Resources), Buryl Payne, Ph.D., urges caution in the application of magnetic fields and advises against home treatment. He states that unless the proper polarity and configuration are selected, serious harm could result. "Incorrect polarity could make a tumor grow more vigorously." Payne warns, "Do not treat tumors, cancerous conditions, or infections with biomagnetic south pole fields." He says magnetic therapy is not a substitute for medical treatment but may serve as an adjunct to dietary, biochemical, or physical forms of treatment. Payne describes a doctor in North Carolina who "successfully treated three cases of breast cancer using super strong Neomax magnets from Japan."[6]

William Philpott, M.D., of Choctaw, Oklahoma, has found negative (north pole) magnetic-field energy of value in treating cancer and other degenerative diseases. (A magnet's true north pole is identified as electromagnetic negative by a magnetometer.) One of Dr. Philpott's cases involved a twenty-year-old male student diagnosed by conventional techniques with a deadly brain tumor, a glioblastoma, that had infiltrated the brain tissue so extensively, it could not be surgically removed. The north pole of a solid-state ceramic magnet was placed on the back of the patient's head where the tumor had initially started growing, and the negative magnetic-field treatment was continued twenty-four hours a day. When first seen by Philpott at the American Biologics hospital in Tijuana, Mexico, this patient was incapable of making any response to environmental stimuli. After three days of magnetic treatment, he was able to wiggle his fingers in response to questions. In three weeks, he walked out of the hospital with the assistance of only a walker. The patient was reported to be well six months later except for a residual imbalance problem, and he continues magnetic-field exposure of the brain five hours a day, according to Philpott. "We cannot say the magnetic therapy was the only thing done to this patient, but all persons involved were convinced that magnetic therapy reversed the tumor."[7]

Philpott writes, "If I had cancer, I would make sure the cancerous area was in a negative magnetic field as many hours of the day and night as I could arrange, and never less than one hour three times a day. This negative magnetic field exposure can be arranged by using a flat magnet poled on opposite sides which thus allows the capacity of exposure to one magnetic pole only." Like other biomagnetic practitioners, Philpott has found that negative (north pole) magnetic energy heals. He makes no claim of statistical or scientific proof that this energy can reverse cancer, but he cites the work of the late Dr. Albert Roy Davis, who claimed to use the same energy from a bar magnet to destroy transplanted tumors in animals. Walter Rawls, Jr., who was Davis's collaborator, now heads Biomagnetics International of Orange Park, Florida, which is continuing research into the use of magnetic fields to arrest and kill cancer cells.

Proponents believe that magnetic fields promote healing by operating simultaneously on many levels—at the subatomic, atomic, ionic, molecular, and cellular levels—and in the organs, the circulatory and nervous systems, and the electrical biofield surrounding the body. Experiments with biomagnetic fields have demonstrated such effects as increased blood flow, more oxygen in the blood, changes in the rate of cell division, and enhanced enzyme activity. Magnetic-field therapy is also said to stimulate the thymus and the lymphatic system to produce more T-lymphocytes, vital to immune defense.

From Russia comes Microwave Resonance Therapy (MRT), a high-frequency, low-intensity electromagnetic treatment that is applied to specific acupuncture points to treat an entire acupuncture meridian. (In Chinese acupuncture, meridians are channels that carry chi, or subtle energy, to the various blood vessels, nerves, and organs of the body.) MRT treatment is said to lead the body to regulate itself into *homeostasis,* or physiological equilibrium. Developed by Professor Sergei Sitko, Ph.D., a physicist, MRT has reportedly been used to treat over 8,000 people in what was the USSR for various illnesses, including peptic ulcer, cancer, cerebral palsy, infectious diseases, diabetes mellitus, and chronic pain. For more information, contact the World Research Foundation (see page xviii for the address and phone number).

Electromagnetic fields can have either a positive or a harmful effect. Used correctly, they can be healing in certain conditions. On the other hand, the abnormal, manmade electromagnetic radiation from high-voltage transmission lines, broadcast towers, and other sources in our increasingly polluted environment has been linked to cancer. The hazards of environmental electropollution are real. People with cancer who live in close proximity to electric power cables, radio or television broadcast towers, or other major sources of electropollution should give serious consideration to moving away from the unhealthy exposure. Electromagnetic radiation from common household appliances and wiring may also pose risks.

Many studies have linked exposure to manmade electromagnetic fields with increases in the incidence of certain cancers, developmental abnormalities in embryos, and increases in the rate of cancer-cell division. Recent books dealing with electropollution include *Currents of Death,* by Paul Brodeur (Simon and Schuster, 1230 Avenue of the Americas, New York, NY 10020, 800-223-2336), *Cross Currents: The Perils of Electropollution, the Promise of Electromedicine,* by Robert O. Becker (see Resources), and *The Healthy House: How to Buy One, How to Build One and How to Cure a "Sick" One,* by John Bower (Carol Publishing Group, 600 Madison Avenue, New York, NY 10022, 212-486-2200).

Resources

Björn Nordenström, M.D.
Solnav, 1
S104-01
Stockholm, Sweden
Phone: 011 46 834-0560

For further information on Nordenström's electrotherapy and details on treatment.

American Biologics–Mexico
    Hospital and Medical Center
1180 Walnut Avenue
Chula Vista, CA 92011
Phone: 619-429-8200
        800-227-4458

For further information on accelerated-charge neutralization and details on treatment.

Bio Health Enterprises, Inc.
P.O. Box 628
Murray Hill, KY 42071
Phone: 502-753-2613
        800-626-3386

For magnets, books, and other materials as well as a subscription to Bio Energy Health Newsletter, *information on workshops, and seminars on magnetism and health topics.*

Phoenix Books
3110 North High Street
Columbus, OH 43202
Phone: 614-268-3100

For books on bioelectric therapies, magnetism, and many other health topics.

Reading Material

Cross Currents: The Perils of Electropollution, the Promise of Electro-medicine, by Robert O. Becker, M.D., Jeremy P. Tarcher (5858 Wilshire Boulevard, Suite 200, Los Angeles, CA 90036; 800-225-3362), 1990.

Vibrational Medicine: New Choices for Healing Ourselves, by Richard Gerber, M.D., Bear and Company (506 Agua Fria Street, Santa Fe, NM 87501; 800-932-3277), 1988.

Energy Medicine, by Laurence Badgley, M.D., Human Energy Press (1020 Foster City Boulevard, Suite 205, Foster City, CA 94404; 415-349-0718), 1987.

The Cancer Cure That Worked: Fifty Years of Suppression, by Barry Lynes, Marcus Books (distributed in the United States by Vitamart, K-Mart Plaza, Route 10, Randolph, NJ 07869; 201-366-4494), 1987. The story of the Rife microscope and Rife generator.

The Body Magnetic, written and published by Buryl Payne, Ph.D., (Santa Cruz, California), revised edition, 1990. Available at health-food stores and alternative book stores.

Cancer Prevention and Reversal, by William Philpott, M.D., Philpott Medical Services (distributed by Envirotech Products, 17171 Southeast 29th Street, Choctaw, OK 73020; 800-445-1962), 1990.

What Your Doctor Won't Tell You, by Jane Heimlich, HarperCollins Publishers (10 East 53rd Street, New York, NY 10022; 800-242-7737), 1990. Includes sections on electrodiagnostics and energy medicine.

"Healing Cancer With Electricity," by Albert Huebner, *East West Journal,* May 1990. On Nordenström's electrotherapy.

"An Electrifying Possibility," by Gary Tauber, *Discover,* April 1986. On Dr. Nordenström.

Chapter 26

HOMEOPATHY

Homeopathy is a medical system that uses microdoses, or minute dilutions, of natural substances from the plant, mineral, and animal kingdoms to stimulate a person's natural healing response. The word *homeopathy,* coined by the system's founder, German physician Samuel Hahnemann (1755–1843), comes from the Greek *homois* and *pathos,* meaning "similar sickness." The basic principle of homeopathy is the Law of Similars, or "like is cured by like." According to this law, a natural substance that causes the symptoms of a sickness in a healthy person can *cure* the same sickness in an unhealthy person when used in a highly diluted form.

A common example is ipecac, a preparation made from the dried roots of a tropical plant. Taken in large quantities, ipecac causes vomiting—but taken in minute quantities, it stops vomiting. Homeopaths often prescribe microdoses of ipecac for women intending to become pregnant in the near future. During pregnancy, these same women very rarely experience the nausea and vomiting of morning sickness.

Disease, from the homeopathic perspective, is an expression of the life process, not a separate entity or an isolated target. A disease is the manifestation of a constitutional weakness coming through the weakest point in the body. A person is not "an asthmatic"; rather, he or she has a fundamental disequilibrium that manifests as respiratory trouble involving the lungs. Likewise, cancer is viewed as a symptom of an underlying imbalance that may be the result of poor diet, chronic exposure to toxins, genetic disposition, repressed emotions, repressive ideas, or other factors. With all sickness, the aim of homeopathic treatment is to strengthen the whole organism's ability to heal itself and to regain homeostasis, or equilibrium.

Symptoms, to the homeopath, are adaptive responses, natural reactions produced by the body in its efforts to heal itself. Symptoms are the body's way of externalizing disease; they dissipate energy like ripples on a pond and enable harmony to be restored. Homeopaths attempt to "go with" these natural reactions by strengthening the body's defenses, instead of attempting to suppress the symptoms.

Hahnemann coined the term *allopathy* (derived from the Greek words meaning "different from the sickness") to describe orthodox medicine, which aggressively attempts to suppress disease symptoms with drugs. From the homeopathic standpoint, when conventional drugs suppress symptoms, they also suppress the body's defense mechanisms. While the symptoms may vanish, the underlying imbalance that created them will often manifest itself somewhere else—much like pushing down on one area of a balloon causes it to bulge out in another spot.

In treating a patient, a homeopath attempts to determine which one substance produces effects that most closely resemble the symptoms of the disease and therefore is most capable of reversing the condition. By means of a thorough interview, the homeopath builds a constitutional picture of the individual, taking into account his or her habits, temperament, and mental attitude, along with the exact nature of the physical complaint. The specific remedy prescribed is matched to this picture. Often, as the person responds to the medicine, a new fundamental picture will emerge, so that a new medicine, or series of medicines, will be required to complete the curative process.

A mysterious and controversial aspect of homeopathy is that the more a medicine is diluted, the greater is its potency. Hahnemann developed the process of *potentization,* in which a medicine is diluted a number of times with distilled water or ethyl alcohol and vigorously shaken between dilutions. Over the past 200 years, homeopaths have observed that the more a medicine is diluted in this fashion, the longer it generally acts, the deeper it heals, and the fewer doses tend to be needed.[1] A highly diluted remedy may not contain even a single molecule of the original substance. The power of the "infinitesimal dose" has subjected homeopathy to ridicule from mainstream medicine. However, homeopaths reply that even if a substance contains no molecules of the original solution, *something* remains—an essence of the original substance, its resonance, energy, or pattern. Besides, they say, even if they don't fully understand the mechanism of the microdose, *it works,* as confirmed by two centuries of clinical experience and a growing body of scientific evidence.

In one remarkable experiment, Australian physicist Paul Callinan demonstrated that a substance leaves behind "footprints" even after it has been greatly diluted. After he froze homeopathic-remedy tinctures to −200°C (−328°F), they crystallized into snowflake patterns that differed for each remedy. The more he diluted a tincture, the *clearer* its pattern became. Quantum physics has discovered that substances leave behind energy fields, and this may provide a clue to the workings of potentization. Dr. Callinan recently presented his theory of the infinitesimal-dose phenomenon to the Australian parliament. He speculates that homeopathic dilution (potentization) imparts energy to the body's water molecules, restructuring body fluids, which in turn modifies enzyme activity.[2]

Homeopaths speak of medicines "resonating" with the patient's "vital force," or "life force." Each person is conceived as being a bioenergy system, vibrating at a certain frequency on both a bodily and a cellular level. An imbalance in vibration represents a disturbance of the life force, the self-healing process of the organism. The correct remedy is a "booster shot" of subtle energy, returning the organism to its proper vibrational frequency by imprinting an energy pattern on the body's fluids or cells. If the prescribed remedy does not have a "resonant frequency" matching the disturbance, it misses the "center of gravity" of the illness and supposedly nothing happens.

The vital force of homeopathy is similar to the force called *chi* in Chinese medicine, *ki* in Japan, *bioplasm* in Russian laboratories, and *prana* in Indian Ayurvedic medicine. Homeopathy, a form of bioenergetic medicine, is actually the oldest holistic system in the modern scientific era. Using nontoxic substances, it attempts to heal in a gentle and profound manner by stimulating the body's vital force to cure itself.

Mainstream, or allopathic, medicine has not only borrowed many remedies from homeopathy but also applies homeopathic principles to treat disease. Immunization is based on the Law of Similars. Smallpox, for example, can be prevented by administering small doses of a similar but less serious disease, cowpox, to people. The "father of immunology," Dr. Emil Adolph von Behring, directly acknowledged the roots of immunology when he asserted, "By what technical term could we more appropriately speak of this influence than by Hahnemann's word 'homeopathy'?"[3]

Nitroglycerine, used by conventional doctors today to treat heart conditions and migraine headaches, was introduced for these purposes around 1850 by Dr. Constantine Hering, the "father of American homeopathy." Today, allergists unknowingly practice the Law of Similars by treating patients allergic to ragweed with a diluted solution of ragweed. Homeopathic physicians have long used minuscule doses of ergot, a poisonous fungus of rye, to treat gangrene, Raynaud's disease, and other circulatory disorders as well as migraines. An alert pharmaceutical company developed Hydergine, an ergot-based proprietary drug, to treat disease caused by arterial constriction. Recently, ergot made its way into "modern medicine" in two proprietary synthetic drugs to treat migraines, methysergide maleate and ergotamine tartrate. Many more examples of allopathy's borrowings from homeopathy could be given.

Cancer can be treated homeopathically and halted, or even cured, depending on how far the disease has progressed, according to various practicing homeopaths. Homeopathic treatment is intended to restore the cancer patient's immune apparatus to maximum health. Some patients have shown regression or disappearance of tumors and control of metastatic processes. Homeopathic medication has reportedly turned inoperable tumors into operable masses.[4] In many cases, it has prolonged survival, affording symptomatic relief, reduced pain, and a better quality of life.

There is no single remedy for treating cancer in homeopathy. A homeopath treats the patient, as shown by the totality of his or her symptoms, instead of treating the disease. Prescribing is a highly individualized science and art, based on the homeopath's assessment of the patient's major symptoms, minor complaints, and other physical and psychological factors. Yet the homeopathic practitioner does draw on an extensive body of research literature, which includes *drug provings*. Provings provide a detailed record of the pattern and range of symptoms that each medicine produced in healthy individuals, along with the therapeutic action on sick individuals. As an aid to prescribing, some homeopaths use computer programs that match a patient's symptoms to medicines that can cause (and cure) the majority of these symptoms.

People with cancer should seek professional homeopathic (or other) care. Homeopathy is *not* recommended as a self-care option for cancer patients. Homeopathic medicines may not be appropriate for some severe or life-threatening conditions. Surgical intervention may be indicated in many cases. At a minimum, the cancer patient interested in homeopathy should first consult an oncologist to determine his or her prospects under conventional treatment.

Homeopathy can serve as a complementary treatment in cancer and other chronic or acute illnesses. Some patients use individualized homeopathic remedies to minimize the side effects of the conventional treatment methods. A homeopath might administer medicines to alleviate pain, nausea, and other reactions.

Alternately, a potentized (diluted) dose of the allopathic chemotherapy drug is sometimes given to patients. With proper instructions, a patient can self-administer it. However, according to Dana Ullman, director of Homeopathic Educational Services in Berkeley, California, "There is not enough clinical experience to know how helpful this procedure is. Some homeopaths say it's beneficial because it inhibits the harmful side effects of the chemotherapy drug, but it may also inhibit the drug's anti-cancer action."

Opinions differ over whether patients have a better chance for survival if they use only homeopathy. "There are risks of using homeopathy alone, just as there are risks of using conventional medicine alone, or of combining the two approaches," says Ullman. "It's important for the patient to understand the risks and potential benefits of each approach before deciding on what treatment or treatments to follow." Some practitioners argue that combining homeopathy with other healing modalities can cloud the overall picture of symptoms, thereby preventing an accurate appraisal of the person and of the healing process. In contrast, eclectic homeopaths combine their craft with other approaches such as nutritional programs and vitamin therapy.

Just how successful is homeopathy in treating cancer patients? According to homeopath William Gray, M.D., of the Hahnemann Medical Clinic in Berkeley, homeopathy's "cure rate of early stage cancer runs around eighty percent. If it's later stage, that drops to forty or fifty percent."[5] If the cancer becomes metastasized, treatment is more difficult and few patients are cured. In persons already treated by radiation, chemotherapy, or surgery, Dr. Gray says, homeopathy can build up health and resistance. In terminal cases, he claims, homeopathy can improve the patient's condition, prolong life, and relieve suffering "without clouding the patient's mind with dope."

Dr. Gray points out that the Hahnemann Medical Clinic does not treat cancer "because in California, non-toxic treatment of cancer is illegal. . . . In California, the only legal treatment for cancer—by *any* physician—is radiation, surgery, and chemotherapy—all of which are poisonous or violently destructive to the body. . . . In California we have to wait until the damage has been done and the cancer has been removed or poisoned. For people who can't leave the state, I'm forced to recommend surgery, then offer to help them pick up the pieces with homeopathy."

Dr. Gray's claimed remission rates for homeopathy are met with skepticism by many people—including many homeopaths who believe that homeopathy is of limited value in curing cancer. The figures he cites resemble those given over forty years ago by Arthur Grimmer, M.D., a Chicago homeopath who treated many cancer patients. In a 1950 article in the *Journal of the American Institute of Homeopathy*, Dr. Grimmer claimed that "at least 95 percent" of patients in a precancerous condition could be cured, approximately 75 percent of people in early or incipient stages of the disease could get well, and about 10 percent of patients in advanced stages could be restored to health. Many advanced or terminal patients given homeopathic medication "will respond to treatment and live in apparent health and comfort for ten or fifteen years, and then die of cancer but without suffering," Dr. Grimmer stated.[6] His article presents a number of case histories, including that of a cancer patient whom he brought to complete remission for seven years after initial diagnosis and that of another patient whom he brought to complete remission for twelve years after diagnosis. He observed that "homeopathic literature abounds with accounts of notable cures" of cancer.

Earlier, Dr. Grimmer had reported on a study of 225 cancer patients treated strictly by homeopathic methods. Two-thirds of them had survived six years at the time of writing, and these patients "give every sign of living many years."[7] Grimmer emphasized the importance of good diet and avoidance of all irritating or harmful foods, a prescription echoed by many contemporary homeopaths.

Another view of the cancer patient's prospects under homeopathic treatment comes from a study of 27 cancer victims.[8] A total of 10 of these patients was diagnosed with terminal cancer of the breast or the intestine before the start of homeopathic treatment. Most had prior surgery, X-ray therapy, or radium treatment. Of the 10 terminal cases, 1 patient, who had a skin melanoma, lost all signs of cancer under homeopathic care alone and had survived five years at the time of writing. In the group of 27 patients, 14 died of their cancer. Most patients experienced subjective relief.

A fifty-nine-year-old man was diagnosed in the early 1980s with small-cell lung cancer, an especially lethal form of the disease. The average survival if the patient is left untreated is six to seventeen weeks from the time of diagnosis. As reported in *Thorax* in 1989, the man lived for five years seven months after diagnosis as a result of homeopathic medicine and the use of the herb mistletoe.[9] Mistletoe extract, or Iscador (Chapter 11), is used by many homeopathic doctors in the treatment of solid tumors. It is potentized according to the homeopathic rules for dilution. It is usually administered by injection, whereas most homeopathic medicines are in tablet form and are dissolved slowly under the tongue.

Symptoms of terminal cancer and of AIDS were eliminated in groups of patients treated homeopathically in various studies undertaken in Greece, as reported at the Second International Symposium on Cancer and AIDS, held in Cyprus in September 1989.[10] The homeopathic medicines were used alone or as part of "parallel" therapy with orthodox approaches. In one study, twenty-one cases with pancreatic cancer—a particularly deadly form of the disease— were given parallel therapy; 48 percent of the patients were alive after two years, whereas no patients (0 percent) had a two-year survival in a matched control group of twenty-one pancreatic cancer patients treated with orthodox medicine alone.

The treatment of twelve HIV-infected patients by homeopathy alone was reported by Drs. Petroula Drossou and Athos Othonos. Three of the patients had full-blown AIDS, four had ARC, and five were HIV-positive with swollen lymph glands. The patients, who were followed over a two-year period, had no prior therapy and received no conventional treatments during the course of their homeopathic programs. All twelve showed a complete remission of symptoms, and all returned to normal numbers of T4 ("helper") cells, indicating restored immune functioning.

Another speaker at the Cyprus conference, Dr. Spiro Diamantidis, described how a patient with liver cancer achieved remission through homeopathy alone, with each change in the patient's predisposition dictating a change in the specific remedy used. Dr. Diamantidis is president of the Medical Institute for Homoeopathic Research and Application (MIHRA) in Athens. MIHRA documents and computerizes homeopathic results in cooperation with the Greek government.

According to Diamantidis, "Many cases of significant relief, inhibition of the disease, and cure" have been reported, "mainly in cases of early-stage breast cancer, cancer of the uterus, primary cancer of the lungs, the stomach, the intestine and the liver."[11]

Research conducted by MIHRA over the last few years has convinced Dr. Diamantidis that the majority of cancer patients have personalities that fall into one of two categories. One personality type is strong and rigid. These people tend to dominate their environment. They lead intense lives, whether professionally, socially, or sexually, and usually exceed their limits. At some point, they break down, or react to a severe psychological shock, and this collapse, according to Diamantidis, creates the prerequisite conditions for cancer to develop.

The second cancer-prone personality type adopts a passive social profile, such as the "good and sympathetic fellow" who never protests and always behaves with dignity. People like this tend to hide their emotions. Prolonged suppression of the emotions and an inability to let off steam, according to Dr. Diamantidis, predisposes them to pathological processes including cancer.

Belgian homeopath Dr. Bernard Marichal developed a homeopathic treatment called Immujem therapy, which he has used against cancer and AIDS. Immujem therapy includes homeopathically potentized doses of RNA, DNA, the immunosuppressant Cyclosporine, and a rabbit antibody called Polypeptide Anti-Atypies (PAA). PAA reportedly helps destroy abnormal cells in cancer patients, and in AIDS patients, it combats the AIDS virus. Dr. Marichal and his team of Belgian doctors have treated over 450 HIV-positive patients with Immujem therapy. They have found it to be effective in boosting the immune system, eliminating fever and diarrhea, and greatly reducing the opportunistic infections associated with AIDS.[12]

For a fuller discussion of the homeopathic treatment of AIDS, read Dana Ullman's *Discovering Homeopathy: Your Introduction to the Science and Art of Homeopathic Medicine* (see Resources).

In 1989, Professor N. Ramayya of India published a compilation of the case reports of fifty cancer patients successfully treated with homeopathy.[13] The majority of these persons were treated during the 1970s and '80s, though some cases went back as far as 1949. "Homeopathy is elegant in therapeutics and radical in symptom analysis, if the results are periodically analyzed and reviewed," comments Dr. Ramayya. However, the editor of *Homoeopathic Heritage,* in which Ramayya's detailed report appears, states in an introductory note, "I am sorry I have not been lucky to *cure* cancer cases, though quite a number have been remarkably helped."

Most mainstream doctors in the United States still hold homeopathy to be highly suspect if not outright quackery. Yet, in 1900, nearly one-fourth of all American physicians subscribed to the homeopathic discipline. Homeopathy was taught in 22 American homeopathic medical colleges and practiced in over 100 homeopathic hospitals, with more than 1,000 homeopathic pharmacies filling prescriptions across the nation. The homeopathic physician enjoyed the same status as the allopathic doctor. Over 30 homeopathic medical journals were published, and state homeopathic medical societies regulated practice, including licensing.

Among the supporters of homeopathy were Mark Twain, Henry James,

Louisa May Alcott, Horace Greeley, William James, and Henry Wadsworth Longfellow. Especially popular among the educated, the science of microdoses was also in wide use among the poor. Among the rich, John D. Rockefeller, who was ninety-eight when he died in 1937, never allowed anyone except homeopathic physicians to treat him.

A major reason homeopathy became popular in the United States and Europe in the 1800s was its success in treating that era's severe infectious epidemics, including cholera, typhoid, yellow fever, and scarlet fever. Compared with those of conventional medicine, the homeopathic death rates were lower and the successful therapeutic results were always greater. In American homeopathic hospitals, the death rates from these epidemics were often one-half to one-eighth those in orthodox hospitals.[14] Homeopaths' success in combating the yellow fever epidemic of 1878 that ravaged the South was so impressive that homeopathy gained a foothold in the region. Skeptics often dismiss effective homeopathic treatments as the result of a placebo effect, but it is hard to imagine how placebos could have successfully treated these deadly infectious diseases.

By the 1840s, homeopathy was successfully competing with orthodox medicine. In 1844, the first national medical association in the United States, the American Institute of Homeopathy, was formed. However, in 1847, the American Medical Association followed suit. A trade union of allopathic doctors, the AMA was organized with the undisguised goal of smashing homeopathy in the United States. According to its charter, one of its goals is "to eliminate the competition, specifically homeopathy."

In 1855, the AMA established a "consultation clause" in its "code of ethics" whereby members would be expelled if they even so much as consulted with a homeopath or any other "nonregular" practitioner. In some states, doctors who were thus blackballed in effect had no legal status to practice medicine, and members of the medical monopoly would then arrange to have them arrested for practicing medicine without a license.

The AMA labeled homeopathy "a delusion" and stepped up its witchhunt against homeopaths, who were booted out of state medical associations in what the *New York Times,* on June 7, 1873, called "unjust, unfair, and abusive" expulsions. By this time, an alliance had been forged between allopathic medicine and the chemical (drug) industry, which would prove to be the most profitable arrangement of modern times. The pharmaceutical industry fully supported the AMA's campaign to destroy homeopathy, well aware that enormous profits could be made from the manufacture and marketing of proprietary medicines. By 1906, all but one medical journal was subsidized by drug companies' advertising, and the allopathic physician in effect became a conscripted sales representative.

Homeopathy, in contrast, was not a lucrative business. Microdoses are very small, and individualizing remedies to meet a patient's specific symptoms is time-consuming.

In 1910, the Carnegie Foundation issued the Flexner Report, an appraisal of American medical schools written by Abraham Flexner in collaboration with the AMA. While seemingly objective, the report laid down guidelines that sanctioned orthodox schools over the homeopathic colleges. The report gave low marks to the homeopathic schools, whose graduates were then barred from taking medical licensing exams. The homeopathic schools lost their federal and private funding, and the gentle but powerful medical science of microdoses faded into oblivion, practiced by a tiny minority of lay and allopathic physicians.

Meanwhile, homeopathy continued to flourish in Europe and elsewhere. Great Britain's Royal Family is still treated by a homeopathic physician, and Queen Elizabeth II travels everywhere with a homeopathic first-aid kit. A 1986 survey in the *British Medical Journal* revealed that 42 percent of the British doctors surveyed refer patients to homeopathic physicians. A similar survey by the *Times* of London put the figure at 48 percent. In France, one-third of the population has tried, or is presently using, homeopathic medicines, and six French medical schools offer courses in homeopathy leading to a degree. Homeopathy is also widely practiced in Germany, the Netherlands, Italy, Brazil, Argentina, Greece, and South Africa. India has over 100 homeopathic medical colleges, which, like their allopathic counterparts, offer a four- or five-year program of study.

Homeopathy is currently enjoying a resurgence of interest in the United States. There are an estimated 1,500 physicians who specialize in homeopathy and another 1,000 health professionals—including dentists, podiatrists, nurses, naturopaths, and veterinarians—who use homeopathic medicines. In most states, there is no licensing per se for homeopaths. Homeopathy as a medical practice is performed under the license of one of the other accepted forms of medicine, so a homeopath must also have qualified for a chiropractic, osteopathic, or acupuncture license, or else be a Doctor of Medicine (M.D.). In Arizona, Connecticut, and Nevada, homeopathy is recognized and regulated by state homeopathic boards, which are independent of the boards that regulate conventional medical practitioners. Everyone who applies to one of these three state boards must be a Doctor of Medicine.

The efficacy of homeopathic medicine has been observed in practice with severely ill people and animals as well as in experiments with animals, plants, yeast, and bacteria. New research on the action of microdoses is being done by scientists in such fields as quantum mechanics, biophysics, and electromagnetic energy.

The prestigious British medical journal *The Lancet* recently reported on a double-blind study that showed *nearly twice as many patients* given a homeopathic medicine recovered from the flu within forty-eight hours as did patients given a placebo. One study involved 487 subjects. After the study's original publication in 1989 in the *British Journal of Clinical Pharmacology*,[15] the editors of *The Lancet* were so impressed with how rigorously it had been conducted, they reported on the results in detail in their own journal.

An immune-response experiment conducted in four countries in the 1980s also seems to support homeopathy. In this research, an antibody solution so diluted that not a single molecule of it could still be present altered the chemistry and internal structure of white blood cells. This series of experiments, led by French immunologist Jacques Bienveniste of the University of Paris, was reported in the respected British journal *Nature* in 1988.[16] The article carried an unprecedented disclaimer by the journal's editors. Peter Newmark, *Nature*'s deputy editor, said that if the reported results were true, "we will have to abandon two centuries of observation and rational thinking about biology, because this can't be explained by ordinary physical laws." He added that the results of the experiment were particularly objectionable because they seemed to "symbolically" support homeopathy.

Nature then sent a team of "ghostbusters"—among them the outspoken magician James Randi—to investigate Bienveniste's laboratory. Under this team's close observation, the experiment was completed seven times. In four runs out of the seven (including three test runs), the microdoses *did* have action. However, based on this, the debunking team announced that the microdoses had *no* action. They overlooked a central fact of experiments in immunology: white blood cells are not always sensitive to large doses of antibodies, let alone to microdoses of them. Bienveniste presented fresh experiments supporting the action of infinitesimal microdoses in an article published in the journal of the French Academy of Sciences in early 1991.

Persons interested in a homeopathic practitioner should determine the amount of training the homeopath received and what kind of results he or she enjoys. Homeopathy is a rigorous art and science that requires many years of disciplined study. Find out, if possible, how much experience the practitioner has had in treating cancer patients and what the outcomes have generally been. If the homeopath also practices conventional medicine, find out what percentage of patients he or she treats with homeopathy—the higher the percentage, the better.

It is important to determine how much time the practitioner spends with patients. The first visit should last roughly one hour to an hour and a half. The initial interview should consist of inquiries and probes designed to reveal a detailed picture of symptoms. Follow-up interviews should last approximately half an hour. If the homeopath spends less time than this, careful individualizing of the correct medicine is not possible.

A good practitioner may ask all sorts of seemingly inconsequential questions that in fact will provide important clues to selecting your constitutional remedy. Seek a practitioner who is interested in your functioning on all levels, including the physical, emotional, and mental.

Resources

Homeopathic Educational
  Services
2124 Kittredge Street
Berkeley, CA 94704
Phone: 510-649-0294

For further information on home-opathy, books, tapes, software, and a directory of licensed health professionals in the United States who practice homeopathy.

International Foundation
  for Homeopathy
2366 Eastlake Avenue East
Suite 301
Seattle, WA 98102
Phone: 206-324-8230

For further information on home-opathy.

National Center for
  Homeopathy
801 North Fairfax
Suite 306
Alexandria, VA 22314
Phone: 703-548-7790

For books, pamphlets, and educational materials on homeopathy as well as a directory of licensed health professionals in the United States who practice homeopathy.

Reading Material

Discovering Homeopathy: Your Introduction to the Science and Art of Homeopathic Medicine, by Dana Ullman, North Atlantic Books (2800 Woolsey Street, Berkeley, CA 94705; 510-652-5309), 1991. The best introduction to homeopathy for the general reader.

Catching Good Health With Homeopathic Medicine, by Raymond Garrett and TaRessa Stone, CRCS Publications (P.O. Box 1460, Sebastopol, CA 95472; 707-829-0735), 1990.

Homeopathy: Medicine That Works! by Robert S. Wood, Condor Books (Pollock Pines, California), 1990. Out of print; available from Homeopathic Educational Services (see page 291 for address and phone number).

The Science of Homeopathy, by George Vithoulkas, Grove Press (841 Broadway, New York, NY 10003-4793; 800-521-0178), 1980.

Bioenergetic Medicines East and West: Acupuncture and Homeopathy, by Clark A. Manning and Louis Vanrenen, North Atlantic Books (2800 Woolsey Street, Berkeley, CA 94705; 510-652-5309), 1988.

Cancer: Its Causes, Symptoms, and Treatment, by Eli G. Jones, M.D., B. Jain Publishers Ltd. (New Delhi, India), reprinted, 1989. Available by special order from Homeopathic Educational Services (see page 291 for address and phone number).

Homeopathic Insight Into Cancer: Causes, Treatment and Cure, by Dr. Sultan Alam M. Bihari, B. Jain Publishers Ltd. (New Delhi, India), 1982. Available by special order from Homeopathic Educational Services (see page 291 for address and phone number).

Chapter 27

AYURVEDA

Ayurveda, perhaps the oldest existing medical system, has been practiced in India for over 6,000 years. Ayurveda literally means "the science of life." This mind-body healing system recognizes that most diseases involve both physical and mental factors and require a holistic treatment of the entire human being. Its branches encompass general medicine, surgery, pediatrics, gynecology, obstetrics, ophthalmology, geriatrics, and otorhinolaryngology (ears, nose, and throat). Part of the ancient Vedic science, which includes yoga and meditation, Ayurveda combines a variety of methods such as herbal medicine, therapeutic diet, massage, detoxification, and breathing exercises.

Although Ayurveda was, until recently, almost unknown in the West, a growing number of medical doctors in the United States have incorporated it into their clinical practice, usually as an adjunct to their basic services. In India, where over 300,000 doctors are registered to practice Ayurvedic medicine, 150 Ayurvedic colleges grant a degree after a five-year program, with postgraduate specialization offered at many, much as in Western allopathic medical schools.

At Benares Hindu University in India, doctors use an age-old Ayurvedic herbal remedy to break up and remove kidney stones without surgery. At Hyderabad's National Institute of Nutrition, doctors advise diabetics to eat a diet rich in *methi seeds* (fenugreek), which decreases insulin dependency in many patients. At the Jawaharlal Nehru Centre for Ophthalmology in Sitapur, Indian scientists use plant extracts to cure trachoma (a viral infection of the cornea and conjunctiva) and to treat glaucoma. Reserpine, the antihypertensive drug familiar to many in the West, is derived from a native Indian climbing shrub *(Rauwolfia serpentina)*, which was described in ancient Ayurvedic texts as a remedy for hypertension and insomnia. Dr. B. S. Blumberg, winner of a Nobel

Prize in medicine, recently published a study in *The Lancet* reporting
an effective treatment for the hepatitis B virus using a plant "described in Indian Ayurvedic literature more than 2,000 years ago" to
treat jaundice.[1]

Ayurveda is a lifestyle and a philosophy as well as a medicine. Its
emphasis is on preventing disease, maintaining good health by enhancing immune function, and promoting longevity. Besides preventing illness, Ayurveda is also used to treat a wide range of
ailments, including cancer, AIDS, digestive and respiratory disorders, heart disease, nervous-system disorders, and mental illness.
There are documented cases of cancer patients brought into remission through Ayurveda, either as a primary or a complementary
therapy. In many other cases, tumors were reduced in size and
patients experienced relief from pain.

Ayurveda, which mostly uses plant substances in its medicines, is
a noninvasive, nontoxic approach free from the adverse side effects
that so often accompany chemotherapy and radiation. There are no
statistics available on what percentage of patients in the United States
recover or benefit from Ayurvedic treatment. In Bombay, India, Dr.
Natwarlal Joshi, an allopath who also practices Ayurveda, has treated
some 460 cancer patients since 1973 using Ayurvedic herbal remedies. In a paper presented in 1989 at the Fifth Biennial Conference
of the Indian Association of Cancer Chemotherapists, Dr. Joshi
reported on 422 cancer patients who had been "given up as terminal
cases" by conventional medicine after treatment with surgery, radiation, chemotherapy, or a combination of these modalities. He said
he obtained "complete relief with prolongation of life" in 70 patients,
fair results (symptomatic relief) in 262 cases, and poor results (no
response) in 90 patients. The plant extracts were ingested, applied
externally, administered by intramuscular injection, or given in enemas. No patients had any harmful side effects. Among those whom
Dr. Joshi treated successfully were a man with a deadly brain tumor
(astrocytoma, Stage III) who had been rejected for further treatment
by Tata Hospital in Bombay; a woman with advanced carcinoma of
the larynx; and patients with advanced lung cancer, osteosarcoma,
cervical metastatic tumor, and cancer of the pancreas, stomach,
breast, and esophagus. Dr. Joshi's results are documented in a twenty-
four-page paper with clinical photographs, reproductions of X-rays
and CAT scans, and hospital records.[2]

In Ayurveda, cancer represents a negative life energy, something
like a parasite that has taken hold in the body. Cancer cells, lacking

oxygen, constitute a growth asserting itself outside the rule of the life force. In their mindless multiplication, cancer cells have lost touch with their basic intelligence, the know-how at the genetic level that regulates cell division. From the Ayurvedic perspective, cancer has many causes, including our toxic environment, devitalized foods, negative emotions, sedentary lifestyle, and lack of spiritual purpose or fulfillment. Suppressed emotion or emotional stagnation is thought to aggravate the accumulation of toxic material in the cells and to gravely weaken the immune system.

At the Sky Mountain Clinic in Santa Fe, New Mexico, Ingrid Naiman and colleagues offer a cancer-treatment program that incorporates many Ayurvedic principles. Naiman says that she frequently receives letters from patients who report that their latest checkup showed them to be in remission. She believes that people consist of spiritual, rational, and subconscious or psychological components. "These three selves may have quite different natures and agendas, but it is essential that they learn to work together towards the fulfillment of the life purpose," she says. "This is difficult in a society as imbalanced and dysfunctional as ours. In simple terms, this means that parts of ourselves have been blocked in their expression and need encouragement to unfold." To facilitate communication with the higher self, Naiman uses guided visualization or classical music "to induce a slightly altered state of consciousness in which the soul can freely display its nature to the observing patient."

Naiman explains, "Many people are not truly individualized. This results in a poor self-image. Cancer patients often have such self-doubt and lowered esteem. Part of them has been in servitude to others who have claimed their identities." One of Naiman's colleagues, Helga Sager, says that "cancer patients wear themselves out being good."

Naiman, who is also a medical astrologer, says that all disease either stems from the subconscious or arises out of the conflict between the three selves. She studies the position of the Moon in the horoscope to determine the issues and needs of "the child within," and using this information, she helps patients "explore those facets of themselves that got blocked, the energies that were never nurtured."

The Sky Mountain program includes diet and herbs as well as a variety of salves called escharotic treatments. The salves have deep roots in herbalism. They are used to draw tumors out through the skin. Biopsy reports confirm that malignant tissues are removed in this manner. "It eases the burden on the body to dispose of toxic debris when neoplasms are drawn out this way rather than dissolved internally," explains Naiman. "The salves are particularly useful when the tumors are visible or palpable, such as with skin and breast tumors, but my information is that these salves have been used by other practitioners on brain and other tumors that are deeply imbedded in the body."

The suppressed or negative emotions that cancer patients harbor are believed to create excess *humors,* or bioforces. Ayurveda sees human beings as entities made up of unique combinations of humors called *doshas,* which interact to create all biologic activities. The three doshas are *Vata* (air), *Pitta* (fire), and *Kapha* (water). *Vata* controls motion and flow. It governs respiration, circulation, neuromuscular activity, and acuity of the senses. *Pitta* directs metabolism, energy exchange, and digestion. It is catabolic, concerned with the metabolic processes of destruction. *Kapha* represents structure, cohesion, and fluid balance. It is anabolic, involved with processes that build up the organism and control bodily stability.

The dynamic interaction of these bioforces creates our *prakriti* (individual constitution). Each individual has a unique constitution and ways of keeping the three humors in balance for optimum health. The three doshas, and the numerous *subdoshas* into which they are divided, correspond to different organ systems. When out of balance, the humors accumulate at specific sites in the body and give rise to the disease process. The humors may increase at their respective sites, overflow into the rest of the body, and relocate to other sites, causing further dysfunctions. By correcting excesses of any of the three humors, the Ayurvedic healer restores the patient to physiological balance and eliminates disease.

In Ayurveda, two people with colon cancer may receive different treatments. Cancer is not a separate disease entity; rather, a person manifests cancer as a result of biologic imbalances and emotional and spiritual factors unique to him or her. The first step in treatment is to determine the patient's particular constitutional type and current state of bioenergetic balance. There are seven major constitutional types, reflecting the different proportions of the three doshas. Some people are strongly predominant in one of the humors. Ayurvedically speaking, there are *Vata,* or air, types; *Pitta,* or fire, types; and *Kapha,* or water, types, in varying combinations and degrees.

Through a detailed analysis of the patient's constitutional predisposition and current health status, the Ayurvedic practitioner creates a therapeutic program integrating all aspects of the individual's life.

Diet, cleansing, herbal therapy, counseling, meditation, and spiritual therapy are all parts of an orchestrated attempt to reverse the condition of *dis-ease*.

An initial consultation may begin with *pulse diagnosis*. According to a recent article in the *Journal of the American Medical Association*, pulse reading enables the skilled Ayurvedic practitioner to diagnose not only cardiovascular disease but also cancers, musculoskeletal diseases, diabetes, asthma, and other conditions.[3] In pulse diagnosis, the combinations of doshas and subdoshas sustaining the person's illness are felt as patterns of vibration in the radial artery. *"Vata, Pitta,* and *Kapha* have different tactile vibratory qualities—as do their sub-doshas," explains the *JAMA* article. "The presence and locations of these vibratory qualities in the pulse alert the practitioner to specific patterns of balance and imbalance that underlie and are responsible for the patient's condition." By touching the patient's wrist, the Ayurvedic doctor can gain comprehensive, valuable information about his or her condition.

Other diagnostic tests may be performed, including close visual analysis of the patient's external features. A consultation also typically involves a probe into the client's emotional status, lifestyle, and outlook. In addition, standard diagnostic tools of allopathic medicine may be used. The physician can correlate the Ayurvedic diagnosis with the disease categories of Western medicine.[4]

Once the analysis is complete, a treatment plan is formulated. Broadly speaking, Ayurvedic treatment follows three stages: removal of accumulated toxins in the body; balancing of the excess biologic humor; and rebuilding of the body, a process of *tonification*, or rejuvenation.

In Western medicine, we know that toxic debris from improper diet and disease processes constantly builds up in every cell of the body. This discolored material is believed to play an active role in causing DNA to make mistakes—a primary cause of many cancers. The waste residues block the assimilation of nutrients, impair cell function, and lead to more rapid aging. The ancient Ayurvedic sages called these waste materials *ama,* which they perceived as a foul-smelling, sticky substance that needs to be evacuated from the body. Most diseases, they maintained, are *ama*-related, including chronic diseases like cancer, arthritis, and allergies.

The first stage of treatment—preliminary detoxification—aims to normalize digestion and eliminate *ama*. The methods include herbs, medicated-oil massages, therapeutic sweating, a diet of raw foods and fresh greens, and juice fasting. Once preliminary detoxification has been achieved, the second phase of clearing the body can begin. This is *pancha karma,* or purification therapy, which may include purgation with strong herbs to flush out the intestines, therapeutic vomiting, or medicated enemas. The aim of these methods is to purge the body and eliminate the disease-causing humors. *Pancha karma* is said to push out the excess humors along with the *ama* that sticks to them.

In Ayurveda, the general rule is, "First reduce, then tonify." Once the toxins and excess humors have been reduced or eliminated, the body can be rebuilt through a radical tonification program called rejuvenation. This includes a diet rich in nutritive foods, as well as herbal therapies. Yogic methods and breathing exercises can also be used to rejuvenate the mind.

Like Chinese medicine (Chapter 28), Ayurveda has a whole class of tonic herbs, including *ashwagandha, shatavari,* and *guduchi,* that have proved their immune-enhancing powers in clinical studies. Additional types of Ayurvedic herbs used in treating cancer are blood-cleansing herbs, such as Indian sarsparilla, and circulatory stimulants, such as *guggul,* which reduce masses and aid in healing the tissues. According to Dr. David Frawley, director of the American Institute of Vedic Studies in Santa Fe, "Such herbs taken with a strong anti-Ama or detoxifying diet may reduce tumors, whether malignant or benign, if the tumors are not large, have not metastasized and the patient is still strong."[5]

Ayurveda has an enormous herbal pharmacopeia and uses many different herbs and herbal combinations in the treatment of disease. Some of these herbs have yet to be identified by Western botanists, and very few have been tested. One popular Ayurvedic herb that has shown clinical value in cancer treatment and control is turmeric. The spice that gives curry its yellow color, turmeric is highly antiseptic and bactericidal, and helps to arrest bleeding. Clinical trials conducted with humans show that an antitumor compound isolated from turmeric is effective against cervical carcinoma and skin cancer. The essential oil of turmeric is composed mainly of curcumol and curdione, both of which are potent anticancer compounds, especially for cervical cancer and lymphosarcoma. Indian and German researchers have found that turmeric rhizomes can prevent a fatty liver from developing and can counteract the accumulation of ingested cholesterol within the liver.[6]

Another Ayurvedic herb used extensively in cancer treatment is *guggul,* made from the resin of the *gum gugal,* also called the *salai tree* or *Indian bedellium.* Guggul is closely related to myrrh. Used either internally or externally to treat cancer, guggul, in India, is passed through an elaborate purification process that is thought to enhance its medicinal benefits.

Dr. Frawley, a Vedic teacher who holds a degree in Oriental medicine (O.M.D.), believes that wrong diet is the main physical cause of disease. In his book *Ayurvedic Healing* (see Resources), he notes that animal products produce toxins in the body and advises the person with cancer to strictly avoid meat and dairy products as well as too much protein. He generally recommends a diet emphasizing raw vegetables and juices made from greens such as wheatgrass (Chapter 14), barley grass, celery, and dandelion, along with alfalfa and sunflower sprouts. Juices made from raw greens are full of *prana* (the life force) and help cleanse negative life energy. Dairy products, observes Dr. Frawley, are mucus-forming and contribute to the body's accumulated toxins. White refined sugar is "a dead or *tamasic* food" that leaches vital minerals out of the body. Dr. Frawley points out that there is no standard diet for everyone in Ayurveda; the food we eat should be in harmony with our individual nature.

Diseases can arise not only from an imbalance of the doshas but also from karmic causes: wrong actions, wrong occupation, emotional difficulties, problems in relationships, transgressions against Nature's laws, and crimes against inner wisdom. To deal with the karmic roots of disease, Ayurveda uses yoga and a system of spiritual therapy that can include meditation, prayers, mantras, music, controlled breathing, and gem therapy.

Yoga helps practitioners maintain their health and reduce anxiety. Yoga-like methods are now routinely employed at major hospitals to induce a "relaxation response." The practice of yoga increases the supply of oxygen to the cells, which potentially enhances immune function and supports the body's ability to neutralize harmful free radicals. *Pranayama,* the yogic control of the breath, promotes circulation, increases strength, and augments prana, the life force. Yogic positions are said to simultaneously train the entire neurological network and the immune system to interact for optimal functioning.

Mantras are healing sounds such as "Om," "Shrim," and "Ram" used in mental chanting and meditation. "Mantra therapy is excellent for cancer," states Frawley. The simple chanting of "Om" is held to balance the *aura*, the vital energy field surrounding the body that wards off disease and maintains the integrity of the whole organism. Other mantras, according to Ayurvedic sages, control the humors, aid detoxification, and promote peace and calm.

Gem therapy is another facet of Ayurveda. Certain gems, it is believed, protect and energize the body's aura, or energy field, while others are held to strengthen the immune system or even to exert antitumor properties.

Aided by Ayurveda, Eleanor, a woman in her early forties, recovered from advanced breast cancer that had metastasized to her lymph nodes. Diagnosed with cancer in 1983 by her orthodox doctors, she faced a grim prognosis after two radical mastectomies, unsuccessful chemotherapy, and further spread of the cancer to twelve different sites in her bones. The five-year survival rate for this type of cancer is about 1 percent. In1986, at the suggestion of her doctor, Eleanor began practicing Transcendental Meditation (TM), a mental technique brought from India to the United States in 1959 by Maharishi Mahesh Yogi. While continuing radiation and chemotherapy, Eleanor received Ayurvedic treatment at a retreat in Lancaster, Massachusetts— the Maharishi Ayur-Veda Health Center—under the care of its medical director, Deepak Chopra, M.D.

To trigger Eleanor's natural healing response, Dr. Chopra prescribed a regimen that included herbal preparations, meditation, altered diet and sleep patterns, massages, and even exposure to "primordial sounds" and aromas. Primordial sounds, which are prescribed for certain illnesses, can be used internally as a "mental sound" during meditation. This technique is said to exert a healing influence on the body and to "bring an awareness of bliss" to the diseased area. For Eleanor, "the results were remarkable," according to Chopra, who relates that his patient's severe bone pain disappeared and that whenever she went home to be X-rayed, her radiologist found fewer and fewer pockets of bone cancer.

Eleanor had to go off chemotherapy temporarily because her blood counts were consistently bad. Once off the chemo and no longer suffering from its multiple side effects, she immediately started feeling better, so she decided to end the chemotherapy, "even at the risk of dying," as she put it. Dr. Chopra, an endocrinologist and president of the American Association of Ayurvedic Medicine, states that it was "far too late" for Eleanor's bone-cancer regressions to have been caused by her earlier radiation or chemotherapy. Several months after beginning her Ayurvedic regimen, Eleanor's blood chemistry returned to the normal range and her bone cancer dwindled until only one small shadow, not proven cancerous, remained on her X-rays.

Many people remember Indian spiritual teacher Maharishi Mahesh Yogi as the guru with a gleeful laugh who promoted Transcendental Meditation in the 1960s and made temporary converts of the Beatles. Few people realize that TM has been the subject of over 500 scientific studies during the past twenty years and that the National Cancer Institute is currently funding a series of studies to determine the cancer-prevention properties of Ayurvedic herbal compounds developed as part of Maharishi Ayur-Veda, the Indian seer's updated version of ancient Ayurvedic practice. Two herbal supplements in particular, *MAK-4* and *MAK-5*, have attracted attention from the scientific community for benefits demonstrated in experimental studies on tumor regression, enhancement of immune response, cancer prevention, and promotion of longevity.

To critics, Ayur-Veda is the brand name of a line of health-food products and medical services offered by the TM movement. According to the National Council Against Health Fraud (NCAHF), these products and services are "of limited, questionable, or unproved value" and "may serve as gateways into the TM cult which has a sordid history." The *NCAHF Newsletter* calls Deepak Chopra "the chief promoter of Ayur-Veda" and points out that the Maharishi "has ceremoniously given [Chopra] the title 'Dhanvantari' [Lord of Immortality], the keeper of perfect health for the world." In 1984, the Maharishi named Philippine dictator Ferdinand Marcos the "Founding Father of the Age of Enlightenment."[7]

The self-appointed "quackbusters" of the NCAHF have close ties to the most conservative factions within the American Medical Association. "NCAHF is staunchly opposed to nutritional medicine, vitamin and herbal supplementation, and organic produce, not to mention *all* alternative AIDS and cancer therapies, reflexology, naturopathy, homeopathy, and chiropractic," writes Sharon Bloyd-Peshkin in *Vegetarian Times*.[8]

It should be noted that there are Ayurvedic practitioners not connected in any way with the Maharishi's TM movement. Some of them consider Maharishi Ayur-Veda to be a cult that uses a nonclassical imitation of Ayurvedic medicine—not the form of Ayurveda taught and practiced in India. Some of the TM movement's statistical studies have also come under sharp criticism. And critics charge that MAK-4 and MAK-5 are not specifically anticancer medicines but general tonics that Maharishi Ayur-Veda prescribes for almost everything.

Nevertheless, the clinical and laboratory studies of Ayur-Veda seem impressive. For example, in a 1987 study of Transcendental Meditation, participants in a stress reduction program who regularly meditated with TM were compared with 600,000 members of an insurance carrier. The TM group had a 63 percent lower rate of hospital admissions for tumors.[9] Other studies have reported links between the use of TM and increased longevity, lowered cholesterol levels, and reduced anxiety and hypertension.

MAK-4 and MAK-5, the herbal compounds developed by Maharishi Ayur-Veda, are *rasayanas,* preparations described in the ancient Ayurvedic texts as increasing resistance to disease and promoting longevity. Professor Hari Sharma, M.D., of Ohio State University and colleagues found that MAK-4 and MAK-5 provide protection against breast cancer in animals during both the initiation and promotion phases of the disease. (In the initiation phase, DNA is damaged and mutation occurs; in the promotion phase, mutated cells proliferate and the cancer establishes itself.)

In one study, rats with mammary tumors induced by DMBA (a potent carcinogen) were given MAK-4 in their diets for four weeks. In 60 percent of the animals, the tumors shrank or disappeared entirely. In a subsequent study, Sharma and colleagues fed MAK-4 and MAK-5 to experimental animals that had been given DMBA. Only 15 percent of the animals developed tumors, compared with 60 percent of the control animals, which had not been fed the Ayurvedic herbs. In summary, Sharma found that MAK-4 and MAK-5 shrank or eliminated tumors in 60 percent of subjects by causing cancer cells to change into normal cells. Overall, 85 percent of animals fed MAK did not develop tumors.[10] Dr. Sharma is director of Ohio State University's Division of Cancer Prevention and Natural Products Research.

MAK-4 has also been shown to prevent metastasis in lung cancer. Animals fed MAK-4 in their diet showed a 60 percent reduction in the number of metastatic nodules and a 60 percent reduction in the size of the nodules.[11] In a 1991 study funded by the National Cancer Institute, MAK-4 and MAK-5 significantly inhibited cancer-cell growth in both human tumors and rat tracheal epithelial cell systems treated in vitro.[12]

Neuroblastoma is a generally incurable form of childhood neurological cancer. The second most common childhood cancer, it can originate in and spread to many parts of the body. Treatment of neuroblastoma with chemotherapy and radiation generates horrendous side effects. However, some preliminary findings on MAK may offer some hope. Dr. Kedar Prasad, radiology professor at the University of Colorado, treated neuroblastoma cells in vitro with MAK-5. The cancer cells differentiated into mature neurons; in other words, they were transformed into normal, healthy cells.[13] "MAK is the only herbal product I know that can do this. These findings are very exciting, since no toxicity of MAK has been reported as yet," says Dr. Prasad, who is also director of the Center for Vitamins and Cancer Research at the University of Colorado Health Sciences Center.

The ingredients of MAK-4 include Indian gallnut, Indian gooseberry, dried catkins, Indian pennywort, nutgrass, white sandalwood, butterfly pea, shoeflower, aloewood, licorice, cardamom, cinnamon, cyperus, turmeric, honey, raw sugar, and *ghee*, or clarified butter. The herbs in MAK-5 are meda milkweed, black musale, heart-leaf moonseed, East Indian globe thistle, butterfly pea, licorice, vanda orchid, elephant creeper, and Indian wild pepper. These herbal mixtures have additionally been shown to inhibit colon cancer and skin tumors in experimental animals.

Research on MAK-4 and MAK-5 suggests that these herbal preparations are extremely effective free-radical scavengers. In Japan, Dr. Yukie Niwa, an immunologist and authority on free-radical generation, conducted in vitro research with human white blood cells to investigate MAK-4 and MAK-5 as potential free-radical scavengers. Niwa found MAK to be more effective in binding to and removing free radicals than any of the 500 known free-radical scavengers previously studied. MAK also reduced levels of lipid peroxide by over 40 percent. Lipid peroxides are known to contribute to coronary artery disease by damaging arterial linings.[14] Dr. Jeremy Fields, associate professor of pharmacology at Loyola University, has investigated Niwa's findings, and he too has found that MAK, like the enzyme superoxide dismutase (SOD), was able to completely scavenge superoxide, a cancer-causing free radical. Unlike administered doses of SOD, the MAK herbal supplements are nontoxic.[15]

The Ayurvedic herbs also enhance immunity. In animals given MAK, the number of T-lymphocytes shot up by 100 to 160 percent.[16]

In Ayurveda, consciousness is conceived as primary, preceding and giving rise to matter. "The Ayurvedic view is that we are thoughts that have somehow learned to create a body," explains Dr. Chopra.[17] This contrasts with conventional Western medicine, which tends to view the body as a machine, with the mind as a secondary phenomenon. Ayurvedic physicians of India have taught for centuries that the human body is composed of innumerable channels that supply the various tissues of the body. Health is proper flow through these channels; disease is blockage or excessive or deficient flow. These channels, though similar to the physiological systems of Western medicine, also contain subtle energy fields. Ayurveda views the body as a complex magnetic field consisting of larger magnetic centers (*chakras*) and channels radiating from them (*nadis*). These centers appear to form pathways, or lines, through the body similar to the acupuncture points and meridians of Chinese medicine.

In 1930, German electrical engineer Fritz Grunewald demonstrated that the human body is comprised of a complicated magnetic field with many magnetic centers, a finding that lent support to the bioenergy systems of Indian and Chinese medicine.

Recent scientific research on the intersection of thoughts and neurochemicals also tends to validate the Ayurvedic system. Ayurveda teaches that "impulses of intelligence" govern the bodily processes of maintenance, repair, and creation. Such impulses (thoughts, for example) are said to express themselves as chemical molecules in the brain and throughout the body. In the 1970s, Western scientists discovered *neurotransmitters*, molecules that act as "communicator chemicals," bringing messages to and from neurons in the brain. This discovery shattered the prevalent model of the nervous system as a sort of telephone network, with electrical impulses moving along the nerves like electricity through cables connecting remote sites in the body with the brain's "central switchboard."

Researchers have identified dozens of different neurotransmitters, each of which seems to correspond with a particular mental state—anger, drowsiness, joy, schizophrenia, and so on. In the early 1980s, scientists at the National Institute of Mental Health discovered receptors for neurotransmitters in the immune system called monocytes. Remarkably, monocytes are not nerve cells at all but white blood cells that travel freely through the circulatory system to reach every cell in the body. These white blood cells act as "circulating neurons," flooding the body with awareness of the brain's thoughts and vice versa. The emergent Western model coalesces the nervous system with the immune system, the circulatory system, and, in fact, all bodily functions. This model corresponds nicely to the Ayurvedic framework.

Ayurveda can be a lifestyle choice as well as a medicine. Applying its principles in daily living can help to prevent disease and reduce emotional stress. Since Ayurveda is not officially recognized as a medicine in the United States, Ayurvedic practitioners must instead be licensed in some other line of health care such as allopathy, chiropractic, homeopathy, or acupuncture. Their Ayurvedic expertise is offered to the client as consultation, an adjunct to their basic services.

In selecting an Ayurvedic healer, try to determine the practitioner's depth of experience, to what extent he or she uses Ayurveda in treating patients, and with what degree of success.

Resources

American Institute of
Vedic Studies
P.O. Box 8357
Santa Fe, NM 87504-8357
Phone: 505-983-9385

For further information on Ayurveda, correspondence courses, and books.

The Lancaster Foundation
11501 Huff Court
North Bethesda, MD 20895
Phone: 301-984-7030

For research reports and a newsletter on Maharishi Ayur-Veda.

The Ayurveda Institute
11311 Menaul, N.E.
Suite A
Albuquerque, NM 87112
Phone: 505-291-9793

For further information on Ayurveda, classes, and counseling.

Maharishi Ayur-Veda
Medical Center
P.O. Box 282
Fairfield, IA 52556
Phone: 515-472-5866

For further information on Maharishi Ayur-Veda, details on treatment, and referrals to local physicians, health centers, and clinics.

Himalayan International
Institute of Yoga Science
and Philosophy of the U.S.A.
R.R. 1, P.O. Box 400
Honesdale, PA 18431
Phone: 717-253-5551

For further information on Ayurveda, details on treatment, retreats, professional training, and a variety of publications.

Reading Material

Ayurvedic Healing: A Comprehensive Guide, by David Frawley, O.M.D., Passage Press (P.O. Box 21713, Salt Lake City, UT 84121-0713; 800-873-0075), 1989. Excellent introduction for the serious layperson. Includes a section on cancer.

Ayurveda: The Science of Self-Healing, by Dr. Vasant Lad, Lotus Press (available from Lotus Light Publications, P.O. Box 2, Wilmot, WI 53192; 800-548-3824), 1984. Accessible guide for the Western reader.

Perfect Health, by Deepak Chopra, M.D., Harmony Books (400 Hahn Road, Westminster, MD 21157; 800-733-3000), 1991.

Quantum Healing: Exploring the Frontiers of Mind/Body Medicine, by Deepak Chopra, M.D., Bantam Books (666 Fifth Avenue, New York, NY 10103; 800-223-6834), 1989.

Two informative, popularly written introductions to Ayurvedic theory and practice. Both include case histories of cancer patients.

A Handbook of Ayurveda, by Vaidya Bhagwan Dash and Acarya Manfred Junius, Concept Publishing (New Delhi, India), 1983. Available from South Asia Books (P.O. Box 502, Columbia, MO 65205; 314-474-0116). Good presentation of the principles of Ayurvedic medicine.

Chapter 28

CHINESE MEDICINE

Chinese medicine, a system reaching back more than 2,000 years, is practiced by about one-fifth of the world's population. Many people in the United States, Canada, Europe, and Australia regard Chinese medicine as their first line of defense in maintaining health and combating disease. Although acupuncture has captured attention in the United States, traditional herbal medicine plays a far greater role in the Chinese health-care system. Backed by centuries of empirical experience, China's huge pharmacopeia contains thousands of substances of plant, animal, or mineral origin, most of them herbs. At least half of Chinese folk remedies have some kind of scientific basis for their reputed claims, according to a National Academy of Sciences study of 796 Chinese herbal and animal remedies.[1] Chinese medicine utilizes a range of therapeutic methods including herbs, diet, massage, osteopathic-type manipulation, breathing, deep relaxation, and therapeutic exercise in a holistic approach to health.

The leading cause of death in China is cancer, followed by stroke. Conventional Western cancer therapies—chemotherapy, radiation, and surgery—have been increasingly used since the 1960s in Chinese hospitals. However, the side effects of these treatments have been, there as here, often highly debilitating. This has led the Chinese government to fund research into the traditional herbal medicines. One result is the routine use of Fu Zhen therapy, an immune-enhancing herbal regimen, as an adjunct to chemotherapy and radiation. Fu Zhen therapy is reported to protect the immune system from damage and to increase survival rates, sometimes dramatically, when used in conjunction with the modern cancer therapies. The principal Fu Zhen herbs (astragalus, ligustrum, ginseng, codonopsis, atractylodes, and ganoderma) strengthen the body's nonspecific immunity and increase the functions of the T-cells.[2]

Herbal antitoxin therapies, also regularly used, contain many herbs that have been found to inhibit tumor growth by a variety of mechanisms. Kelp and pokeroot are among the herbs known to dissolve tumors in Chinese herbal therapy.

In the United States, it is very rare for a person with cancer to be treated solely by Chinese medicine, even though many practitioners say that traditional Chinese medicine can often handle cancer on its own, with success in cases that proved untreatable by Western medicine.[3] "For patients who desire the expertise of a conventional oncologist as well as the benefits of more natural methods," says Roger Jahnke, a doctor of Oriental medicine and director of the Health Action Clinic in Santa Barbara, California, "Chinese medicine can provide an important collaborative resource to link with conventional cancer treatment. Patients should develop a healing team that could include the oncologist, a practitioner of acupuncture and herbal pharmacology, and perhaps a nutritionist, psychologist and support group of some kind. The result is a more comprehensive and synergistic therapeutic effect." When used in tandem with chemotherapy, Chinese herbal medicine can control and minimize the side effects of chemical drugs and may enhance their therapeutic effects. Herbs also bolster immune-system functions depressed by radiation.[4]

In China, surgery, chemotherapy, and radiation are considered viable treatments for benign and malignant tumors by physicians who are attempting to integrate Eastern and Western methods. Conventional treatments may be required to deal with a situation within the time available to the patient, notes Zhang Dai-zhao, a specialist in cancer treatment in Beijing. Although Chinese energetic therapies such as herbal medicine and acupuncture may be able to eventually dismantle pathologic matter, "they may take more time than the patient has," he states.[5] Many practitioners in China say that the best results against cancer are obtained by means of a joint attack combining Oriental and Western medicine, with the patient pursuing a suitable diet, Chinese yoga, and therapeutic exercise.

In classic Chinese medicine, there is no specific concept of cancer, though there is of tumors. Many nutritive tonics and herbal medicines were developed to alleviate pain and prolong survival by strengthening the body's life forces and arresting tumor progression. Chinese doctors believe the causes of cancer are multiple, including toxins and other environmental factors, called "external causes," as well as "internal causes" such as emotional stress, bad eating habits, accumulated wastes from food, and damaged organs. Two main factors are stagnant blood and a blockage or accumulation of *chi*, or *qi* (pronounced chee), the vital energy said to circulate along the *meridians*, or pathways, linking all parts of the body.

Illness is an energy imbalance, an excess or deficiency of the body's elemental energies. According to the ancient Chinese, chi, the life force, controls the body's workings as it travels along the meridians, completing an energy cycle every twenty-four hours. A person is healthy when there is a balanced, sufficient flow of chi, which keeps the blood and body fluids circulating and fights disease. But if the circulation of chi is blocked for any reason or becomes excessive or deficient, pain and disease can result. The flow of chi may be disrupted by an imbalanced diet or lifestyle, overwork, stress, repressed or excessive emotions, or lack of exercise. Imbalances in *yin* and *yang*—complementary forces in dynamic flux—also disturb the normal, smooth flow of chi.

Cancer, like all other diseases, is regarded as a manifestation of an underlying imbalance. The tumor is the "uppermost branch," not the "root," of the illness. Each patient may have a different imbalance causing what outwardly looks like the same type of cancer. Each person is unique, so the Oriental doctor attempts to identify the exact individual pattern of excess, deficiency, or blockage that led to the disease. The doctor treats the imbalance rather than a condition known as "stomach cancer," or "breast cancer," or so on. The prescribed treatment will vary from one patient to the next, depending on the specific imbalances.

The Chinese doctor makes a diagnosis in terms of yin and yang, chi, *Blood*, and organ imbalance. The term *Blood* refers to much more than the material substance. Blood is the process of nourishing the organism; it occurs in a mutually regulating relationship with chi and *Moisture* (body fluids). In forming a diagnosis, the doctor is guided by the Eight Principles, which are four sets of polar categories (yin and yang, cold and heat, deficiency and excess, and interior and exterior). The Eight Principles serve as the framework for the data gathered through physical examination, tongue and pulse diagnosis, and observation of symptoms. Once the doctor forms a cohesive picture of the pattern of disharmony, he or she can formulate a treatment plan to restore balance.

The tongue is considered a sensitive barometer of human health in traditional Chinese medicine. Subtle changes in its color, texture, and coating indicate specific body imbalances and reveal the progress of the illness to the experienced doctor. In neglecting tongue diagnosis, "The West may be overlooking a highly valuable clinical tool," according to David Eisenberg, M.D., a clinical research fellow at Harvard Medical School. Dr. Eisenberg, who speaks Chinese, worked inside urban Chinese hospitals in 1979 and 1980. He concluded from his firsthand observations that "acupuncture, herbal medicine, and massage may be highly effective therapeutic tools."[6]

The pulse, like the tongue, is also a barometer of harmony or disorder. By feeling positions on each wrist along the radial artery, the well-trained Chinese diagnostician can detect underlying imbalances in internal organs and in the body as a whole.

Herbs and foods in Chinese medical practice are viewed energetically, that is, in terms of their influence on the body's energy field. This is also true of Indian Ayurvedic medicine (Chapter 27). The diet must be aligned with the energetics of the prescribed herbs; otherwise, the foods eaten may inhibit the herbal preparations' beneficial effects. Conversely, a diet in harmony with the herbal therapy will enhance the herbs' healing powers. The Chinese healer recognizes that what we eat can either protect and rebalance our bodies or pollute our systems. Diet is a remedy of prime importance. Chinese food therapy is a sophisticated system that recognizes six different human constitutional types and evaluates foods according to their therapeutic properties. For cancer patients, Chinese doctors frequently recommend a diet based upon whole grains, beans, and fresh vegetables.

Most Chinese healers advise patients undergoing herbal treatment to avoid all raw foods, because they are too "cold," and white sugar, because it is too rich and overstimulates the pancreas and liver. Strong spices, thought to disperse energy from within to the surface of the body, should be avoided. Cancer patients are also advised to shun coffee, because it overtaxes the adrenals; cold dairy foods, because they are too congesting; and shellfish and citrus, because they are too "cold" and "moist."

Most Chinese people prefer herbal medicines to Western allopathic drugs. Herbal preparations are thought to be more natural, much less dangerous, and slower and gentler in action, yet equally or more effective compared to synthetic chemical drugs. Herbs are nearly always used as compound prescriptions, with a single formula containing between six and twelve herbs. Remedies are often complex, combining multiple ingredients to mirror and correct patterns of disorganized chi, Blood, and Moisture. Generally, each formula contains a chief herb, one or more assistant herbs, and a "courier herb" to take the medicine to the site of the "lesion."

Studies of Fu Zhen therapy in the United States and China have demonstrated its value in treating a wide range of immune-compromised conditions, including cancer, leukemia, AIDS and ARC, and chronic Epstein-Barr virus. In a study of seventy-six patients with Stage II primary liver cancer, twenty-nine of the forty-six people receiving Fu Zhen therapy in combination with radiation or chemotherapy survived for a year, and ten survived for three years. Only six of the thirty patients who received radiation or chemotherapy alone survived one year, and all died by the third year.[7] In laboratory studies, Fu Zhen herbs have prevented the growth of transplanted tumors.

The most highly praised blood tonic in the East, *Tang kuei* (*Angelica sinensis*), has been used clinically in China to treat cancer of the esophagus and liver with good results. The Chinese have claimed dramatic success using this herb both alone and in combination with other medicinal agents in treating cervical cancer and, to a lesser extent, breast cancer in women.[8] It can be administered in either infusion or douche form. Many other Chinese herbs could be cited for their documented antitumor effects.[9]

Nearly all of the Chinese herbs used today to treat cancer and other immune-deficient conditions fall into three broad categories. *Tonic herbs* increase the number and activity of immunologically active cells and proteins. *Toxin-clearing herbs* clear the blood of germs and of waste products from the destruction of tumors and germs. *Blood-activating herbs* reduce the coagulation and inflammatory reactions associated with immune response. Herbal therapy in cancer treatment can improve appetite, reduce nausea and vomiting, and alleviate stress.

In Japan, classical Chinese herbal formulas are prepackaged and standardized. *Kanpo,* the Japanese version of Chinese herbalism, has reported many successes in treating cancer. In Tokyo, many kanpo doctors work in conventional hospitals prescribing drugs but moonlight to pursue their private herbal practices. Kanpo doctors dispense with much of the conceptual framework of traditional Chinese medicine such as the division of the body into yin and yang parts.

Another component of Chinese medicine used in cancer treatment is *chi gong,* a 3,000-year-old exercise that combines the slow, symmetrical, graceful movements of tai chi with meditation, relaxation, patterned breathing, guided imagery, and other behavioral techniques. The aim is to enable a person to regulate and direct the flow of chi, or vital force, within his or her own body. The student or patient is taught to focus his or her chi at a point in the center of the body, roughly two inches below the navel, called the *dan tian,* or vital center. From this center, the chi is said to emanate to distant regions of the body. Students reportedly learn to sense the presence of chi at the vital center in the form of localized warmth and then to direct the life energy to specific parts of the body. Based on the experience of students who take chi gong courses for self-treatment purposes, it usually takes about three months for the exercises to show their effect. In cancer therapy, the Chinese practitioner prescribes exercises geared to the individual patient.

Since 1979, "the Chinese have cured hundreds of cancer victims through chi gong," and many thousands have used this practice to prolong their lives, reports Paul Dong, a journalist and chi gong practitioner and teacher based in Oakland, California.[10] Dong, who was born in mainland China, went to China in 1984 to investigate chi gong. Case histories of recovered cancer patients are frequently reported in chi gong magazines. This physical-mental exercise has aided remissions in many lung cancer patients who found conventional Western therapies ineffective. On December 2, 1986, the *New York Times* reported that the twenty-six chi gong clinics in China had successes in treating some cardiac diseases, paralysis, and neurological disorders.

The modern use of chi gong to treat cancer originated with Guo Lin (1906–1984), a Chinese painter who was afflicted with uterine cancer in 1949 and was treated by surgery. The cancer recurred in 1960, with metastasis to the bladder. After another operation, Guo Lin had another recurrence and doctors told her she had six months to live. Turning to ancient chi gong manuals left to her by her grandfather, a Taoist priest, she practiced chi gong two hours every day, and in six months, the cancer had abated. Convinced that chi gong was responsible for her recovery, Madame Guo, in 1970, began giving lessons in what she called New Chi Gong Therapy. By 1977, cancer patients from all over China were pouring into Beijing to take part in her chi gong therapy classes. Guo Lin reportedly helped hundreds of cancer sufferers attain remissions while prolonging the lives and easing the pain of thousands more.[11]

Among the first masters of chi gong were Taoist and Buddhist monks. China's great scholars and philosophers, including Confucius and Lao Tse, were also students of this discipline, which predates all the martial arts and gave birth to tai chi, kung fu, and tai kwan do.

Today, millions of Chinese rise every morning at dawn to practice the ancient technique of chi gong to promote mental and physical well-being. *Chi gong* translates as "manipulation of vital energy" or, simply, "breathing skill" (since the character for *chi* means both "vital energy" and "breath").

How chi gong achieves healing effects is not fully understood, though several mechanisms of action have been proposed. From the standpoint of traditional Chinese medicine, chi gong energizes the body's vital forces, balances yin and yang, strengthens blood circulation, and improves the patient's emotional and mental states. From the viewpoint of Western medicine, chi gong increases the absorption and utilization of oxygen from the blood, as does yoga. Nobel Prize–winner Otto Warburg found that oxygen deficiency is typical of cancer cells and that when the body is rich in oxygen, cancer cells die. Practicing chi gong exercises has a positive effect on certain enzymes that play key roles in the body's maintenance of health and in *phosphorylation,* a basic biochemical process that supplies the energy necessary for cell work.[12] Phosphorylation is central to oxygen provision for all of the body's cells and is vitally important to immune response.

Exercise can mobilize the body's natural killer cells, which seek out and destroy cancer cells and cells infected by viruses. An increased oxygen uptake from the blood can also neutralize free radicals. The slow, deep breathing and moderate body motion of chi gong (or yoga) can cause the newly available oxygen to bind with free radicals, rendering them harmless.[13] Research in China indicates that after a chi gong exercise lasting about forty minutes, the body's internal regional blood volume increases by 30 percent, which greatly improves the supply of oxygen available to the cells.[14]

Through intensive practice of chi gong, "a whole set of beneficial psychological and spiritual conditions emerge," observes Paul Dong in his book *Chi Gong: The Ancient Chinese Way to Health.* Besides promoting emotional well-being, chi gong exercises build patients' confidence and steel their will to defeat cancer. Dong, who has practiced chi gong since 1980, notes that positive attitude plays a role in curing disease. He likens chi gong's apparent immune-boosting effects to Western mind-body healing approaches such as the new field of psychoneuroimmunology (see page 327).

In addition to *internal chi gong,* the manipulation of energy flow within one's own body, there is also *external chi gong,* the reputed ability to project one's internal chi toward another body. In external chi therapy, widely accepted in China for the treatment of many disorders, no physical contact is required. The advanced chi gong expert simply projects his or her chi energy through the fingers or palm toward the patient, thereby purportedly killing cancer cells. External chi gong practitioners in China claim that through this technique, they can destroy bacteria and transmit health-promoting energies. They believe they have proven the existence of chi as a physical reality evident in psychokinetic (mind-over-matter) powers, clairvoyance, and healing effects. To skeptics, these assertions spring from self-deception and heightened suggestibility.

Paul Dong tells of a Japanese cancer victim, with a tumor the size of an egg deeply imbedded in his nasal cavity, who made a trip to a Beijing hospital to undergo external chi therapy. After twelve days of treatment, the man's tumor had shrunk and his pain had considerably eased.[15] Dr. Feng Li-da, professor of immunology at Beijing College of Traditional Chinese Medicine, has done many experiments on external chi transmission and claims that a chi gong expert can destroy uterine cancer cells, gastric cancer cells, flu virus, and colon and dysentery bacilli with varying degrees of success. In *The Scientific Basis of Chi Gong,* Professor Xie Huan-zhang of Beijing Industrial College states that chi effects detected with scientific instruments include magnetic fields, infrared radiation, infrasound, and ion streams of visible light and superfaint luminescence.[16]

Dong stresses that external chi treatment should only be considered a temporary measure. But he also suggests that if a patient is too weak or otherwise unable to practice chi gong regularly, external chi should be tried. Combinations of internal and external chi treatment can also be attempted.

Acupuncture is another Chinese therapeutic method for changing the flow or quality of the life force and rebalancing body energies. The Chinese say that chi circulates within fourteen major meridians, or energy channels, traversing the body from the top of the head to the tips of the fingers and toes. Each meridian is connected to an internal organ. Specific points on each invisible channel, when stimulated, affect the flow of chi in that and other channels or in the associated organs. By stimulating these points with extremely fine needles or massage, acupuncture unblocks energy or adjusts its flow. Inserting and manipulating the needles—hairlike slivers of stainless steel—is believed to correct the imbalances that underlie disease.

Acupuncture has been used to treat persistent pain, arthritis, asthma, infertility, and acute and chronic diseases. In cancer, it can alleviate the pain and functional disorders associated with the illness, for example, improving the ability to swallow in victims of esophageal cancer. Acupuncture is also used to mitigate the side effects of chemotherapy and radiation, and has been employed as a primary treatment for very early signs of breast and cervical cancer, though the Chinese are more likely to utilize herbal remedies to support immunity and control malignant growth. Acupuncture can also be helpful in stress reduction and the alleviation of pain following surgery.

Some practitioners advise against acupuncture in the treatment of cancer, arguing that the increased energy flow and circulation pose a risk of spreading the disease. Most others disagree, however, pointing to the benefits already cited. Leukemia has been successfully treated with acupuncture therapy.[17] In addition, acupuncture has exhibited a wide range of actions in boosting immunity, including increasing the number of white blood cells,[18] boosting natural killer cell activity,[19] and increasing the amount of B-cells, which manufacture antibodies, chemicals that help destroy foreign invaders in the body.[20] Acupuncture also elevates the levels of circulating immunoglobulins and stimulates the production of red blood cells.

A major use of acupuncture, at least in China, is as an alternative to anesthesia during surgery. Dr. David Eisenberg of Harvard Medical School assisted with the acupuncture during a surgical operation performed on a fifty-eight-year-old man who had a chestnut-sized tumor located in the center of his brain. The successful surgery was done without anesthesia at the Beijing Neurosurgical Institute. The patient remained totally awake and responsive during brain surgery and felt no pain. He laughed and talked with Dr. Eisenberg during the four-hour operation while a few well-placed, ultrathin needles protected him from pain.[21]

Since acupuncture needles are extremely fine, minimal or no pain is experienced when they are inserted. Many people feel a slight pinprick when the needle goes in, followed by another mild sensation as the needle goes deeper. The response to acupuncture treatment is highly individual; many patients report a dreamy sense of relaxed well-being and elation. The needles are often left in place for twenty to thirty minutes.

For those who feel uncomfortable with the idea of needles being stuck in them, other techniques are available to stimulate the acupuncture points and balance the body's energy system. The points can be activated by *acupressure,* a term encompassing several massage techniques, such as *tui na,* a traditional Chinese system to mobilize chi and promote blood circulation. In *shiatsu,* a Japanese equivalent of Chinese massage, the practitioner presses his or her fingers into the acupuncture points and massages them. The points are held for just three to five seconds. In another technique, *moxibustion,* the glowing tip of a tiny cone of smoldering moss is held next to the acupuncture point. When the patient finds it too hot, the moxa stick, made of compressed dried leaves of Chinese mugwort, is withdrawn. Finally, *electroacupuncture devices* stimulate the points without any needles or bodily invasion.

The energy meridians and acupuncture points are invisible—if they exist, they do not correspond to any known anatomical entities. Critics dismiss acupuncture as a placebo effect. However, it is now known that acupuncture triggers a significant release of morphinelike substances called endorphins and enkephalins, natural painkillers that also promote healing and relieve depression. Some scientists speculate that the needles cause an anesthetic effect in surgery by closing "gates" to the brain along the spinal cord, blocking the pain message so it isn't felt. Nobel Prize–nominee Robert Becker, M.D., a pioneer in tissue repair and regeneration through electrotherapy, has theorized that the meridians are electrical conductors and the acupuncture points, amplifiers. With the help of a biophysicist, Dr. Becker proved to his satisfaction that "at least the major parts of the acupuncture charts had, as the jargon goes, 'an objective basis in reality.'"[22]

Two French physicians have done a series of intriguing experiments that they claim make visible the acupuncture meridian system. Jean-Claude Darras, M.D., and Professor Pierre de Vernejoul, M.D, injected radioactive isotopes into the acupoints of patients and traced the isotopes' uptake by gamma-camera imaging. They found that the isotopes migrated along the classical Chinese meridian pathways. In contrast, injecting the isotopes into random points on the skin produced no such results. Further tests demonstrated that the migration was not through the vascular or lymphatic system. The research, conducted at the Nuclear Medical Section of Neckar Hospital in Paris, was reported at the World Research Foundation Congress in 1986.

When seeking a doctor in the United States who practices Oriental medicine, cancer patients need to be aware of what doctors can do and what patients can learn to do for themselves. According to Dr. Roger Jahnke, "There are four basic things that the doctor of Chinese medicine can do for you: herbal prescriptions, acupuncture, massage, and external chi gong. At least as important, however, are the things the doctor can teach you to do for yourself. These include guidance in the use of tonic or wellness herbs, in proper nutrition, and in devising a suitable exercise program that may involve activities like swimming or walking. A competent practitioner can also teach the patient self-applied massage, meditation and relaxation techniques, and chi gong exercises. Finally, the doctor can offer guidance to help patients fulfill their unique spiritual purpose. Prospective patients should look for a doctor who provides all of these things, or one who can help patients network to all of these things, from body care up to the spiritual components of health."

Resources

Health Action Clinic
Roger Jahnke, L.Ac., O.M.D.
19 East Mission Street
Suite 102
Santa Barbara, CA 93101
Phone: 805-682-3230

For further information on Oriental medicine.

Quan Yin Healing Arts Center
1748 Market Street
San Francisco, CA 94102
Phone: 415-861-4964

For referrals to local practitioners of Oriental medicine as well as a training program for health professionals in the treatment of AIDS and HIV infection.

Oriental Healing Arts Institute
1945 Palo Verde Avenue
Suite 208
Long Beach, CA 90815
Phone: 213-431-3544

For further information on Oriental medicine.

American College of
  Traditional Chinese Medicine
455 Arkansas Street
San Francisco, CA 94107
Phone: 415-282-7600

For further information on Oriental medicine.

American Association of
  Acupuncture and
  Oriental Medicine
c/o National Acupuncture
  Headquarters
1424 16th Street, Northwest
Suite 501
Washington, DC 20036
Phone: 202-265-2287

For further information on Oriental medicine and acupuncture.

American Academy of
  Medical Acupuncture
2520 Milvia Street
Berkeley, CA 94704
Phone: 415-841-7600

For further information on acupuncture.

Traditional Acupuncture
  Institute
American City Building
Suite 100
Columbia, MD 21044
Phone: 301-997-4888

For further information on acupuncture.

Institute for Traditional
  Medicine
2442 Southeast Sherman
Portland, OR 97214
Phone: 503-233-4907

For further information on Fu Zhen therapy and herbal healing.

Reading Material

Chinese Herbal Therapies for Immune Disorders, by Subhuti Dharmananda, Ph.D., Institute for Traditional Medicine (2017 Southeast Hawthorne, Portland, OR 97214; 503-233-4907), 1988.

Between Heaven and Earth: A Guide to Chinese Medicine, by Harriet Beinfield, L.Ac., and Efrem Korngold, L.Ac., O.M.D., Ballantine Books (201 East 50th Street, New York, NY 10022; 800-638-6460), 1991.

The Web That Has No Weaver: Understanding Chinese Medicine, by Ted J. Kaptchuk, O.M.D., Congdon and Weed (298 Fifth Avenue, Seventh Floor, New York, NY 10001; 212-736-4883), 1983.

Part Eight

THE MIND-BODY CONNECTION

For this is the great error of our day,
that physicians separate the soul from the body.
—Plato

Part Eight of *Options* focuses on two central questions: First, to what extent do emotions and attitudes influence the onset of illness, specifically cancer? Second, if psychological factors do play a role in cancer, can therapeutic approaches that emphasize the link between mind and body actually benefit the patient? Part Eight reviews some of the latest studies in this area and examines such techniques as visualization, meditation, hypnosis, and psychoneuroimmunology.

Chapter 29

MIND-BODY APPROACHES

The role of emotions, behaviors, and faith in recovery from serious illness is the basis for mind-body approaches to cancer. Hate, suppressed anger, depression, sorrow, and frustration can produce powerful, harmful changes in the body's biochemistry that may possibly set the stage for illness. Conversely, positive emotions—will to live, trust, love, hope, determination—may also possibly affect biologic states and restore a person to wellness.

Cancer patients are now offered a wide range of services to help them deal with the emotional and psychological aspects of the disease. Almost every hospital serving cancer patients offers some form of psychosocial support, and many independent groups provide counseling, psychotherapy, and instruction in meditation, relaxation, and guided imagery or visualization. Biofeedback, hypnosis, and audio cassettes are other techniques. A common belief underlying these approaches is that patients' efforts to promote their emotional and spiritual well-being may tip the balance toward recovery.

Some mind-body practitioners go further and claim that the use of these techniques can actually change the course of the disease, causing tumor regression and, in some cases, bringing about remission of cancer. For example, in discussing visualization and meditation, Dale Figtree, Ph.D., a nutritional health practitioner in Laguna Beach, California, reported, "There are people who have healed themselves, or were healed, solely on the use of this practice, after all traditional approaches to healing their cancer had failed." In Figtree's own experience with cancer, "Visualization was an important and valued part of my healing process, as was diet, a change in lifestyle and attitude."

Treated for six months with chemotherapy and radiation for a lymphatic tumor attached to his heart, main arteries, and lung,

Figtree was given a guarded prognosis and told there was nothing else that could be done after the tumor had shrunk from the size of a grapefruit to the size of a grape. That was in 1977. Three years later, after practicing visualization and making major dietary and lifestyle changes, Figtree had a CAT scan that found no trace of cancer.[1]

Critics warn that mind-body approaches often instill a false sense of hope in patients desperately looking for a miracle. "Mind-body techniques are just so many Band-Aids unless healing takes place on a deep biological level," says Susan Silberstein, executive director of the Center for Advancement in Cancer Education, an information, counseling, and referral agency in Wynnewood, Pennsylvania. Silberstein leans strongly toward biologic, metabolic, and nutritional approaches to treating cancer. Yet, she says that she herself knows of two remarkable cases of people who apparently healed themselves of cancer through the exclusive use of mind-body techniques. While the number of such individuals may be extremely small, their existence attests to the fact that there are no absolutes in dealing with cancer.

Mind-body practitioners argue that there is no such thing as false hope since hope is the image of, and desire for, a positive outcome. They point out that when cancer patients are diagnosed as terminal or hopeless, their immune function often drops precipitously. "To argue for the *absence* of a mind-body connection could be viewed as offering the patient *false despair* in contrast to the much feared problems of offering false hope," notes B. O'Regan in a 1989 issue of *Noetic Sciences Review*.[2]

In fact, studies have shown that feeling hopeful, positive, and in control of one's battle against cancer goes hand-in-hand with a strong immune response. Cancer patients who adopt an optimistic fighting stance against their illness do better than those who react with passive acceptance or helpless despair.

"The concept of false hope is one of the most ridiculous things I know of," commented Bernie Siegel, M.D., founder of the Exceptional Cancer Patients (ECaP) program in New Haven, Connecticut, and author of bestselling books. "Why should we try to authorize hope according to the statistics? Hope is the variable that can *change* the statistics. If only 99% die of a condition, then let's stress the fact that that person has a chance of not dying. If you tell a group of those people that they are the 10% who will survive, you may find that 30% or 40% or 50% get better."[3]

Siegel, a surgeon who teaches at Yale University, supports the conventional methods used in cancer therapy—chemotherapy, radiation, and surgery. But he stands somewhat apart from the cancer establishment because of his strong belief in the vital link between consciousness and healing. The ECaP program of "carefrontation" includes individual and group psychotherapy intended to "facilitate personal change and healing." He asks patients five important questions to call attention to hidden problems:

1. Do you want to live to be 100?
2. What happened to you in the year or two before your illness?
3. What does illness mean to you?
4. Why do you need the illness? "Sickness gives people permission to do things they would otherwise be inhibited from doing."
5. Describe your disease and what you are experiencing. "There is more to disease than just physical illness."

The ECaP program includes meditation, visualization, art therapy, relaxation, nutrition, exercise, play and laughter, focusing of the mind, and faith. Siegel's popular books are full of "exceptional patients"—feisty, self-reliant people who take charge and live life to the fullest. ECaP supplies books, audio and videotapes, and the names of other centers that offer similar services.

A study of the ECaP program conducted in the early 1980s by Hal Morgenstern and colleagues in collaboration with Siegel attempted to assess the impact of the program on survival of patients with breast cancer. The study found a small—but not statistically significant—increase in survival time among ECaP participants compared to nonparticipants.[4]

The whole question of whether psychosocial intervention can affect cancer patients physically—and if so, to what extent—is wrapped in controversy. One of the studies most frequently cited in support of mind-body approaches involved eighty-six women with metastatic breast cancer. Half of the women received medical treatment alone; the other half received medical treatment plus one year of weekly group therapy sessions and lessons in self-hypnosis exercises combining imagery and relaxation. The women who received the psychosocial support survived nearly twice as long as those who received medical treatment alone. Some researchers called the findings "marvelous" and "provocative"—and in need of replication.

David Spiegel, M.D., the Stanford University psychiatry professor who conducted the ten-year study,[5] warns against drawing far-reaching conclusions from it. "Of 86 women in my study, 83 died. We are not wishing away cancer here." The patients who received group therapy survived a mean of 36.6 months; the control patients survived a mean of 18.9 months. Spiegel's cautionary comment reflects a realistic attitude that patients need to adopt as they consider mind-body approaches. Summing up the known benefits of psychosocial support, Dr. Spiegel says, "It's life-enhancing. It's comparatively inexpensive. It helps patients cope with a difficult but important time in their lives. It does no harm."[6]

While some studies suggest that psychological factors affect the longevity of people with cancer, other studies show no such relationship at all. "There is evidence, but there is also contrary evidence," says Bernard Fox, Ph.D., professor of psychiatry at Boston University School of Medicine and author of many surveys in this field.[7]

Is there a "cancer-prone personality?" Lawrence LeShan, Ph.D., a New York psychotherapist, evaluated hundreds of patients using Rorschach blots, questionnaires, and personal interviews. In the mid-1960s, he declared that a cancer-prone personality does exist. Such people, he said, are long-suffering, tend to repress anger or resentment, and have a low sense of self-worth. He found that certain psychosocial factors often accompany the development of malignancy, including self-dislike and the loss of an emotionally important relationship. Many of his patients with cancer recalled a bleak childhood in which they felt lonely and isolated. They reported having had a tense or hostile relationship with their mother, father, or both. Often these people had made a tremendous emotional investment—in a job, a cause, or an individual—that became the centerpiece of their lives but was eventually destroyed. In the aftershock, they succumbed to feelings of hopeless despair and helplessness. Prior to their diagnoses with cancer, many of LeShan's patients experienced a major personal loss such as death or divorce.

In his therapeutic practice, LeShan attempts to uncover the roots of the psychological orientation that presumably prevents many cancer patients from harnessing all their resources to fight the disease. He believes these mental blockages are linked to the development of the cancer in the first place. LeShan seeks ways to help patients make the cancer a turning point in their lives rather than a sign of its ending. He encourages patients to delve deeply into their past in order to analyze the blocks that prevent them from living out their true nature. The goal is to unlock patients' self-healing ability and creative potential, allowing them to fulfill their individual purpose rather than conforming to what they believe they are supposed to be.

LeShan claims that his psychotherapeutic approach has dramatically lengthened the lives of many patients. After some twenty years of practice, he maintains, "Approximately half of my 'hopeless,' 'terminal' patients have gone into long-term remission and are still alive. The lives of many others seemed longer than standard medical predictions would see as likely. Nearly all found that working in this new way improved the 'color' and the emotional tone of their lives and made the last period of their lives far more exciting and interesting than they had been before."[8]

Other investigators, among them Scottish oncologist David Kissen, have also found definite links between personality attributes and cancer. A psychological profile of the person likely to develop cancer can be pieced together from all these studies. Cancer-prone individuals, it can be generalized, are rigid and conforming, with an overly critical attitude toward themselves. Their relationship with their parents is disturbed or emotionally sterile. They tend to bottle up strong emotions such as anger, fear, anxiety, and jealousy. Unable to cope with stress, they sink into feelings of hopelessness and depression. Many experience the loss of an important relationship, position, or something similar prior to the onset of the cancer.

The only trouble with this theory is that it is just a theory. Many other studies have found *no* association between cancer and personality traits. "There is no scientifically defensible research to conclude that there is a 'cancer personality,'" asserts Dr. Merlin Leach, an El Segundo, California, psychologist who does recognize the "depressed-helpless-hopeless condition" as a major contributing factor in many cases.[9] In *Cancer and Emotion* (see Resources), Jennifer Hughes, senior research fellow in the department of psychiatry at England's University of Southampton, finds the case for a cancer-prone personality to be extremely weak. Not all cancer patients possess the presumed traits, she notes, and many healthy people do possess them but never develop cancer. She also states that there is "little evidence" cancer patients have experienced more stressful events in their lives than other people—but she concedes that stressful events may encourage the growth of cancer in predisposed people.

A proponent of the view that emotional stress contributes to cancer is O. Carl Simonton, M.D. "Effects of emotional stress can suppress the immune system, thus lowering our resistance to cancer and other diseases," he writes in *Getting Well Again* (see Resources). A radiation oncologist, Simonton, along with his former wife, Stephanie Matthews-Simonton, developed a visualization technique intended to help patients enhance the potency of their immune systems. First, patients achieve deep relaxation by means of specific techniques that relieve tension and stress. Then patients visualize their white blood cells attacking and killing the cancer cells.

People are instructed to visualize the tumor as a weak, confused, soft mass of cells. They see their conventional treatment (chemotherapy or radiation) as powerful and effective, capable of shrinking tumors. They imagine their white blood cells as a vast army easily overwhelming the weak cancer cells. The specifics of the imagery depend on each person's imagination. Some people prefer to visualize the white blood cells and cancer cells in their natural forms, picturing the struggle as it actually occurs inside the body. Some imagine the confrontation symbolically, with the white blood cells as voracious sharks devouring the cancer cells, which are small, frightened fish. Other patients see an army of white-knight lymphocytes mowing down slow-moving malignant creatures. Patients then imagine dead and dying cancer cells flushed out of the body by natural processes until no more tumor cells remain. For people who aren't comfortable with the "killer" image of white blood cells, the whole process can be visualized as a "whisking away" of the cancer cells.

The Simontons, together and independently, have expanded their method into a comprehensive program that includes group psychotherapy, discussion of diet and exercise, and guidance in dealing with recurrence of the disease and facing the prospect of death. Generally, they have claimed that their cancer patients live twice as long as typical cases mentioned in the cancer literature. Dr. Simonton's studies have found that his patients' survival rates are "two times the survival times seen in the best cancer centers and three times the expected national norms, with significantly improved quality of life and quality of death."[10] He also claims that repeated practice with visualization is associated with remission in a highly select group of cancer patients.

The Simontons' claim of significant life extension has been widely challenged and their studies faulted. At times, colleagues' criticisms have been biting, with one physician alleging that Simonton is "perpetuating a cruel hoax on cancer patients."[11] In one pilot study, Simonton found that breast cancer patients who participated in his program lived an average of 38.5 months as compared to an average of 29 months for patients with similar cancers. However, since Simonton matched his cases against only general health statistics, "his pilot study makes an interesting, but scientifically weak point," according to Steven Locke, M.D., a psychiatrist at Harvard Medical School. "Comparing real people to statistical averages . . . does not produce persuasive data: it is the weakest form of controlled experiment."[12]

Another "contaminating factor" in Simonton's research is the kind of cancer patient who seeks out his program. "They are not typical cancer patients," notes Locke. They tend to be a self-selected group: well-educated, intelligent, highly motivated to get well, mostly white and middle-class, and probably in better physical and financial shape than the average patient. These factors may also contribute to Simonton's claimed higher survival rates.

For some cancer patients, the idea that they were in some sense responsible for the onset of the disease and can help reverse its course is hope-giving and inspirational. But there is a flip side to this. When patients do not get better, they may blame themselves for past situations and present medical conditions beyond their control. Feelings of guilt can result, dragging the patient down further. Simonton and other mind-body practitioners have been criticized for giving cancer patients a massive "guilt trip."

In reply, mind-body therapists point out that there is a big difference between "blaming oneself" and "accepting responsibility." Patients are encouraged to go beyond simple concepts like "blame" and "guilt"—to work with those factors that can be changed and to take responsibility for them, while accepting those phenomena beyond their control. Dr. Simonton has adjusted his therapy in an effort to avoid guilt and foster feelings of hope. His emphasis is on helping patients set easy-to-attain, low-level goals. To demonstrate the untapped resources within each of us, Simonton also gives firewalking demonstrations, walking barefoot across a fifteen-foot-long bed of live coals. Through mental discipline and the power of the mind, successful firewalkers emerge unharmed. Those cancer patients who feel so inclined are invited to try a firewalk themselves. The aim of this dramatic demonstration of the mind's latent powers is to mobilize patients' hope, faith, and will power to fight the disease.

There is now "pretty good evidence" that psychosocial factors can affect the immune system, according to Harvard psychiatrist Steven Locke. Studies have demonstrated that stress can significantly lower our ability to manufacture T-cells. People under increased stress from major life-changing events also show a decreased activity of natural killer cells.

Exploring possible links between the emotions and the immune system is the central focus of a new field, *psychoneuroimmunology* (*PNI*). PNI researchers chart the complex interactions between the mind (psycho), the brain and central nervous system (neuro), and the body's biochemical resistance to abnormal cell development and disease (immunology). PNI adherents believe that the patient's positive emotions are physiological factors in healing. They maintain that depression is a cause of ill health due to its suppression of the immune system. They assert that the best depression-blockers are a strong will to live and a sense of purpose expressed in interesting, useful activity. But critics of PNI point out that no one knows whether behaviorally induced changes in immune function actually have any clinical effect—especially in cancer, where the relationship between the immune system and disease is mysterious and complex.

Promising efforts to translate PNI insights into viable treatment techniques for people with cancer and other chronic diseases are underway. Richard Sheldon, a retired real estate broker, used PNI combined with chemotherapy and radiation to gain remission in an inoperable, two-inch-wide tumor in the left lung with primary and secondary metastasized sites. He practiced meditation, relaxation, guided imagery, and visualization along with nutrition, exercise, and the cultivation of healthy mental attitudes. "My newly acquired Walkman accompanied me to all my medical visits, creating my own chosen environment (sounds of the sea), instead of the hospital world filled with its depressing sights, sounds, and smells."

Sheldon describes his change of outlook in these terms:

> Like others, I had forced myself to adapt to the world, hoping to impress others and by so doing be accepted—but at the expense of my true self. Now I am learning to get the world to adapt to me (it's harder work, but much more rewarding). . . . Let's face it, we are all going to die someday. But I've come to the conclusion that the quality of my death will be determined by the quality of my life. Now I know that I can control the quality of both, with my choices of how I decide to live my life and by accepting my cancer as a challenge and opportunity to change my lifestyle.[13]

By January 15, 1991, twelve weeks after Sheldon started conventional treatment, the large tumor in his lung had completely disappeared. Five weeks later, a CAT scan showed no lymph-node involvement. Sheldon and his wife, Betty, a registered nurse, founded the Center for Cancer Survival, an educational resource center in Santa Barbara, California. Their six-week Cancer Survival Training Program teaches PNI "to augment traditional cancer protocols and perhaps enhance the immune system" as well as psychosocial techniques to help survivors "create their future" and develop their own cancer rehabilitation program. Sheldon's philosophy is, "Cancer is not to be viewed as a failure. The failure is in not living, not pursuing your dreams and not choosing life."

Hypnosis is a frequently overlooked mind-body technique that some people have used with reported success in coping with cancer. Albert Marchetti, M.D., a pathologist who spent four years researching adjunct cancer therapies, states that contemporary medical literature contains "innumerable examples of a variety of mental ailments and physical problems that have responded well to hypnotic cures." Generally, he notes, hypnosis is used as an adjunct to other, more conventional therapies. "Nevertheless, the results have been real, greater than what normally would have been expected," he asserts in *Beating the Odds* (see Resources).[14] Like psychotherapy, hypnotherapy is meant to desensitize patients to stressful situations, to help them work through feelings of depression and anxiety over death, to encourage effective coping strategies, and to change defeatist attitudes.[15] Marchetti's book explains how to use meditation, visualization, hypnosis, and diet in conjunction with surgery, chemotherapy, and radiation.

Resources

Cancer Survival Training
104 West Anapamu Street
Suite B
Santa Barbara, CA 93101-3126
Phone: 805-962-6221

For lessons in psychoneuroimmunology skills and for patient support.

Exceptional Cancer Patients
1302 Chapel Street
New Haven, CT 06511
Phone: 203-865-8392

For programs based on the work of Bernie Siegel, M.D.

Commonweal Cancer Help
  Program
P.O. Box 316
Bolinas, CA 94924
Phone: 415-868-0970

For week-long retreats combining stress reduction, health education, and group support.

Lawrence LeShan, Ph.D.
263 West End Avenue
New York, NY 10023

For evaluation and referral to an appropriate psychotherapist.

Simonton Cancer Center
P.O. Box 890
Pacific Palisades, CA 90272
Phone: 213-459-4434

For intensive group psychotherapy programs developed by Dr. O. Carl Simonton.

Wellness Community
1235 Fifth Street
Santa Monica, CA 90401
Phone: 213-393-1415

For patient support groups around the United States.

For a listing of other support groups and related services, see *Third Opinion: An International Directory to Alternative Therapy Centers for the Treatment and Prevention of Cancer and Other Degenerative Diseases,* by John Fink (see Appendix A for description).

Reading Material

You Can Fight for Your Life: Emotional Factors in the Treatment of Cancer, by Lawrence LeShan, M. Evans and Company (216 East 49th Street, New York, NY 10017; 212-688-2810), 1977.

Cancer as a Turning Point: A Handbook for People With Cancer, Their Families, and Health Professionals, by Lawrence LeShan, Penguin Books/Plume (375 Hudson Street, New York, NY 10014; 212-366-2000), 1990.

Getting Well Again, by O. Carl Simonton, Stephanie Matthews-Simonton, and James Creighton, Bantam Books (666 Fifth Avenue, New York, NY 10103; 800-223-6834), revised edition, 1980.

Love, Medicine, and Miracles, by Bernie S. Siegel, Harper and Row (10 East 53rd Street, New York, NY 10022; 800-242-7737), 1986.

Peace, Love and Healing, by Bernie S. Siegel, Harper and Row (10 East 53rd Street, New York, NY 10022; 800-242-7737), 1989.

The Healer Within: The New Medicine of Mind and Body, by Steven Locke and Douglas Colligan, New American Library/Mentor (375 Hudson Street, New York, NY 10014; 212-366-2000), 1987. A summary of the research into the mind's influence on health. Includes a good list of resources and organizations.

Cancer and Emotion, by Jennifer Hughes, John Wiley and Sons (605 Third Avenue, New York, NY 10158; 212-850-2272), 1987. A thorough, skeptical inquiry into purported mind-body connections in cancer.

Beating the Odds: Alternative Treatments That Have Worked Miracles Against Cancer, by Albert Marchetti, Contemporary Books (180 North Michigan Avenue, Chicago, IL 60601; 800-691-1918), 1988.

Healing Yourself: A Step-by-Step Program for Better Health Through Imagery, by Martin L. Rossman, Pocket Books (1230 Avenue of the Americas, New York, NY 10020; 800-223-2336), 1987.

CONCLUSION

Many different promising approaches to curing cancer now exist, urgently in need of further research to bring out their full potential. Yet many of these approaches and their practitioners have been persecuted, harassed, straitjacketed, or driven out of the country by a medical establishment that puts profits before people and cares mainly about preserving its business monopoly. Dr. Robert C. Atkins, well-known nutrition author and an advocate of complementary medicine, puts the matter succinctly when he says, "There have been *many* cancer cures, and all have been ruthlessly and systematically suppressed with a Gestapo-like thoroughness by the cancer establishment. The cancer establishment is the not-too-shadowy association of the American Cancer Society, the leading cancer hospitals, the National Cancer Institute, and the FDA." He adds, "The shadowy part is the fact that these respected institutions are very much dominated by members and friends of members of the pharmaceutical industry, which profits so incredibly much from our profession-wide obsession with chemotherapy."[1]

A lot of people simply can't believe that the deliberate suppression of lifesaving, valid therapies—especially *cancer* therapies—is possible in modern America. Unfortunately, they are dead wrong. To cite a few examples, chosen at random from this book:

- Royal Rife's Frequency Instrument, a bioelectric device that cured terminal cancer and many other diseases in the 1930s, was smashed and eliminated by the American Medical Association.
- Stanislaw Burzynski, M.D., Ph.D., has cured many cancer patients

333

with his nontoxic antineoplaston therapy, a cancer treatment using harmless peptides that occur naturally in humans. However, the American Cancer Society dismisses him as a "quack," and the FDA illegally raided his institute in 1985 and seized his medical and scientific records, which it still holds. Meanwhile, Japan and Russia are eagerly developing antineoplaston therapy—but in the United States, Dr. Burzynski can only practice in Texas.

- Lawrence Burton, Ph.D., made worldwide headlines in 1966 when his serum caused large tumors in mice to vanish totally within a few hours in a demonstration done under ACS auspices. He went on to cure cancer patients in Great Neck, New York, in the 1970s, but was then driven out of the country by FDA and ACS harassment. He now practices his Immuno-Augmentative Therapy in the Bahamas.

- Harry Hoxsey, using an herbal cancer remedy with possible roots in Native American and folk medicine, cured thousands of patients and, by 1955, operated the world's largest private cancer-treatment center, in Dallas. His clinics and his therapy were banned, and his chief nurse was forced to open a clinic in Mexico, even though a 1953 federal report to Congress found the AMA, FDA, and NCI guilty of a "conspiracy" to "suppress" an impartial assessment of his methods.

The cancer establishment has a fifty-year history of corruption, incompetence, and deliberate suppression of cancer therapies that actually work. This includes the rigging of clinical trials at major institutions in order to discredit nontoxic, natural therapies (as Barry Lynes has documented in his invaluable book *The Healing of Cancer*). Even distinguished medical doctors who "play by the rules" of modern science—publishing their results and making their alternative methods available for inspection—are condemned by the cancer establishment because those methods, if widely adopted, would directly compete with the money-intensive modalities of toxic chemotherapy, radiation, and surgery, invasive treatments that often do more harm than good.

Today, treating cancer is a megabillion-dollar industry. Every thirty seconds, another American is diagnosed with the disease. Half a million Americans die of cancer annually, yet there are even more people making a living off cancer than there are people dying of it—and many of them are making a very good living indeed. Just getting a new anticancer drug approved takes ten to twelve years and $120 million. This process in itself excludes many promising alternatives from ever being tested. Cancer patients typically spend $30,000 to $50,000 on toxic, often devastating therapy and get very little for their money. Cancer is the single most lucrative segment of the medical industry, which eats up a fat chunk of the Gross National Product.

Given the high stakes, what are the chances the medical-pharmaceutical complex would welcome an innovative outsider who came up with a safe, nontoxic, inexpensive cancer cure—a diet, an herbal compound, a bioelectric energy, or a naturally occurring bodily chemical? Practically nil. As Barry Lynes bluntly states, "The American Cancer Society is not interested in a cure. It would go out of business."[2]

Unlike so many other countries, the United States supports only one kind of medicine. Because of this, Americans have been denied many vital aspects of the science and art of healing. "Your family doctor is *no longer free* to choose the treatment he or she feels is best for you, but must follow the dictates established by physicians whose motives and alliances are such that their decisions may not be in your best interests," says Alan Levin, M.D.[3] Patients' most fundamental right—medical freedom of choice—has been lost in this country. The medical monopoly's right to make money comes before your right to decide—in consultation with your doctor—which cancer therapy would be best for your particular condition. The dilemma faced by the cancer patient is movingly illustrated by the following letter. The author is a psychologist.

> My wife was diagnosed as having terminal ovarian cancer five years ago. She is alive, well, and healthy because of non-approved and unconventional cancer treatment.
>
> I am writing this as a letter of protest and in an attempt to educate you and possibly save your life or that of your wife or child. I am not a crazy fanatic, but I am a 48-year-old man who, five years ago, had to decide what to do in order to try and save my wife's life. We investigated and researched our options and made an informed and intelligent decision to seek something other than what was offered by traditional medicine in this country.
>
> I am angry, frustrated, and mad as hell that I have had to take my wife out of this country, had to struggle with my health insurance company because her treatment was "not approved," and had to struggle to obtain her medications because they are "not approved" and subject to confiscation. It has been a battle to provide her with alternative cancer treatment.
>
> I now know that there is a financial war going on, and the victims are the millions of people who have been denied

alternative cancer treatments because the AMA or FDA or someone has decided that we can only undergo an approved treatment. . . . There are no rights to life or liberty in this country when it comes to freedom of choice in medicine. There is only coercion and subversion and greed—and people dying. We are the financial prisoners of the AMA and FDA, and they are killing us in the name of approved treatment.

My wife was almost a victim; and if you allow this to continue, then one day you will become a victim, too.

Please help to do something to bring truth, sanity, and morality back to health care in America. [4]

Only the rich or the well-off middle-class person can take advantage of many of the effective alternative cancer therapies by going out of the country—or else by seeking an American alternative practitioner, who is not likely to be covered by medical insurance. This is highly undemocratic and unfair. "Nothing could be more obscene than the spectacle of dying Americans denied freedom of choice in therapy having to go underground, go abroad, or do without," says Michael Culbert of the Committee for Freedom of Choice in Medicine. "The vicious system, which on the one hand says, 'We cannot cure you,' and on the other, 'But don't try some unproven remedy,' must come to an end. It is blatantly immoral."

What Americans call alternative medicine is simply part of the legal medical system in many European countries. For instance, in England, Germany, and Switzerland—countries with high-quality medical care— doctors and therapists who use nondrug approaches to healing are practicing freely in lively competition with conventional doctors. "To deny someone freedom to seek a therapy which they believe would save their life is a denial of every moral principle," declares Frank Wiewel of People Against Cancer, based in Otho, Iowa. He adds, "The United States government, in suppressing alternative cancer therapies, is in direct violation of the international Helsinki Accords to which this country is signatory." The 1964 Helsinki Declaration, approved by the United States Congress, stipulates that "the doctor must be free to use a new therapeutic measure, if in his judgment it offers hope of saving life, reestablishing health, or alleviating suffering."

Chemotherapy at most prevents "perhaps 2 or 3 percent" of the nearly half-a-million cancer deaths per year, as Dr. John Cairns of the Harvard School of Public Health documented in the November 1985 issue of *Scientific American*. If this fact were widely publicized, the cancer-treatment centers would close down tomorrow and the public would loudly demand both the freedom to use alternative therapies as well as massive funding to research nontoxic approaches. Prominent American cancer specialist Albert Braverman, M.D., called for "scaling back the whole chemotherapeutic enterprise." In the April 13, 1991, issue of *The Lancet*, he says, "Chemotherapy should be prescribed only when there is a reasonable prospect either of cure or of benefit in quantity and quality of life. Our oncology trainees should be taught that chemotherapy is not part of the management of every cancer patient; for many or most patients, medical intervention should be confined to symptom management and enrolment in a hospice programme."

Chemotherapy is incapable of extending in any appreciable way the lives of patients afflicted with the most common cancers—and even the palliative effect of these toxic drugs, which supposedly improve the quality of life, "rests on scientifically shaky ground." That was the conclusion of West German cancer biostatistician Ulrich Abel, Ph.D., in the most comprehensive study ever undertaken on cancer chemotherapy. In his 1990 book,[5] Dr. Abel wrote, "There is no evidence for the vast majority of cancers that treatment with these drugs exerts any positive influence on survival or quality of life in patients with advanced disease." The advanced cancers to which Dr. Abel is referring are those malignancies responsible for over 80 percent of the cancer deaths in the Western industrial countries. "Among others, they include nearly all malignant tumors of trachea, bronchus, lung, stomach, colon, rectum, esophagus, breast, bladder, pancreas, ovary, cervix and corpus uteri, head and neck, and liver. . . . Tumors are called advanced if they are recurrent, disseminated, or not radically resectable."

Chemotherapy does shrink tumors, at least initially, in many patients. Unfortunately, this partial or complete "reduction of tumor mass does not prolong expected survival," Dr. Abel found, because the cancer usually returns, often more aggressively than before. Only in small-cell lung cancer is there any "good direct evidence of a survival improvement by chemotherapy"—a whopping three months! Otherwise, for the common killer cancers, chemotherapy remains a blind alley. Abel polled hundreds of cancer doctors while investigating the world medical literature to produce his study. Indeed, he learned that many oncologists would not take chemotherapy themselves if they had cancer. Germany's major news magazine, *Der Spiegel*, gave Abel's important research extensive, mostly favorable coverage. But it was almost completely suppressed in the United States, where the media, manipulated by vested interests, maintains a virtual blackout about the true nature of the abortive "war on cancer."

Calling chemotherapy "another unproven cancer remedy," Alan Gaby, M.D., medical editor of the *Townsend Letter for Doctors*, writes, "Until cancer researchers start answering the important questions, we should all refuse to contribute to the American Cancer Society and other bastions of misinformation. And don't forget to explain, to the little old lady standing out in the cold in front of the drugstore collecting money for cancer research, exactly why you refuse to contribute."

The American Cancer Society lobbies vigorously to suppress new ideas and promising new approaches to treating cancer. It instigates government persecution and harassment of independent researchers and imposes its narrow views on government-funded research, all the while soaking the public for money through its deceptive public-relations image as the nation's vanguard cancer fighter. Founded by John D. Rockefeller, Jr., and his business associates, the ACS collects around $400 million a year from the unenlightened American public, then spends less than 30 percent of this huge cash hoard on research. No major breakthrough in treating cancer has ever resulted from an ACS grant. In 1988, the ACS spent a mere 26 percent of its $336 million income on research. Most of its money goes into fat salaries and other nonresearch expenses—land, buildings, and bank accounts (its "fund balance" in 1988 was $426 million). The ACS's "failure to dedicate the major portion of [its] income" to research "borders on dishonesty. It also fits perfectly with the highly politicized agendas of today's health charities," writes Dr. James Bennett, an economist at George Mason University, in his exposé on health charities that rip off gullible Americans.[6]

"In other words," concludes journalist Peter Barry Chowka in a 1978 probe, "ACS is hoarding and investing for profit many millions of dollars contributed by the public to fight cancer, while the Society claims that vital research is going begging for funds."[7]

Most people, notes Barry Lynes, are surprised to learn that "the ACS does not meet the standards of the National Information Bureau, the charity watchdog. How could they? Most of their money goes into salaries, public relations campaigns, publications which attack legitimate if unorthodox therapies, and lobbying federal officials in Washington."[8]

Two-time Nobel laureate Linus Pauling summed up the situation well when he said, "Everyone should know that the 'war on cancer' is largely a fraud, and that the National Cancer Institute and the American Cancer Society are derelict in their duties to the people who support them." According to Barry Lynes, "At a minimum, the American Cancer Society . . . should be investigated by the U.S. Justice Department for fraud, false advertising, conspiracy and a variety of other anti-trust, monopolistic crimes."[9]

Furthermore, the ACS's Unproven Methods list is a self-serving blacklist. This unscientific compendium is used to smear effective or promising alternative cancer therapies as "quackery" (see Chapter 1). How ironic that a vice president of Memorial Sloan-Kettering Cancer Center admitted to Ralph Moss that the ACS blacklist was "where they got all their best ideas."[10]

Closely linked to the ACS through interlocking directorates is the National Cancer Institute, a government-funded agency that goes begging to Congress every year for a bigger budget—now at *$1.5 billion.* The NCI should be a catalyst for innovation, openly encouraging any new technique or method that might slow the death count in a cancer epidemic claiming 10,000 American lives each week. Instead, NCI is just the opposite, a repressive guardian of the status quo that funds an "old boys' network" committed to chemotherapy and radiation, while actively conspiring with other federal agencies to harass or thwart innovative alternative cancer therapies. NCI helped suppress the Hoxsey therapy (Chapter 9) and is thus directly responsible for the deaths of millions of people who might have been cured had this treatment option remained legal in the United States. Instead of serving the public, "NCI created a bureaucratic haven for scientism, filled with committee procedures, payoffs, collusion with drug companies and interminable roadblocks for the truly innovative cancer fighters," as Barry Lynes observed in *The Healing of Cancer.*[11]

What NCI does with your $1.5 billion in taxes is a unique form of corruption in the history of science. NCI distributes these billions in research grants and, together with the ACS, sets the dominant trends in research. Incredibly, 90 percent of the members of NCI's peer review committee get NCI money for their own research, while 70 percent of the ACS's research budget goes to individuals or institutions with which the ACS board members are personally affiliated. "In any other part of government, it would be a corrupt practice for the persons giving out the money and the persons getting it to be the same people," says Irwin Bross, Ph.D., former director of biostatistics at the famed Roswell Park Memorial Institute, the nation's oldest cancer-research hospital. Testifying before a congressional subcommittee, Dr. Bross added, "It is a corrupt practice even when it is called 'peer review' or 'cancer research' . . . This set-up is not worth revamping and should simply be junked."

"Cancer, Inc.," the group of vested, interlocking interests that preserves the status quo in cancer treatment and research, includes the ACS and NCI along with the giant pharmaceutical companies, insurance firms, hospitals, and medical schools. The insurance companies provide third-party reimbursements to doctors, making up 70 percent of doctors' incomes. Spearheading the medical cartel is the American Medical Association, a trade union with an extremely powerful lobby. The AMA, which represents less than half of the allopathic doctors in the United States, wages a megabuck campaign in Congress and the state legislatures to push laws that strengthen its stranglehold on American health-care policies. Over the course of its history, the AMA has denounced midwifery, self-care, optometry, homeopathy, osteopathy, acupuncture and lay analysis as being dangerous, fraudulent, or both. In 1987, the AMA was found guilty of restraint of trade in a "conspiracy to destroy and eliminate" the chiropractic profession, a legitimate competitor. Today, the AMA coordinates harassment campaigns against alternative doctors who may have their licenses revoked and their careers destroyed for practicing valid nonorthodox healing methods.

Does a conspiracy exist to actively suppress effective and promising alternative cancer therapies? In 1953, a United States Senate investigation into the cancer industry concluded that the AMA, NCI, and FDA had entered into a conspiracy to promote radiation, chemotherapy, and surgery while suppressing alternative cancer therapies *that were highly praised by the cured patients themselves.* Attorney Benedict Fitzgerald of the United States Justice Department, who led the investigation, called for a full-scale probe to expose the lethal bureaucracy thwarting advances in cancer treatment and research. For this, he was fired.

The same lethal bureaucracy is alive and well today, as can be seen from a 300-page report on alternative cancer therapies released in September 1990 by the Office of Technology Assessment. Heavily slanted toward negative preconclusions, the report, titled *Unconventional Cancer Treatments,* dismisses any positive data in support of alternative therapies as "anecdotal" but presents negative data as "proof" that the therapies are worthless. Important clinical studies and documented case material attesting to the effectiveness of specific therapies are either totally ignored or dismissed as "unacceptable" or minimized. The thousands of human beings with advanced cancer who were cured by alternative methods do not exist in the report except as fleeting statistics, grudgingly mentioned. The misleading, sanitized OTA report, which cost well over half a million dollars in taxpayers' money, is "a mostly meaningless mishmash of misinformation," wrote Michael Culbert, who appeared before two of the OTA advisory meetings, in an article in the Winter 1990 issue of *The Choice*.

Nevertheless, buried within the OTA report are over 180 positive medical and scientific studies supporting the efficacy of alternative therapies. And Roger Herdman, M.D., OTA assistant director, said the report urges researchers "to take a sympathetic and thoughtful look at some of these treatments." Yet, when the OTA in late 1990 recommended that the National Cancer Institute devote a tiny part of its research budget to alternative treatments, the NCI was incredulous and rejected every one of OTA's recommendations, as *Z Magazine* reported in June 1991. In other words, it's business as usual at NCI and ACS. About 10,000 American cancer victims will continue to die on schedule every week. And the "unproven" alternative methods will continue to be condemned and banished without a fair evaluation.

Meanwhile, the "proven" methods of toxic chemotherapy, carcinogenic radiotherapy, and surgery are a failure for the majority of patients. The death rates from the six major killer cancers—cancers of the lung, colon, breast, prostate, pancreas, and ovary—have either stayed the same or increased during the past sixty years. The American Cancer Society's publicity staff knows that people will not give money to a hopeless cause, so it regularly announces "breakthroughs," talks about "winning" the "war on cancer," and inflates the statistics. "The Society also fails to tell us that the 'improved' survival rate seen over the past 80 years . . . is largely the result of earlier detection—*not* more effective treatment," explains John McDougall, M.D. "Finding the cancer earlier does allow more people to live 5 years after the time of diagnosis. Thus, more people will fit the definition of 'cured.' However, in most cases, early detection does not increase a person's life span but only the length of time a person is aware that he or she has cancer."[12]

Cancer is this century's Black Plague—1,400 people die from it every day in the United States, with over 500,000 dying from it per year, and the death rates are mounting. To reverse this cruel epidemic, a multiplicity of therapeutic approaches is urgently needed. Patients and their doctors need immediate information on the therapies—alternative, experimental, and conventional—that will work best for a specific type of cancer at a particular stage. And they need immediate access to these therapies. Many cures now exist, waiting to be perfected.

People with AIDS deserve credit for exposing the harmful effects of medical politics in this country. The AIDS epidemic has produced a sense of urgency, a willingness to cut through bureaucratic red tape and to encourage experimental treatments. Where is the sense of urgency in the cancer epidemic?

Only a grassroots movement can restore the patient's freedom to choose, the doctor's freedom to prescribe, and the researcher's ability to experiment. Only a nationwide movement of informed cancer patients and their families and friends has the potential to break the stranglehold of the medical monopoly, to end the great waste of dollars, and to focus on real cures. Until this happens, no change is possible on a national scale, and millions will continue to die. Change will require massive citizen participation, major legislative reform, protests to politicians, pressure on the mass media, and guaranteed commitments from whichever Democratic and Republican candidates run for president. Groups like People Against Cancer, Project CURE, and the Foundation for the Advancement of Innovative Medicine (FAIM) are working to build a democratic, nationwide movement for medical freedom and health-care reform.

The following are a few modest proposals that would benefit cancer patients and health-care consumers in general:

First, restore to all patients the recognized right to choose the therapies they believe might help them. Polls show that most Americans want the freedom to decide on their own cancer-treatment options instead of having a Big Brother government dictating their most personal health decisions.

Second, let doctors treat their patients as they see fit, without the meddlesome interference and threats of a medical orthodoxy that represents a minority of all doctors.

Third, put medical freedom of choice into the United States Constitution as a health-care rights amendment to the Bill of Rights. The necessity of doing this was recognized over 200 years ago by Dr. Benjamin Rush, a signer of the Declaration of Independence. His farsighted words are worth heeding:

> Unless we put Medical Freedom into the Constitution, the time will come when medicine will organize into an undercover dictatorship. To restrict the art of healing to one class of men and deny equal privileges to others will constitute the

Bastille of medical science. All such laws are un-American and despotic. . . . The Constitution of this Republic should make special provisions for Medical Freedom as well as Religious Freedom.

If Dr. Rush's advice had been followed, 10,000 Americans might not be dying of cancer every week. The Healthcare Rights Amendment guaranteeing self-determination in the choice of health care has garnered nearly 100,000 signatures. (See Appendix C.) It should be revived and circulated widely until a congressperson introduces it as legislation.

Fourth, "abolish the American Cancer Society and distribute its shameful and colossal bank accounts to cancer patients," as Patrick McGrady, Jr., advises in his article, "The Cancer Patient's Quandary," in the June 1984 *Townsend Letter for Doctors.* "Nobody can point to a single major research development from the billions we've given them. That institution is a disgrace."

Fifth, dismantle the National Cancer Institute bureaucracy and purge it of corrupt officials. Appoint "a hound dog of a director who will drive the agency into areas it has avoided and who has some kind of direct, ongoing reporting obligation to the American public," as Barry Lynes suggests in *The Healing of Cancer.* Make the NCI a true clearinghouse of innovative treatment approaches.

Sixth, earmark at least 50 percent of NCI's billions of dollars of our tax money toward research into promising, nontoxic alternative cancer treatments that have shown some efficacy. Examples, chosen at random, include the Essiac and Hoxsey herbal remedies, Burzynski's antineoplaston therapy, the Naessens 714-X compound, Royal Rife's bioelectric treatment, Kelley's metabolic therapy, Burton's Immuno-Augmentative Therapy, and ozone therapy. This step alone could dramatically improve the nation's health by slowing the course of the cancer epidemic.

Seventh, set up a national databank or intelligence service that cancer patients can readily tap for unbiased, up-to-date information about alternative, experimental, and orthodox treatments. The current establishment services are extremely limited because of their built-in political bias. Although there are a number of valuable patient-referral services in the alternative field, a coordinated, scientific system is needed that goes beyond any one person's individual perspective. Patients would be able to get information on which therapy or combination of therapies is most likely to help their particular cancer at its specific stage.

Eighth, conduct fair, objective, in-depth tests of alternative cancer therapies to find out whether they work, how well, and for which types of illness. A major obstacle to such testing has been the cancer establishment's insistence on double-blind random trials—in which half the patients are guinea pigs who do *not* receive the treatment being tested. This procedure is immoral since the guinea pigs being deprived of the medication are human beings dying of severe or terminal cancer. Furthermore, double-blind clinical trials are wholly unnecessary. "As proof of efficacy, they are entirely superfluous for tumors which normally fail to respond at all but which, in statistically significant numbers, do respond to the new agent," states Patrick McGrady, Jr., of CANHELP. (*Note:* Up to 90 percent of *orthodox* medical procedures have never been tested by double-blind controlled trials, according to a 1987 OTA study.)

Ninth, "scale back the whole chemotherapy enterprise," as suggested by respected oncologist Albert Braverman, M.D., of the State University of New York, in a major *Lancet* editorial on April 13,1991. The overprescription of chemotherapy drugs is a national scandal—a system that enriches the few while countless patients are killed by the chemo drug rather than by the cancer. Chemotherapy and radiation should have a limited, strictly defined role in cancer treatment.

Tenth, get the FDA out of the cancer field altogether. Its testing procedures are a parody of science. The Food and Drug Administration was founded to ensure purity and safety in our food and medicines. It has not fulfilled that purpose. Instead, it functions as a government police force, approving experimental studies for the giant companies it favors while blocking approval for those it dislikes. There is "a very lethal and dangerous partnership between the drug companies and the FDA," reported Sidney Wolfe, M.D., Washington health advocate, on the television news show *Frontline* in 1989. Mired in corruption, with close ties to the industries it is supposed to regulate, the FDA has a long history of approving dangerous drugs and carcinogenic chemical food additives—while using harassment, unconstitutional procedures, illegal break-ins, endless delays, and even falsified evidence to suppress promising cancer treatments.

Abolish or drastically modify the 1962 Kefauver efficacy amendments to the Food and Drug law. The *Wall Street Journal* has waged a campaign to abolish the Kefauver amendments. These amendments give police powers to the FDA far beyond the agency's original purpose. And the FDA regularly uses its police powers to stamp out alternative therapies, to block medical research, and to prevent patients and doctors from using safer medications of their choice. The FDA should stick to its original function of ensuring safety. It is not capable of determining efficacy.

Protecting cancer patients from quacks who sell worthless nostrums is certainly a legitimate public-health concern. But this has been used as a pretext to suppress alternative therapeutic approaches and to deny patients the fundamental right to choose treatments they think are best for them. In a competitive health-care marketplace, alert, educated citizens will soon differentiate the worthless cures from the ones that work. This process will allow innovations to emerge.

Eleventh, change the insurance-reimbursement policies. Cancer patients who use alternative, experimental, or orthodox therapies prescribed by competent practitioners should be promptly reimbursed by their insurance company, Medicare, or health maintenance organization (HMO) plan. There is now a clear-cut, across-the-board policy to deny insurance and Medicare reimbursement for alternative treatment. This must stop. Patients must not be financially punished for choosing alternative medical care, which is usually less expensive than conventional care.

Finally, organize a massive public effort focusing on cancer prevention. The great majority of cancers are preventable, as Samuel Epstein, M.D., pointed out in his 1978 book, *The Politics of Cancer.* Among the major culprits in the cancer epidemic are chemical and industrial wastes, radioactive debris, work-place chemicals, medical X-rays, food additives, air pollution, tobacco, improper diet, and chlorinated water. Each of these items represents powerful, highly profitable vested interests that will not give up their "right to pollute" without a struggle. When it comes to diet, the implicated cancer-causing factors are "principally fat and meat intake, excessive caloric intake, and the hormonal and metabolic factors affected by nutrition," as Dr. Gio Gori, deputy director of the National Cancer Institute's Division of Cancer Cause and Prevention, told Congress in 1976.[13] Simple dietary changes are something everyone can do to greatly reduce their cancer risk. For specific suggestions, see *Everyday Cancer Risks and How to Avoid Them*, by Mary Kerney Levenstein (Avery Publishing Group, Garden City Park, NY, 1992).

A range of therapy options is available when cancer does strike. However, the time between diagnosis of cancer and initiation of treatment can be filled with stress, confusion, and fear, and many people never look at the options. Instead, patients turn to their doctor, nearly always an allopathic practitioner, and hand over total control of their life and illness and therapy. Why? Because they don't know they have options, or how to seek them out. And they're afraid that if they question their doctor's decisions, he will brand them a "bad patient"—a label that will be echoed by family and friends.

Patients, especially American cancer patients, need to regain control over their own life, over their own therapy and survival. One way to accomplish this is to ask those feared questions. Another way is to learn about cancer in general, about your cancer in particular, and about all the treatment possibilities available. Hopefully, this book will help you begin the process, by teaching you what kind of questions to ask and by reviewing the alternative treatment options available. Then you can actively work toward your most important options of all: health and life.

NOTES

Chapter 1
Alternative Cancer Therapies

1. Gary Null, "Medical Genocide Part 16," *Penthouse*, 1987, quoted in Barry Lynes, *The Healing of Cancer* (Queensville, Ontario: Marcus Books, 1989), p. 10.
2. John Cairns, "The Treatment of Diseases and the War Against Cancer," *Scientific American*, November 1985.
3. W.H. Cole, "Opening Address: Spontaneous Regression of Cancer and the Importance of Finding Its Cause," *Conference on Spontaneous Regression of Cancer*, U.S. Department of Health, Education and Welfare, Public Health Service, National Institutes of Health, Monograph 44, Department of Health, Education and Welfare Pub. No. (NIH) 76-1038, 1976, pp. 5-9.
4. Judith Glassman, *The Cancer Survivors* (Garden City, NY: Dial Press, 1983), pp. 323-324.
5. Harold D. Foster, "Lifestyle Changes and the 'Spontaneous' Regression of Cancer: An Initial Computer Analysis," *International Journal of Biosocial Research*, vol. 10, no. 1, 1988, pp.

17-33, reprinted in *Healing Newsletter*, vol. 5, no. 3, available from the Gerson Institute.
6. Peter Barry Chowka, "The National Cancer Institute and the Fifty Year Cover Up," *East West Journal*, January 1978, cited in Lynes, op. cit.
7. Hardin B. Jones, "A Report on Cancer," speech delivered to the American Cancer Society's 11th Annual Science Writers' Conference, New Orleans, Louisiana, 7 March 1969, published in *The Choice*, May 1977.
8. Barrie Cassileth et al., "Contemporary Unorthodox Treatments in Cancer Medicine," *Annals of Internal Medicine*, vol. 101, 1984, pp. 105-112.
9. Robert Houston, *Repression and Reform in the Evaluation of Alternative Cancer Therapies*, Project CURE, Washington, D.C., 1987, p. 13.
10. Ralph Moss, *The Cancer Industry* (New York: Paragon House, 1989), p. 98.
11. Houston, op. cit., p. 7.
12. "Assessing the Efficacy and Safety of Medical Technologies," U.S. Congress, Office of Technology Assessment, PB 286-929, 1978, p. 7.
13. Ken Wilber, *Grace and Grit:*

Spirituality and Healing in the Life and Death of Treya Killam Wilber (Boston: Shambhala, 1991), chap. 15.

14. *New York State Journal of Medicine*, March 1971, p. 554.

15. John Laszlo, *Understanding Cancer* (New York: Harper and Row, 1987).

16. Dick Richards, *The Topic of Cancer: When the Killing Has to Stop* (Oxford, England and New York: Pergamon Press, 1982).

17. T.J. Powles et al., "Failure of Chemotherapy to Prolong Survival in a Group of Patients With Metastatic Breast Cancer," *The Lancet*, 15 March 1980, p. 580.

18. *Dissent in Medicine: Nine Doctors Speak Out* (Chicago: Contemporary Books, 1985).

19. Robert C. Atkins, *Dr. Atkins' Health Revolution: How Complementary Medicine Can Extend Your Life* (New York: Bantam Books, 1990), p. 332.

20. Lucien Israel, *Conquering Cancer* (New York: Random House, 1978), p. 95.

21. Jan Stjernsward, "Decreased Survival Related to Irradiation Postoperatively in Early Operable Breast Cancer," *The Lancet*, 30 November 1974; and Mark Fuerst, "Doctors Persist With Outmoded Cancer Therapies," *Cancer Forum*, vol. 9, no. 7-8, Winter 1988-1989, p. 11.

22. Israel, op. cit., p. 95.

23. Ben Fitzgerald, *Congressional Record*, 28 August 1953; and see Lynes, op. cit.

24. Quoted in Moss, op. cit., p. 72.

25. "Primary Treatment Is Not Enough for Early Stage Breast Cancer," *Update*, National Cancer Institute, Office of Cancer Communications, 18 May 1988.

26. William D. Kelley, *Dr. Kelley's Answer to Cancer* (Winthrop, WA: Wedgestone Press, 1986), p. 11.

27. Patrick McGrady, Jr., "The Cancer Patient's Quandary," *Townsend Letter for Doctors*, no. 16, June 1984, p. 99.

Part One
Biologic and Pharmacologic Therapies

1. Robert C. Atkins, *Dr. Atkins' Health Revolution: How Complementary Medicine Can Extend Your Life* (New York: Bantam Books, 1990), p. 52.

2. Erik Enby with Peter Gosch and Michael Sheehan, *Hidden Killers: The Revolutionary Medical Discoveries of Professor Guenther Enderlein* (Saratoga, CA: Sheehan Communications, 1990), available from Michael Sheehan, Sheehan Communications, P.O. Box 706, Saratoga, CA 95071, 408-741-0235; and Michael Sheehan, "What Your Doctor Doesn't Know Can Kill You," *Townsend Letter for Doctors*, July 1991, pp. 575-576.

Chapter 2
Antineoplaston Therapy

1. S.R. Burzynski, E. Kubove, and B. Burzynski, "Phase II Clinical Trials of Antineoplaston A10 and AS2-1 Infusions in Astrocytoma," 17th International Congress of Chemotherapy, Berlin, Germany, 1991.

2. Ralph W. Moss, *The Cancer Industry* (New York: Paragon House, 1989), pp. 307-308.

3. Burzynski et al., op. cit.

4. S.R. Burzynski, M.D., Ph.D., "The Body Itself Has a Treatment for Cancer," lecture presented at the 1990 World Research Foundation Congress, Los Angeles, 7 October 1990, published in *Health Consciousness*, June 1991, pp. 31-32.

5. Avis Lang, "The Disease of Information Processing: An Interview With Stanislaw R. Burzyn-

ski, *Townsend Letter for Doctors,* June 1989, p. 294.

6. Dvorit Samid, Lin Ti Sherman, and Donata Rimoldi, "Induction of Phenotypic Reversion and Terminal Differentiation in Tumor Cells by Antineoplaston AS2-1," abstract, Ninth International Symposium on Future Trends in Chemotherapy, Geneva, 26–28 March 1990.

7. T.G. Muldoon, J.A. Copland, A.F. Lehner, and L.B. Hendry, "Inhibition of Spontaneous Mouse Mammary Tumour Development by Antineoplaston A10," *Drugs Under Experimental and Clinical Research,* vol. 13 (supp. I), 1987.

8. Lang, op. cit., p. 292.

Chapter 3
Gaston Naessens

1. Interview with the author.

2. Peter Tocci, "Views on the 1991 Symposium: From Béchamp's Microzyma to the Somatid Theory," *Health Consciousness,* October 1991, p. 39.

3. Christopher Bird, *The Persecution and Trial of Gaston Naessens* (Tiburon, CA: H.J. Kramer, 1991).

4. Ibid., p. 4.

5. Christopher Bird, "Gaston Naessens' Symposium on Somatidian Orthobiology: A Beachhead Established," *Townsend Letter for Doctors,* vol. 99, October 1991, p. 797.

6. Raymond Keith Brown, *AIDS, Cancer and the Medical Establishment* (New York: Robert Speller Publishers, 1986).

7. Christopher Bird, "In Defense of Gaston Naessens," *New Age Journal,* September–October 1989, p. 119.

8. Tocci, op. cit., pp. 33–40.

9. Gaston Naessens, "714X—A Highly Promising Non-Toxic Treatment for Cancer and

Other Immune Deficiencies," C.O.S.E., Quebec.

10. Bird (note 3), op. cit., pp. 136–140.

11. Bird (note 7), op. cit., p. 123.

12. Bird (note 5), op. cit., p. 799.

13. Victor Penzer, "Gaston Naessens: La Nouvelle Biologie," *Health Consciousness,* December 1990, p. 20.

Chapter 4
Revici Therapy

1. Gerhard N. Schrauzer, Ph.D., letter to the Board of Regents, Department of Education, State of New York, 14 February 1986.

2. Barry Bryant, *Cancer and Consciousness* (Boston: Sigo Press, 1990), p. 147.

3. *The Cancer Chronicles,* vol. 2, no. 1, Summer 1990, p. 2; and Seymour Brenner, M.D., letter to Guy V. Molinari, 24 March 1988.

4. Dwight L. McKee, M.D., *Emanuel Revici M.D.: A Review of His Scientific Work* (New York: Institute of Applied Biology, 1985), p. 14.

5. Richard A. Passwater, *Cancer and Its Nutritional Therapies* (New Canaan, CT: Keats Publishing, 1983), p. 149.

6. Marcus A. Cohen, "On Emanuel Revici, M.D.," unpublished manuscript, 1988.

7. Ibid., pp. 1, 6.

8. Ibid., p. 12.

9. Ibid., pp. 4, 14.

10. Robert Ravich, "Revici Method of Cancer Control. Evaluation of 1047 Patients With Advanced Malignancies Treated From 1946–1955," unpublished manuscript, undated.

Chapter 5
Hydrazine Sulfate

1. Lawrence Linderman, "Finding a Magic Bullet," *Penthouse,* July 1989, p. 110.

2. Quoted in Ralph W. Moss, *The*

Cancer Industry (New York: Paragon House, 1989), pp. 192–193.

3. Robert G. Houston, *Misinformation From OTA on Unconventional Cancer Treatments*, invited review for the U.S. Congress, Office of Technology Assessment (Otho, IA: People Against Cancer, 1990), p. 27.

4. Moss, op. cit., p. 205.

5. Joseph Gold, "Hydrazine Sulfate: A Current Perspective," *Nutrition and Cancer*, vol. 9, nos. 2 and 3, 1987, pp. 64–65.

6. Joseph Gold, M.D., "Cancer Therapy With Hydrazine Sulfate," *Cancer Control Journal*, vol. 1, no. 4, November–December 1973, p. 16.

7. Linderman, op. cit., p. 112.

8. Jeff Kamen, "Finally, Attention for Cancer Wonder Drug," *West Side Spirit*, New York, 24 July 1990, pp. 9, 34.

9. Kamen, op. cit., p. 34.

10. Naomi Pfeiffer, "Studies Spur New Look at Low-Cost Anti-Cachexia Drug," *Oncology Times*, vol. 12, no. 6, June 1991, p. 14.

Part Two
Immune Therapies

1. Linda Edwards Hood, "Interferon," *American Journal of Nursing*, April 1987, pp. 459–463.

2. *Science*, 9 January 1987.

3. Charles G. Moertel, "On Lymphokines, Cytokines, and Breakthroughs," *Journal of the American Medical Association*, vol. 256, 12 December 1986, p. 3141; and *Fortune*, November 1985.

4. *Business Week*, 22 September 1986; *Toronto Globe and Mail*, 28 May 1988; *Wall Street Journal*, May 1988; and *Science*, 20 December 1985.

5. *Cancer Victors Journal*, vol. 21, no. 1, Spring 1987, p. 5.

6. *Cancer Facts and Figures*, 1988.

7. Raymond Keith Brown, *AIDS, Cancer and the Medical Establishment* (New York: Robert Speller Publishers, 1986), pp. 171–172.

Chapter 6
Burton's Immuno-Augmentative Therapy

1. Robert Houston, "The Burton Syndrome," *Our Town*, 22 April 1979.

2. R. John Clement, Lawrence Burton, and Gerald N. Lampe, "Peritoneal Mesothelioma," *Quantum Medicine*, vol. 1, no. 1–2, 1988, pp. 68–73.

3. Robert Houston, *Analysis of a Survey of Patients on Immuno-Augmentative Therapy* (Otho, IA: People Against Cancer, 1988).

4. Dick Jacobs, "Patient's Research Pays Off, Cancer Under Control," *Cancer Victors Journal*, Summer–Fall 1988, pp. 26–27; Dick Jacobs, "How I Beat Cancer," *Cancer Control Society Newsletter*, vol. 6, no. 1, March 1990; and interview with the author.

5. Arlin J. Brown, "Dr. Lawrence Burton—Cancer Researcher in Exile," *Cancer Victory Bulletin*, vol. 7, no. 2, February 1981, pp. 1–2.

6. Jane Riddle Wright, *Diagnosis: Cancer–Prognosis: Life* (Huntsville, AL: Albright and Co., 1985), p. 94.

Chapter 7
Livingston Therapy

1. Raymond Keith Brown, *AIDS, Cancer and the Medical Establishment* (New York: Robert Speller Publishers, 1986), p. 92.

2. *Cancer Chronicles*, vol. 2, no. 2, August 1990, p. 5.

3. Michael Lerner, *Varieties of Integral Cancer Therapy* (Bolinas, CA: Commonweal, 10th ed., 1990); and news article in *Townsend Letter for Doctors*, May 1987, p. 100.

4. Irene Diller and William Diller, "Intracellular Acid-Fast Organisms Isolated From Malignant Tissues," *Transactions of the*

American Microbiological Society, vol. 84, 1965, pp. 138–146.

5. Virginia Livingston-Wheeler and Owen Wheeler, eds., *The Microbiology of Cancer: Compendium* (San Diego, CA: Livingston-Wheeler Clinic, 1977), p. 9.

6. Virginia Livingston-Wheeler and Owen Wheeler, *Food Alive* (San Diego, CA: Livingston-Wheeler Clinic, 1977).

7. V. Wuerthele-Caspe (Livingston) et al., "Cultural Properties and Pathogenicity of Certain Organisms Obtained From Various Proliferative and Neoplastic Diseases," *American Journal of Medical Science*, vol. 220, 1950, pp. 638–646.

8. Brown, op. cit., p. 96.

9. Gary Null, *Gary Null's Complete Guide to Healing Your Body Naturally* (New York: McGraw-Hill, 1988), p. 93.

10. Jules Vautrot, "The Search for Cure in Cancer—Part IV: An Organism and Vaccines: The Work of Dr. Virginia Livingston," *The Challenge*, vol. 13, no. 3, July 1991, pp. 19–20.

11. Barrie Cassileth et al., "Survival and Quality of Life Among Patients Receiving Unproven as Compared With Conventional Cancer Therapy," *New England Journal of Medicine*, vol. 324, no. 17, 25 April 1991, pp. 1180–1185.

12. Jules Vautrot, "Cover Commentary," *The Challenge*, July 1991, p. 1.

Chapter 8
Issels' Whole-Body Therapy

1. Jack Tropp, *Cancer: A Healing Crisis* (Los Angeles: Cancer Resource Center, 1980), p. xiii.

2. Barry Lynes, *The Healing of Cancer* (Queensville, Ontario: Marcus Books, 1989), p. 182.

3. Ibid., p. 181.

4. Josef Issels, *Cancer: A Second Opinion* (London: Hodder and Stoughton, 1975).

5. Josef Issels, "Cancer—Whole-body Approach and Immunotherapy," lecture given in New York, 1980.

6. Ibid.

7. Judith Glassman, *The Cancer Survivors* (Garden City, NY: Dial Press, 1983), pp. 250–251.

8. Tropp, op. cit., pp. 8–9.

9. F. Fuller Royal, "When Traditional Oriental or Modern Medicine Fail: Could Dental Amalgams Be Contributing to Our Declining Health?" *American Journal of Acupuncture*, vol. 18, no. 3, 1990, p. 210.

10. Ibid., pp. 208–209.

11. A. Elkadi et al., "Nigella Sativa and Cell-Mediated Immunity," *Archives of AIDS Research*, vol. 1, 1987, pp. 232–233; and A. Elkadi and O. Kandil, "The Black Seed (Nigella Sativa) and Immunity: Its Effect on Human T-Cell Subsets," a paper presented at the 71st Annual Meeting of the Federation of American Societies for Experimental Biology, Washington, D.C., March 1987, published in *Federation Proceedings*, vol. 46, no. 4, 1987, p. 1222.

Chapter 9
Hoxsey Therapy

1. Ken Ausubel, "The Troubling Case of Harry Hoxsey," *New Age Journal*, July–August 1988, p. 79.

2. *Surgery, Gynecology and Obstetrics*, vol. 114, 1962, pp. 25–30; and see Walter H. Lewis and Memory P.F. Elvin-Lewis, *Medical Botany: Plants Affecting Man's Health* (New York: John Wiley and Sons, 1977).

3. F.E. Mohs, "Chemosurgery: A Microscopically Controlled Method of Cancer Excision," *Archives of Surgery*, vol. 42, 1941, pp. 279–295, cited in Patricia Spain Ward, "History of Hoxsey Treatment," contract report submitted to U.S. Congress, Office of Technology Assessment, May 1988, pp. 2–3.

4. Ward, op. cit., p. 8.
5. Kazuyoshi Morita, Tsuneo Kada, and Mitsuo Namiki, "A Desmutagenic Factor Isolated From Burdock (*Arctium Lappa* Linne)," *Mutation Research*, vol. 129, 1984, pp. 25–31, cited in Ward, op. cit., p. 7.
6. Harry Hoxsey, *You Don't Have to Die* (New York: Milestone Books, 1956), pp. 44–48.
7. Ibid., p. 59.

Chapter 10
Essiac

1. C.A. Dombrádi and S. Földeák, "Screening Report on the Antitumor Activity of Purified *Arctium Lappa* Extracts," *Tumori*, vol. 52, 1966, p. 173, cited in Patricia Spain Ward, "History of Hoxsey Treatment," contract report for the U.S. Congress, Office of Technology Assessment, May 1988.
2. Kazuyoshi Morita, Tsuneo Kada, and Mitsuo Namiki, "A Desmutagenic Factor Isolated From Burdock (*Arctium Lappa* Linne)," *Mutation Research*, vol. 129, 1984, pp. 25–31, cited in Patricia Spain Ward, "History of Hoxsey Treatment," contract report for the U.S. Congress, Office of Technology Assessment, May 1988.
3. Sheila Snow Fraser and Carroll Allen, "Could Essiac Halt Cancer?" *Homemaker's*, June–July–August 1977, p. 19.
4. "Essiac as an Aid in Surgery," *Bracebridge Examiner*, 13 March 1991.
5. Gary L. Glum, *Calling of an Angel* (Los Angeles: Silent Walker Publishing, 1988), p. i.
6. "Essiac Added 18 Years to Her Mother's Life," *Bracebridge Examiner*, 6 February 1991.
7. "Cancer Commission Was Nothing But a Farce," *Bracebridge Examiner*, 9 January 1991.
8. Glum, op. cit., p. 136.

9. Ibid.

Chapter 11
Mistletoe (Iscador)

1. Tibor Hajto and K. Hostanka, "An Investigation of the Ability of *Viscum Album*-Activated Granulocytes to Regulate Natural Killer Cells *In Vivo*," *Clinical Trials Journal*, vol. 23, no. 6, 1986, pp. 345–358; and Peter Heusser, "Immunological Results of Mistletoe Therapy," in *Iscador: Compendium of Research Papers 1986–1988*, edited by Paul W. Scharff, M.D. (Spring Valley, NY: Mercury Press, 1991).
2. Robert G. Houston, *Repression and Reform in the Evaluation of Alternative Cancer Therapies*, Project CURE, Washington, D.C., 1989, p. 15.
3. Rita Leroi, M.D., *An Anthroposophical Approach to Cancer* (Spring Valley, NY: Mercury Press, 1982), p. 44.
4. Rita Leroi, M.D., *The Mistletoe Preparation Iscador in Clinical Use* (Arlesheim, Switzerland: Society for Cancer Research, 1987), pp. 34–35.
5. Leroi (1982), op. cit., p. 23.
6. Friedrich Lorenz, M.D., *Cancer: A Mandate to Humanity* (Spring Valley, NY: Mercury Press, 1982), p. 23.
7. Ibid., p. 26.
8. Leroi (1982), op. cit., pp. 30–31.
9. Ibid., pp. 33–34.
10. Leroi (1987), op. cit., pp. 35–36.
11. Leroi (1982), op. cit., pp. 41–42.
12. Tibor Hajto et al., "Increased Secretion of Tumor Necrosis Factor α, Interleukin 1, and Interleukin 6 by Human Mononuclear Cells Exposed to β-Galactoside-Specific Lectin From Clinically Applied Mistletoe Extract," *Cancer Research*, vol. 50, 1 June 1990, pp. 3322–3326.

Chapter 12
Pau D'Arco

1. Wayne Martin, "Pau D'Arco in Cancer Treatment," *Cancer Victors Journal*, Winter–Spring 1991, pp. 27–28.
2. Bill Wead, *Second Opinion: Lapacho and the Cancer Controversy* (Vancouver: Rostrum Communications, 1985), pp. 161–162.
3. Ibid., pp. 171–196.
4. R.T. Chlebowski, S.A. Akman, and J.B. Block, "Vitamin K in the Treatment of Cancer," *Cancer Treatment Reports*, vol. 12, 1985, p. 49.
5. Wead, op. cit., pp. 152, 159–161.
6. See also Hye Koo Yun with John Heinerman, *East/West Cancer Remedies for Wellness and Recovery*, unpublished manuscript (San Ysidro, CA: EastWest Wellness Center,1990), pp. 231–232.
7. *Reviews of the Institute of Antibiotics*, University of Recife, Brazil, vol. 20, no. 1-2, 1980–1981.
8. M.C.F. Linardi et al., *Journal of Medicinal Chemistry*, vol. 18, 1975, pp. 1159–1161.
9. *36th Annual Congress of the Society for Medicinal Plant Research*, 12–16 September 1988.
10. David Moikeha and Y. Hokama, University of Hawaii, paper presented to the Minority Biomedical Symposium, New Orleans, Louisiana, April 1986.
11. *Cancer Research*, vol. 28, 1968, pp. 1952–1954.
12. *Reviews of the Institute of Antibiotics*, University of Recife, Brazil, vol. 12, 1972, pp. 3–12.
13. Yun and Heinerman, op. cit., p. 229; and C.H. Burgstaller, *La Vuelta a los Vegetables*, Buenes Aires, 1968.
14. Varro Tyler, *The New Honest Herbal* (Philadelphia: George F. Stickley Co., 2nd ed., 1987), pp. 176–177; and Michael Lerner, *Varieties of Integral Cancer Therapy* (Bolinas, CA: Commonweal, 1983, 1990).
15. D.V.C. Awang, "Commercial Taheebo Lacks Active Ingredient," *Canadian Pharmaceutical Journal*, vol. 121, no. 5, 1988, pp. 323–326.
16. Martin, op. cit., pp. 27–28.

Chapter 13
Chaparral

1. Ronald S. Pardini et al., "Inhibition of Mitochondrial Electron Transport by Nor-dihydroguaiaretic Acid (NDGA)," *Biochemical Pharmacology*, vol. 19, 1970, p. 2699.
2. Dean Burk and N. Woods, "Effect of Nordihydroguaiaretic Acid and Other Antioxidants in Relation to X-Ray Action on Cancer Cells. (NIH)," *Radiation Research Supplement*, vol. 3, 1963, pp. 212–246; and Charles R. Smart et al., "Clinical Experience With Nordihydroguaiaretic Acid," *Rocky Mountain Medical Journal*, vol. 11, 1970, pp. 39–43.
3. Douglas Rigby, "Desert Drugstore," *Arizona Highways*, January 1959, p. 28.
4. *Journal of the American Pharmaceutical Association*, vol. 34, 1945, p. 82.
5. *Rocky Mountain Medical Journal*, vol. 67, November 1970, pp. 39–43.
6. John Heinerman, *The Treatment of Cancer With Herbs* (Orem, UT: BiWorld Publishers, 1984), p. 205.
7. Smart et al., op. cit.
8. "Chaparral Tea," *Cancer*, vol. 20, 1970, p. 113.
9. *Parallax View*, no. 1, 1975, p. 10; and Heinerman, op. cit., pp. 206–210.
10. Arlin J. Brown, *March of Truth on Cancer* (Fort Belvoir, VA: Arlin J. Brown Information Center, 7th ed., 1986), p. 116.
11. Michael Tierra, *The Way of Herbs* (New York: Pocket Books, 1983); and Michael Tierra,

Planetary Herbology (Santa Fe, NM: Lotus Press, 1988).

12. *Cancer Victory Bulletin*, vol. 5, no. 6, June 1979.

Part Four
Nutritional Therapies

1. G.W. Hepner, "Altered Bile Acid Metabolism in Vegetarians," *American Journal of Digestive Diseases*, vol. 20, no. 10, October 1975, p. 935; and M.J. Hill, "Bacteria and the Aetiology of Cancer of the Large Bowel," *The Lancet*, vol. 1, 1971, pp. 95–100.

2. E.L. Wynder, "The Dietary Environment and Cancer," *Journal of the American Dietetic Association*, vol. 71, 1977, pp. 385–392.

3. T. Hirayama, paper presented at the Conference on Breast Cancer and Diet, U.S.-Japan Cooperative Cancer Research Program, Fred Hutchinson Cancer Center, Seattle, Washington, 14–15 March 1977.

4. *Cancer Research*, vol. 35, 1975, pp. 3513–3522.

5. "'Vegetarians Do Better Than Carnivores'—Study," *The Choice*, vol. 16, no. 2–3, Summer 1990, p. 24.

Chapter 14
Wheatgrass Therapy

1. Eydie Mae Hunsberger with Chris Loeffler, *How I Conquered Cancer Naturally* (Garden City Park, NY: Avery Publishing Group, 1992).

2. Ann Wigmore, *Be Your Own Doctor* (Garden City Park, NY: Avery Publishing Group, 1982).

3. Kristine Nolfi, M.D., *My Experiences With Living Foods: The Raw Food Treatment of Cancer and Other Diseases* (Mokelumne Hill, CA: Health Research, no date), p. 14.

4. Otto Warburg, "On the Origin of Cancer Cells," *Science*, vol. 123, 1956.

5. Yoshihide Hagiwara, *Green Barley Essence: A Surprising Source of Health* (Tokyo: Association of Green and Health Distributors, 1981).

6. Tsuneo Kada et al., "Detection and Chemical Identification of Natural Bio-Antimutagens. A Case of the Green Tea Factor," *Mutation Research*, vol. 150, 1985, pp. 127–132.

7. Yasuo Hotta, "Preliminary Report on How the Juice of Young Green Barley Grass Plants Can Normalize and Rejuvenate Cells and Tissue, Can Repair Damaged DNA, Restore Cellular Activity, and Prevent Aging of Tissue," Green Foods, Carson, California, 1981.

8. Chiu-Nan Lai, "Chlorophyll: The Active Factor in Wheat Sprout Extract Inhibiting the Metabolic Activation of Carcinogens in Vitro," *Nutrition and Cancer*, vol. 1, 1978, pp. 27–30.

9. Robert A. Good et al., "The Influence of Nutrition on Development of Cancer Immunity and Resistance to Mesenchymal Diseases," in *Molecular Interrelations of Nutrition and Cancer*, edited by M.S. Arnott (New York: Raven Press, 1982), p. 85.

10. Gerald T. Keusch et al., "Nutrition, Host Defenses, and the Lymphoid System," in *Advances in Host Defense Mechanisms*, edited by John Gallin and Anthony Fauci (New York: Raven Press, 1983), vol. 2, p. 345.

11. Eduardo N. Siguel, "The Cancerostatic Effect of Vegetarian Diets," *Nutrition and Cancer*, vol. 4, 1983, pp. 285–289.

12. Herbert M. Shelton, *Health for All* (Mokelumne Hill, CA: Health Research, no date), pp. 213–215.

13. Louise Greenfield, "Raw Diet

Beats Cancer," *Cancer Forum*, vol. 6, no. 7–8, Summer 1982.

Chapter 15
Macrobiotics

1. "Heal Thyself," interview with Michio Kushi, *East West Journal*, March 1983, pp. 39–40.
2. Vivien Newbold, "Complete Remission of Advanced Medically Incurable Cancer in Six Patients Following a Macrobiotic Approach to Healing," *Townsend Letter for Doctors*, October 1990, pp. 638–642, published in expanded form in *Cancer Free: 30 Who Triumphed Over Cancer Naturally*, compiled and edited by the East West Foundation with Ann Fawcett and Cynthia Smith (Tokyo and New York: Japan Publications, 1991), pp. 235–255.
3. *Cancer Free*, op. cit., p. 237.
4. Ibid., p. 250.
5. Randi Londer, "Cure by Diet?" *Health*, October 1985.
6. Michio Kushi with Edward Esko, *The Macrobiotic Approach to Cancer* (Garden City Park, NY: Avery Publishing Group, rev. ed., 1991), p. 41.
7. Terry Shintani, "Macrobiotics, Nutrition and Disease Prevention," in *Doctors Look at Macrobiotics*, edited by Edward Esko (Tokyo and New York: Japan Publications, 1988), p. 205.
8. Correspondence with Mona Sanders; and *Cancer Free*, op. cit., pp. 160–164.
9. *Doctors Look at Macrobiotics*, op. cit., pp. 37–39.
10. *The World of Science*, Ghent, Belgium, 1983.
11. *Cancer Free*, op. cit., p. 266.

Chapter 16
Moerman's Anti-Cancer Diet

1. Ruth Jochems, *Dr. Moerman's Anti-Cancer Diet: Holland's Revolutionary Nutritional Program for* *Combating Cancer* (Garden City Park, NY: Avery Publishing Group, 1990), pp. xiii–xiv.
2. C. Moerman, *A Solution to the Cancer Problem* (Playa del Rey, CA: International Association of Cancer Victors and Friends, no date), p. 5.
3. Jochems, op. cit., pp. 22–23.
4. Otto Warburg, *Z. Naturforsch*, vol. 25, 1970, pp. 3, 332–333.
5. Kedar N. Prasad, *Vitamins Against Cancer* (Rochester, VT: Healing Arts Press, 1989), pp. 65, 74.
6. Richard A. Passwater, *Cancer and Its Nutritional Therapies* (New Canaan, CT: Keats Publishing, 1983), pp. 108–112.
7. Moerman, op. cit., p. 13.
8. Hye Koo Yun with John Heinerman, *East/West Cancer Remedies for Wellness and Recovery*, unpublished manuscript (San Ysidro, CA: EastWest Wellness Center, 1990), pp. 106–111.
9. Jochems, op. cit., pp. 24–27.
10. "Moerman Therapy Cures!" *Uitzicht: Magazine for the Natural Fight Against Cancer*, no. 3, May 1991, pp. 4–7. (All quotations are translated from the Dutch.)

Part Five
Metabolic Therapies

1. B. Rossi et al., *Proceedings of the Ninth International Cancer Congress*, 1966.
2. Richard A. Passwater, *Cancer and Its Nutritional Therapies* (New Canaan, CT: Keats Publishing, 1983), pp. 156, 182.
3. *New England Journal of Medicine*, vol. 299, 1978, p. 549.
4. "Dr. Linus Pauling Criticizes Consumer Report," *Cancer Victors Journal*, vol. 24, no. 1–2, Winter–Spring 1991, p. 24.
5. Anne Lee and Robert Langer, "Shark Cartilage Contains Inhibitors of Tumor Angiogenesis," *Science*, vol. 221, 16 September 1983, pp. 1185–1187.

Chapter 17
Gerson Therapy

1. Michael Lerner, *Varieties of Integral Cancer Therapy* (Bolinas, CA: Commonweal, 10th ed., 1990.)
2. Steve Austin, correspondence with the author.
3. Raymond Keith Brown, *AIDS, Cancer and the Medical Establishment* (New York: Robert Speller Publishers, 1986), p. 168.
4. Jane Kinderlehrer, "Liver May Hold the Secret of Cancer Prevention," *Prevention,* November 1972; and *Cancer Control Journal,* vol. 3, no. 1-2, 1975, pp. 49-55.
5. See, for example, William Regelson, *Journal of the American Medical Association,* vol. 243, no. 4, 25 January 1980, pp. 337-339.
6. Kedar N. Prasad, *Vitamins Against Cancer* (Rochester, VT: Healing Arts Press, 1989), pp. 27-28.
7. Peter Lechner, "Dietary Regime to Be Used in Oncological Postoperative Care," a paper presented at Graz, Austria, 21-23 June 1984.
8. Harold D. Foster, "Lifestyle Changes and the 'Spontaneous' Regression of Cancer: An Initial Computer Analysis," *International Journal of Biosocial Research,* vol. 10, no. 1, 1988, pp. 17-33, reprinted in *Healing Newsletter,* vol. 5, no. 3, 1989, available from the Gerson Institute.

Chapter 18
Kelley's Nutritional-Metabolic Therapy

1. Nicholas James Gonzalez, M.D., *One Man Alone: An Investigation of Nutrition, Cancer, and William Donald Kelley,* unpublished manuscript, 1987.
2. Robert G. Houston, *Misinforma-tion From OTA on Unconventional Cancer Treatments,* invited review for the U.S. Congress, Office of Technology Assessment (Otho, IA: People Against Cancer, 1990), p. 10.
3. Harold Ladas, "Book Review," *Cancer Victors Journal,* Summer-Fall 1988, pp. 23-24.
4. Interview in *Healthview Newsletter,* vol. 1, no. 5, 1976, pp. 4, 10.
5. For a review of these enzyme studies, see Max Wolf, M.D., and Karl Ransberger, Ph.D., *Enzyme Therapy* (Los Angeles: Regent House, 1972), pp. 135-146.
6. William Donald Kelley, *One Answer to Cancer* (Winthrop, WA: Wedgestone Press, 1974).
7. *Cancer Forum,* vol. 3, no. 5-6, 1980; and interview with the author.
8. Gonzalez, op. cit., pp. 71-72.
9. Robert W. Maver, "Nutrition and Cancer: The Gonzalez Study," *On the Risk,* vol. 7, no. 2, 1991, originally published in *Discoveries in Medicine,* Mutual Benefit Life.

Chapter 19
Hans Nieper, M.D.

1. Hans A. Nieper, *Revolution in Technology, Medicine, and Society* (Oldenburg, Germany: MIT Verlag, 1985), p. 274.
2. Hye Koo Yun with John Heinerman, *East/West Cancer Remedies for Wellness and Recovery,* unpublished manuscript (San Ysidro, CA: EastWest Wellness Center, 1990), pp. 163-164.
3. Hans Nieper, "New Developments in Gene Repair," lecture given in Phoenix, Arizona, May 1985, published in *New Horizons Newsletter,* vol. 2, no. 5-6, September 1986, available from A. Keith Brewer International Science Library.
4. Ibid. Also see Nieper (note 1), op. cit., p. 275.

5. Nieper (note 3), op. cit.
6. Nieper (note 1), op. cit., p. 278.
7. Morton Walker, D.P.M., "Medical Profile: Profile of Helmut Keller, M.D.," *raum und zeit*, vol. 2, no. 4, 1991, p. 21; and Morton Walker, "The Carnivora Cure for Cancer, AIDS, and Other Pathologies," *Townsend Letter for Doctors*, no. 95, June 1991, p. 416.
8. Walker *(Townsend Letter for Doctors)*, ibid., pp. 412–413.
9. Jacqueline Verrett and Jean Carper, *Eating May Be Hazardous to Your Health* (New York: Simon and Schuster, 1974), p. 170.

Chapter 20
Oxygen Therapies

1. Otto Warburg, *The Metabolism of Tumors* (London: Constable and Company, 1930).
2. Otto Warburg, "On the Origin of Cancer Cells," *Science*, vol. 123, 1956, pp. 309–315.
3. Michael L. Culbert, *AIDS: Hope, Hoax, and Hoopla* (Chula Vista, CA: Bradford Foundation, 1989), p. 245.
4. Gerard V. Sunnen, "Ozone in Medicine: Overview and Future Directions," *Journal of Advancement in Medicine*, vol. 1, no. 3, Fall 1988, pp. 159–174.
5. C. Tietz, "Ozontherapie als Adjuvans in der Onkologie," *Ozo-Nachrichten*, vol. 2, no. 4, 1983; and Kurt S. Zanker and Ronald Kroczek, "In Vitro Synergistic Activity of 5-Fluorouracil With Low-Dose Ozone Against a Chemoresistant Tumor Cell Line and Fresh Human Tumor Cells," *International Journal of Experimental and Clinical Chemotherapy*, vol. 36, 1990, pp. 147–154.
6. Siegfried Rilling and Renate Viebahn, *The Use of Ozone in Medicine* (New York: Haug, 1987); and J. Varro, "Die Krebsbehand-

lung mit Ozon," *Erfahr hk*, vol. 23, 1974, pp. 178–181.
7. J. Sweet et al., "Ozone Selectively Inhibits Growth of Human Cancer Cells," *Science*, vol. 209, 1980, pp. 931–933.
8. Keith H. Wells et al., "Inactivation of HIV Type 1 by Ozone In Vitro," *Blood*, vol. 78, no. 7, 1 October 1991, pp. 1882–1890.
9. Ed McCabe, *Oxygen Therapies: A New Way of Approaching Disease* (Morrisville, NY: Energy Publications, 1988), pp. 112–115.
10. Ibid., p. 119.
11. C. Borek, "Ozone Carcinogenesis In Vitro and Its Co-carcinogenesis With Radiation," *Annals of the New York Academy of Science*, vol. 534, 1988, pp. 106–110.
12. M.G. Mustafa et al., "Pulmonary Carcinogenic Effects of Ozone," *Annals of the New York Academy of Science*, vol. 534, 1988, pp. 714–723.
13. P.A. Cerutti, "Prooxidant States and Tumor Promotion," *Science*, vol. 227, no. 4685, 1985, pp. 375–381.
14. C.F. Nathan and Z.A. Cohn, "Anti Tumor Effects of Hydrogen Peroxide In Vivo," *Journal of Experimental Medicine*, vol. 154, 1981, pp. 1539–1553.
15. *Japanese Journal of Cancer Research*, vol. 77, 1986, pp. 188–194.
16. Correspondence, *Health Consciousness*, February 1989, pp. 16–17.
17. Vincent Speckhart, "Hydrogen Peroxide in Malignancy With and Without Radiation Therapy," *Proceedings of the First International Conference on Bio-Oxidative Medicine*, edited by Charles Farr (Dallas/Fort Worth: International Bio-Oxidative Medicine Foundation, 1989), pp. 35–38.
18. Robert Bradford and Michael Culbert, *Hydrogen Peroxide: The*

Misunderstood Oxidant (Chula Vista, CA: Bradford Research Institute, 1989).

19. Bradford and Culbert, "Hydrogen Peroxide," *Health Consciousness*, February 1989, pp. 28–29.

20. Charles H. Farr, "Physiological and Biochemical Responses to Intravenous Hydrogen Peroxide in Man," *Journal of Advancement in Medicine*, Summer 1988.

Chapter 21
Hyperthermia

1. Jack Tropp, "Heat, Wholeness and Health," *Cancer Victors Journal*, vol. 22, no. 2–3, Summer–Fall 1988, p. 5.

2. Haim I. Bicher et al., "Local Hyperthermia for Superficial and Moderately Deep Tumors—Factors Affecting Response," in *Consensus on Hyperthermia for the 1990s*, edited by H.I. Bicher et al. (New York: Plenum Press, 1990).

3. Z. Petrovich et al., "Regional Hyperthermia for Advanced Tumors: A Clinical Study of 353 Patients," *International Journal of Radiation: Oncology-Biology-Physics*, vol. 16, 1989, pp. 601–607.

4. K. Storm et al., "Magnetic Induction Hyperthermia: Results of a 5-Year Multi-institutional National Cooperative Trial in Advanced Cancer Patients," *Cancer*, vol. 55, 1985, pp. 2677–2687.

5. H.I. Bicher et al., "Air-cooled 300 MHz Applicators Used in a Parallel Opposed Phased System (POPAS)," *International Journal of Radiation: Oncology-Biology-Physics*, vol. 11, no. S1, 1985, p. 217.

6. Marilyn Elias, "Heat Therapy May Help Against Cancer," *USA Today*, 31 March 1986.

7. Ned B. Hornback et al., "Radiation and Microwave Therapy in the Treatment of Advanced Cancer," *Radiology*, vol. 130, 1979, pp. 459–464.

8. Ned B. Hornback et al., "Advanced Stage III-B Cancer of the Cervix: Treatment by Hyperthermia and Radiation," *Gynecologic Oncology*, vol. 23, 1986, pp. 160–167.

9. Ronald S. Scott et al., "Local Hyperthermia in Combination With Definitive Radiotherapy: Increased Tumor Clearance, Reduced Recurrence Rate in Extended Follow-up," *International Journal of Radiation: Oncology-Biology-Physics*, vol. 10, 1984, pp. 2119–2123.

10. H.I. Bicher et al., "Clinical Use of Regional Hyperthermia," in *Consensus on Hyperthermia for the 1990s*, edited by H.I. Bicher et al. (New York: Plenum Press, 1990).

11. J.S. Stehlin et al., "Heat As an Adjuvant in the Treatment of Advanced Melanoma: An Immune Stimulant," *Houston Medical Journal*, vol. 4, 1988, pp. 61–82.

12. Maryann Napoli, *Health Facts* (Woodstock, NY: Overlook Press, 1982), pp. 145–146.

13. Hornback et al. (note 8), op. cit.

14. M. Hiraoka et al., "Radiofrequency Capacitive Hyperthermia for Deep-Seated Tumors. II. Effects of Thermoradiotherapy," *Cancer*, vol. 60, 1987, pp. 128–135; and H.I. Bicher et al., "Treatment of Intrathoracic Lesions, Preliminary Results," abstract, presented at the 37th Annual Meeting of the Radiation Research Society, Seattle, Washington, 18–23 March 1989.

Chapter 22
DMSO Therapy

1. Daniel McCabe et al., "Polar Solvents in the Chemoprevention of Dimethylbenzanthracene-Induced Rat Mammary Cancer,"

Archives of Surgery, vol. 121, December 1986.
2. Stanley W. Jacob and Robert Herschler, "Pharmacology of DMSO," *Cryogiology*, vol. 23, 1986, pp. 14–27.
3. *Urology Times*, April 1987.
4. Joel Warren et al., "Potentiation of Antineoplastic Compounds by Oral Dimethyl Sulfoxide in Tumor-Bearing Rats," *Annals of the New York Academy of Science*, vol. 243, 27 January 1975.
5. P.A. Marks and R.A. Rifkind, "Erythroleukemic Differentiation," *Annual Review of Biochemistry*, vol. 47, pp. 419–448; and P.A. Marks et al., "Expression of Globin Genes During Induced Erythroleukemia Cell Differentiation," in *Cellular and Molecular Regulation of Hemoglobin Switching*, edited by G. Staniatory-annopoulos and A.W. Neinhuis (New York: Grune and Stratton, 1979), pp. 437–455.
6. D.G. Volden, E. Thorud, and O.H. Iversen, "Inhibition of Methyl-Cholanthrene-Induced Skin Carcinogenesis in Hairless Mice by Membrane-Labelizing Agent DMSO," *British Journal of Dermatology*, vol. 109 (suppl. 25), July 1983, pp. 133–136.
7. Morton Walker, *DMSO: Nature's Healer* (Garden City Park, NY: Avery Publishing Group, 1992); and Robert Gosselin, *Clinical Toxicology of Commercial Products* (Baltimore: Williams and Wilkins, 5th ed., 1984).
8. Walker, ibid.
9. Bruce Halstead, M.D., and Sylvia Youngberg, R.N., *The DMSO Handbook* (Colton, CA: Golden Quill Publishers, 1981), p. 32.
10. J.G. Cornejo and R.E. Lagos, "Dimethyl Sulfoxide Therapy as Toxicity-Reducing Agent and Potentiator of Cyclophosphamide in the Treatment of Different Types

of Cancer," *Annals of the New York Academy of Science*, vol. 243, 1975, pp. 412–420.
11. Pat McGrady, Sr., *The Persecuted Drug: The Story of DMSO* (New York: Charter Books, 1973).
12. Walker, op. cit.
13. Jonathan Collin, M.D., "DMSO: Its Chemistry and Therapeutic Applications—Part II," *Townsend Letter for Doctors*, no. 26, May 1985, p. 107.

Chapter 23
Chelation

1. Robert C. Atkins, *Dr. Atkins' Health Revolution: How Complementary Medicine Can Extend Your Life* (New York: Bantam Books, 1990), p. 208.
2. Raymond Keith Brown, *AIDS, Cancer and the Medical Establishment* (New York: Robert Speller Publishers, 1986), p. 115.
3. Elmer Cranton and Arline Brecher, *Bypassing Bypass* (Norfolk, VA: Donning Company, 1989).
4. Daniel Steinberg, "Beyond Cholesterol: Modifications of Low-Density Lipoprotein That Increase Its Atherogenicity," *New England Journal of Medicine*, vol. 320, 6 April 1989.
5. Morton Walker, *The Chelation Way: The Complete Book of Chelation Therapy* (Garden City Park, NY: Avery Publishing Group, 1990), p. 109.
6. Walter Blumer and Elmer M. Cranton, "Ninety Percent Reduction in Cancer Mortality After Chelation Therapy With EDTA," *Journal of Advancement in Medicine*, vol. 2, no. 1–2, Spring–Summer 1989, pp. 183–188.
7. Wunderlich, "The Disintegration of Retroviruses by Chelating Agents," *Archives of Virology 1982*, vol. 73, no. 21, pp. 171–183.
8. Brown, op. cit., pp. 116–117.

Chapter 24
Live-Cell Therapy

1. Philip M. Boffey, "Use of Fetal Tissue as Cure Debated," *New York Times*, 15 September 1988.
2. Wolfram W. Kuhnau, M.D., with Michael Culbert, *Live-Cell Therapy: My Life With a Medical Breakthrough* (No city, Mexico: Artes Graficas, 1983).
3. H. Lettré, *Arzneimittelforschg.*, vol. 4, no. 8, 1954, pp. 484–485; *Antibiotica und Chemotherapie*, vol. 8, 1960; and "Versuche zur Klärung der Wirksamkeit der Zellulartherapie nach Niehans," *Umschau in der Wissenschaft und Technik*, vol. 23, 1954, pp. 708 ff.
4. Michael Osband et al., "Histiocytosis-X. Demonstration of Abnormal Immunity, T-Cell Histamine H2-Receptor Deficiency, and Successful Treatment With Thymic Extract," *New England Journal of Medicine*, vol. 304, no. 3, 1981, pp. 146–153.
5. Robert Langer, "Shark Cartilage Contains Inhibitors of Tumor Angiogenesis," *Science*, 16 September 1983.
6. "Cell Therapy Suspended," *The Lancet*, vol. 2, no. 8557, 1987, p. 503.
7. U.S. Department of Health and Human Services, Public Health Service, Food and Drug Administration, "Cell Therapy," Talk Paper T84-78, 5 November 1984.

Chapter 25
Bioelectric Therapies

1. Barry Lynes, *The Cancer Cure That Worked: Fifty Years of Suppression* (Queensville, Ontario: Marcus Books, 1987, 1989), p. 61.
2. Arthur Yale, "Cancer," *Pacific Coast Journal of Homeopathy*, July 1940, cited in Barry Lynes, *The Healing of Cancer* (Queensville,

Ontario: Marcus Books, 1989), pp. 74–75.
3. Robert O. Becker, *Cross Currents: The Perils of Electropollution, the Promise of Electromedicine* (Los Angeles: Jeremy P. Tarcher, 1990), p. 156.
4. Ibid., p. 160; and interview with Robert O. Becker.
5. Ibid., p. 162.
6. Buryl Payne, *The Body Magnetic* (Santa Cruz, CA: self-published, 1988, 1990), pp. 116–154.
7. William Philpott, *Cancer Prevention and Reversal* (Choctaw, OK: Philpott Medical Services, 1990), also published in *Health Consciousness*, June 1991, pp. 37–40.

Chapter 26
Homeopathy

1. Dana Ullman, *Discovering Homeopathy* (Berkeley, CA: North Atlantic Books, 1991), p. 12.
2. Paul Callinan, "The Mechanism of Action of Homeopathic Remedies—Towards a Definitive Mode," *Journal of Complementary Medicine*, July 1985, p. 45.
3. Ullman, op. cit., p. 6.
4. K.N. Kasad, "Cancer: The Therapeutic Dilemma," *Indian Journal of Holistic Medicine*, vol. 25, no. 1, January–March 1990, p. 14.
5. Robert S. Wood, *Homeopathy: Medicine That Works!* (Pollock Pines, CA: Condor Books, 1990), pp. 217–218.
6. A.H. Grimmer, M.D., "Homeopathic Treatment of Cancer," *Journal of the American Institute of Homeopathy*, vol. 43, June 1950, pp. 121–123.
7. A.H. Grimmer, M.D., "Further Results in the Homeopathic Treatment of Cancer," *Homeopathic Recorder*, vol. 46, 1931, pp. 674–679.
8. Elizabeth Wright Hubbard, M.D., and James Stephenson, M.D., "Cancer—27 Consecutive Cases," *Journal of the American*

Institute of Homeopathy, vol. 50, September–October 1957, pp. 267–270.

9. G.W. Bradley and A. Clover, "Apparent Response of Small Cell Lung Cancer to an Extract of Mistletoe and Homeopathic Treatment," *Thorax*, vol. 44, 1989, pp. 1047–1048.

10. "Cyprus Conference: Homeopaths Report Progress vs. Cancer, AIDS," *The Choice*, vol. 15, no. 4, Fall–Winter 1989, pp. 1–7.

11. Spiro A. Diamantidis, M.D., *Homoeopathic Medicine: Theory, Methodology, Applications* (Athens, Greece: MIHRA, no date), pp. 225–226.

12. Bernard Marichal, "Immujem Therapy: Homeopathic Treatment for AIDS," lecture given at the World Research Foundation 1990 Congress, Sherman Oaks, California.

13. N. Ramayya, "Homoeopathic Treatment of Cancer in India—A Review," *The Homoeopathic Heritage*, July 1989, pp. 317–335.

14. Thomas L. Bradford, *The Logic of Figures or Comparative Results of Homoeopathic and Other Treatments* (Philadelphia: Boericke and Tafel, 1900), p. 59; and Harris L. Coulter, *Divided Legacy* (Berkeley, CA: North Atlantic Books, 1975), vol. 3, pp. 298–305.

15. J.P. Ferley et al., "A Controlled Evaluation of a Homeopathic Preparation in the Treatment of Influenza-like Syndromes," *British Journal of Clinical Pharmacology*, vol. 299, March 1989, pp. 365–366.

16. E. Davenas et al., "Human Basophil Degranulation Triggered by Very Dilute Antiserum Against AgE," *Nature*, vol. 333, 30 June 1988, pp. 816–818.

Chapter 27
Ayurveda

1. S.P. Thyagarajan, S. Subramanian, T. Thirunalasundari, P.S. Venkateswaran, and B.S. Blumberg, "Effect of Phyllanthus Amarus on Chronic Carriers of Hepatitis B Virus," *The Lancet*, 1 October 1988, pp. 764–766.

2. N.D. Joshi, M.B.B.S., M.C.P.S., "Indigenous Drug Therapy in Advanced Malignancy," paper presented at 5th Biennial Conference of Indian Association of Cancer Chemotherapists, February 1989, available from Joshi Estate, S.V. Road, Irla, Bombay 400 058, India; and see *Townsend Letter for Doctors*, vol. 93, April 1991, p. 244, and vol. 95, June 1991, pp. 449–450.

3. Hari M. Sharma, Brihaspati Dev Triguna, and Deepak Chopra, "Maharishi Ayur-Veda: Modern Insights Into Ancient Medicine," *Journal of the American Medical Association*, vol. 265, no. 20, 22–29 May 1991, pp. 2633–2637.

4. Ibid., p. 2633.

5. David Frawley, *Ayurvedic Healing: A Comprehensive Guide* (Salt Lake City, UT: Passage Press, 1989), p. 229.

6. *CRC Critical Reviews in Food Science and Nutrition*, vol. 12, June 1980, pp. 291–292; and Hye Koo Yun with John Heinerman, *East/West Cancer Remedies for Wellness and Recovery*, unpublished manuscript (San Ysidro, CA: EastWest Wellness Center, 1990), pp. 80–81.

7. "Ayurvedic Medicine—A Quackbuster View," *NCAHF Newsletter*, available from the NCAHF, Box 1276, Loma Linda, CA 92354, reprinted in *Townsend Letter for Doctors*, October 1991, p. 734.

8. Sharon Bloyd-Peshkin, "The Health-Fraud Cops: Are the Quack Busters Consumer Advocates or Medical McCarthyites?" *Vegetarian Times*, August 1991, p. 51.

9. D.W. Orme-Johnson, "Medical Care Utilization and the Tran-

scendental Meditation Program," *Psychosomatic Medicine,* vol. 49, 1988, pp. 493–507.

10. H.M. Sharma et al., "Antineoplastic Properties of Maharishi 4 Against DMBA-Induced Mammary Tumors in Rats," *Journal of Pharmacology, Biochemistry and Behavior,* vol. 35, 1990, pp. 767–773; and H. Sharma et al., "Effect of MAK (M4 and M5) on DMBA-Induced Mammary Tumors," a paper presented at the Annual Meeting of the Federation of the American Societies for Experimental Biology, Washington, D.C., 1–5 April 1990.

11. Vimal Patel et al., "Reduction of Mouse Lewis Lung Carcinoma (LLC) by M-4 Rasayana," a paper presented at the Annual Meeting of the Federation of the American Societies for Experimental Biology, Washington, D.C., March 1990.

12. Julia Arnold et al., "Chemopreventive Activity of Maharishi Amrit Kalash and Related Agents in Rat Tracheal Epithelial and Human Tumor Cells," *Proceedings of the American Association for Cancer Research,* vol. 32, 15–18 May 1991, p. 128.

13. Kedar N. Prasad et al., "Extracts of Maharishi Amrit Kalash-5, an Ayurvedic Herbal Preparation, Induces Differentiation in Neuroblastoma Cells in Culture," *Neuropharmacology,* 1991.

14. Yukie Niwa, "Variety of Oxidative Disorders Induced by Oxygen Radicals in Modern Polluted Environments and Marked Anti-Oxidant Acitivity Demonstrated in Maharishi Amrit Kalash," a paper presented at the Soviet Academy of Sciences, Moscow, 11 September 1989, and the National Institutes of Health, Bethesda, Maryland, 18 September 1989.

15. Jeremy Fields et al., "Oxygen Free Radical Scavenging Effects of an Anti-Carcinogenic Natural Product, Maharishi Amrit Kalash (MAK)," *The Pharmacologist,* vol. 32, 1990, p. 155.

16. K.N. Dileepan et al., "Priming of Splenic Lymphocytes After Ingestion of an Ayurvedic Herbal Food Supplement: Evidence for an Immunomodulatory Effect," *Biochemical Archives,* vol. 6, August 1990, pp. 267–274.

17. Craig Lambert, "The Chopra Prescriptions," *Harvard Magazine,* September–October 1989, p. 26.

Chapter 28
Chinese Medicine

1. Carl Sherman, "Folk Remedies That Really Work," *Prevention,* August 1979, p. 108.

2. Subhuti Dharmananda, *Chinese Herbal Therapies for Immune Disorders* (Portland, OR: Institute for Traditional Medicine, 1988), pp. 9–25.

3. Hong-Yen Hsu, *Treating Cancer With Chinese Herbs* (Long Beach, CA: Oriental Healing Arts Institute, 1982), p. viii.

4. Zhang Dai-zhao, *The Treatment of Cancer by Integrated Chinese-Western Medicine* (Boulder, CO: Blue Poppy Press, 1989), pp. 126–127.

5. Ibid., p. vi.

6. David Eisenberg with Thomas Lee Wright, *Encounters With Qi: Exploring Chinese Medicine* (New York: Penguin Books, 1987), p. 134.

7. Dharmananda, op. cit., p. 10; and Paul Bergner, "Botanical Medicine," *The Nutrition and Dietary Consultant,* April 1988.

8. John Heinerman, *The Treatment of Cancer With Herbs* (Orem, UT: Bi-World Publishers, 1984), p. 110.

9. Hong-Yen Hsu, op. cit.; Y.K. Hsieh, *Anti-Cancer Chinese Herbs* (Hong Kong: Hsing Hua Books, 1977); and Chinese Anti-Cancer Herb Research Center, *A Collection of Chinese Anti-Cancer Formulas* (Taichung, China: China Medical College, 1975).

10. Paul Dong and Aristide H. Esser, *Chi Gong: The Ancient Chinese Way to Health* (New York: Paragon House, 1990), p. 85.

11. Ibid., pp. 86–87.

12. Wang Chong-xing et al., in *First World Conference for Academic Exchange of Medical Qi Gong*, 1988, p. 85.

13. Roger Jahnke, "The Most Profound Medicine, Part II: Physiological Mechanisms Operating in the Human System During the Practice of Qigong and Yoga/Pranayama," *Townsend Letter for Doctors*, February–March 1991, p. 126.

14. Dong, op. cit., p. 95.

15. Ibid., p. 97.

16. Xie Huan-zhang, *The Scientific Basis of Chi Gong* (Beijing: Beijing Institute of Technology, 1985).

17. S.K. Kaneko, "Acupuncture Therapy for Leukemia," *Journal of the Japan Acupuncture and Moxibustion Association*, vol. 25, no. 2, May 1976, pp. 47–50.

18. M. Brown et al., "The Effect of Acupuncture on White Cell Counts," *American Journal of Chinese Medicine*, vol. 2, no. 4, 1974, pp. 383–398; and T. Craciun et al., "Neuro-Humoral Modification After Acupuncture," *American Journal of Acupuncture*, vol. 1, April 1973, pp. 67–70.

19. Y. Kurono et al., "Effects of Electrical Acupuncture on the Human Immune System (III)," *Journal of the Japan Society of Acupuncture*, vol. 33, no. 1, September 1983, pp. 112–117.

20. Y. Kurono, "The Influence of Acupuncture on the Immune System in the Human Body," *Journal of the Japan Acupuncture and Moxibustion Society*, vol. 29, no. 2, 1980, pp. 22–27.

21. Eisenberg and Wright, op. cit., pp. 68–77.

22. Robert Becker and Gary Selden, *The Body Electric* (New York: William Morrow, 1985), p. 236.

Chapter 29
Mind-Body Approaches

1. Dale Figtree, "Healing Cancer," *Cancer Victors Journal*, vol. 23, no. 3–4, Winter–Spring 1990, p. 21.

2. B. O'Regan, "Barriers to Novelty II," *Noetic Sciences Review*, 1989, p. 13.

3. "Patient As Healer," interview with Bernie Siegel in *Cancer and Consciousness*, edited by Barry Bryant (Boston: Sigo Press, 1990), p. 23.

4. Hal Morgenstern et al., "The Impact of a Psychosocial Support Program on Survival With Breast Cancer: The Importance of Selection Bias in Program Evaluation," *Journal of Chronic Diseases*, vol. 37, no. 4, 1984, pp. 273–282.

5. D. Spiegel et al., *The Lancet*, vol. 2, 1989, pp. 888–891.

6. Flora Johnson Skelly, "Cancer and the Mind," *American Medical News*, Part I, 10 June 1991, p. 33, and Part II, 17 June 1991, p. 22.

7. Ibid. (17 June 1991), p. 22.

8. Lawrence LeShan, *Cancer as a Turning Point* (New York: Penguin Books/Plume, 1990), p. 21.

9. Merlin Leach, "Cancer and the Mind," *Cancer Victors Journal*, vol. 23, no. 3–4, Winter–Spring 1990, p. 9.

10. "Mind Over Illness: O. Carl Simonton Looks to Life's Healing Powers," *Coping*, September–October 1987, p. 19.

11. Ibid.

12. Steven Locke and Douglas Colligan, *The Healer Within* (New York:

New American Library/Mentor, 1986), p. 191.

13. Richard Sheldon, "Cancer: An Unsolicited Gift," *The Challenge*, vol. 13, no. 3, July 1991, pp. 10–14.

14. Albert Marchetti, *Beating the Odds: Alternative Treatments That Have Worked Miracles Against Cancer* (Chicago: Contemporary Books, 1988), p. 183.

15. Daniel P. Brown and Erika Fromm, *Hypnosis and Behavioral Medicine* (Hillsdale, NJ: Lawrence Erlbaum Associates, 1987), pp. 140–141.

Conclusion

1. Robert C. Atkins, M.D., *Dr. Atkins' Health Revolution: How Complementary Medicine Can Extend Your Life* (New York: Bantam Books, 1990), pp. 324–325.

2. Barry Lynes, *The Healing of Cancer* (Queensville, Ontario: Marcus Books, 1989), p. 52.

3. *Dissent in Medicine: Nine Doctors Speak Out* (Chicago: Contemporary Books, 1985), quoted in Christopher Bird, *The Persecution and Trial of Gaston Naessens* (Tiburon, CA: H.J. Kramer, 1991), p. 243.

4. *Cancer Victors Journal*, Winter–Spring 1990.

5. Ulrich Abel, *Chemotherapy of Advanced Epithelial Cancer: A Critical Review* (Stuttgart, Germany: Hippokrates Verlag GmbH, 1990), available from People Against Cancer, P.O. Box 10, Otho, IA 50569-0010. See also "Chemo's 'Berlin Wall' Crumbles," *The Cancer Chronicles*, December 1990, pp. 4–5; and "Chemotherapy: A Dull Weapon," *Innovation*, Spring–Summer 1991 (translation of *Der Spiegel* article), available from Foundation for the Advancement of Innovative Medicine, P.O. Box 338, Kinderhook, NY 12106-0338.

6. James T. Bennett, "Charity Groups Shortchange Research," *Tampa Tribune-Times*, 9 September 1990, p. 6C.

7. Peter Barry Chowka, "The Cancer Charity Rip-Off," *East West Journal*, July 1978.

8. Lynes, op. cit., p. 51.

9. Ibid., p. 53.

10. *Cancer Scandal: The Policies and Politics of Failure*, one-hour videotape featuring Robert Houston, Patrick McGrady, Jr., and Ralph Moss, available from Patient Rights Legal Action Fund, 202 West 78th Street, Suite 3E, New York, NY 10024.

11. Lynes, op. cit., p. 61.

12. John McDougall, M.D., "The Misguided War on Cancer," *Vegetarian Times*, September 1986, pp. 12–13.

13. Vic Sussman, *The Vegetarian Alternative: A Guide to a Healthful and Humane Diet* (Emmaus, PA: Rodale Press, 1978), pp. 56–57.

Appendix A

RESOURCE GUIDE

See "Guidelines for Choosing a Therapy" on page xi for a listing of educational organizations, information centers, and referral services. See the Resources section at the end of each chapter for leads regarding each therapy.

Books

Third Opinion: An International Directory to Alternative Therapy Centers for the Treatment and Prevention of Cancer and Other Degenerative Diseases, by John Fink, Avery Publishing Group (120 Old Broadway, Garden City Park, NY 11040; 800-548-5757), revised edition, 1991.

Provides basic information on about 160 alternative and complementary therapy centers, practitioners, support groups, educational centers, and information services for the treatment and prevention of degenerative diseases, mainly cancer. It contains a concise description of each clinic's approach and method of treatment as well as contact names, addresses, and phone numbers; prices; and a large listing of relevant books. For the cancer patient seriously investigating alternative or adjunctive treatment, this book is a user-friendly, extremely helpful resource.

Gary Null's Complete Guide to Healing Your Body Naturally, by Gary Null, McGraw-Hill (1221 Avenue of the Americas, New York, NY 10020; 212-512-2000), 1988.

Informative chapters cover the following cancer therapies: Livingston, Burzynski, Burton, Issels, and Gerson. Gary Null, well-known advocate of alternative medicine, also covers heart disease, mental illness, arthritis, diabetes, nutrition, and allergies.

The Cancer Survivors and How They Did It, by Judith Glassman, Dial Press (Garden City, New York) 1983.

Inspirational survivor stories along with an in-depth look at various alternative and complementary therapies: Gerson, Kelley, Wigmore, Moerman, macrobiotics, Hoxsey, Livingston, Issels, Burton, hyperthermia, orthodox immunotherapy, and laetrile. Out of print but worth tracking down. The Cancer Control Society (see page xv for the address and phone number) sometimes has copies.

The Healing of Cancer, by Barry Lynes, Marcus Books (distributed in the United States by Vitamart, K-Mart Plaza, Route 10, Randolph, NJ 07869; 201-366-4494), 1989.

A hard-hitting exposé of the medical establishment's fifty-year history of suppressing alternative cancer therapies. American journalist Barry Lynes discusses various alternative treatments in this incisive analysis.

The Cancer Industry: Unravelling the Politics, by Ralph W. Moss, Paragon House (90 Fifth Avenue, New York, NY 10011; 212-620-2820), 1989.

A definitive analysis of the politics of the cancer establishment and its suppression of innovative ideas and alternative therapies. It includes useful cautionary chapters on surgery, radiation, and chemotherapy. The chapters on Burton, Livingston, Burzynski, hydrazine sulfate, laetrile, and so on, though written from a historical perspective, contain information of value to prospective patients.

Magazines

The Cancer Chronicles, c/o People Against Cancer, P.O. Box 10, Otho, IA 50569; 515-972-4444. Editor: Ralph Moss, Ph.D. A newsletter covering developments in the alternative field.

Cancer Victors Journal, a publication of the International Association of Cancer Victors and Friends (see page xviii for the address and phone number). Editor-in-chief: Ann Cinquina. A quarterly magazine with news, articles, and case histories.

The Challenge, a publication of the Cancer Federation, 21250 Box Springs Road, Moreno Valley, CA 92388; 714-682-7989. Editor: John Steinbacher. Research reports, case histories, and articles on alternative and complementary cancer therapies, with emphasis on immunotherapies.

The Choice: The International Newsmagazine of Metabolic Therapy and Freedom of Choice in Medicine, a publication of the Committee for Freedom of Choice in Medicine, 1180 Walnut Avenue, Chula Vista, CA 91911; 619-429-8200. Editor: Michael Culbert. News analyses and case histories, with emphasis on alternative cancer therapies.

Explore (formerly *raum & zeit*), P.O. Box 1508, Mount Vernon, WA 98273; 206-424-6034 or 800-845-7866 (for orders only). Editor: Chrystyne Jackson. Articles and book reviews on alternative medicine and physics.

Health Consciousness: An Holistic Magazine, P.O. Box 550, Oviedo, FL 32765; 407-365-6681. Editor: Roy Kupsinel, M.D. A "forum for accent in credible medicine"; often publishes articles on cancer.

Health Freedom News, a publication of the National Health Federation, 212 West Foothill Boulevard, P.O. Box 688, Monrovia, CA 91017; 818-357-2181. Articles on natural preventive medicine.

Health Victory Bulletin, a publication of the Arlin J. Brown Information Center, P.O. Box 251, Fort Belvoir, VA 22060; 703-752-9511. Articles on cancer, including question-and-answer pieces with specialists.

Innovation, a publication of the Foundation for the Advancement of Innovative Medicine, P.O. Box 338, Kinderhook, NY 12106-0338; 800-462-FAIM. Editor: Monica Miller. Published quarterly for physicians, medical professionals, and patients.

Townsend Letter for Doctors: An Informal Newsletter for Doctors Communicating to Doctors, 911 Tyler Street, Port Townsend, WA 98368-6541; 206-385-6021. Editor-in-chief: Jonathan Collin, M.D. Focuses on alternative and holistic medicine.

Appendix B

THE CANCER PATIENT'S BILL OF RIGHTS

By Patrick M. McGrady, Jr.,
Director, CANHELP, Inc.

Preamble

This Bill of Rights arises from a desperate need to improve the lot of cancer patients, whose situation differs radically from that of other sick people. Life after a cancer diagnosis can be painful and brief: a few months or a year. Most patients are diagnosed too late for surgical cure, or for effective radiation and chemotherapy. Victimized both by disease and an unfriendly system of patient care, they are desperate for real help. And they need that help today.

The system works against the patient. As billions of dollars have been exacted from taxpayers to fund a "War Against Cancer," hospital and doctors' fees have soared to astronomical levels. (A "Medicare-approved" midwestern hospital specializing in cancer treatment, for example, charges its patients over $3000 per day. It is not uncommon for a year's treatment in many hospitals—usually unsuccessful—to run into six figures.) The "war" has enriched phenomenally the health care "providers," with precious little benefit trickling down to cancer patients. Many patients have been bankrupted trying to pay for specious treatments. Still others, unwilling to impoverish their spouses and families, have declined all treatment.

Even patients with advanced, refractory disease have been deprived of the right to fight for their own lives. As ultimate control over treatment has drifted into the hands of an amorphous bureaucracy of regulators, even physicians are forbidden to exercise their professional discretion. True, some patients still have the right to choose their physicians, but fewer and fewer physicians choose to challenge the therapeutic authority emanating from the Beltway. Treatment options have dwindled drastically. More and more, cancer doctors find themselves working exclusively from obsolescent protocols—with results as grotesque as ever.

As Dr. Lucien Israel has noted, the cancer patient has far less to lose than other patients from bold attempts at salvage. Yet, instead of a right to salvage, the patient is given the dubious privilege of participating in risky, low-yield government-sponsored trials of untried agents—often mainly to test fine points of drug activity. A deadly triage begins with a selection process called randomization in which half of the patients are consigned to placebos. Not that it makes that much difference.

Maurie Markman, M.D. reports in *CA–A Cancer Journal for Clinicians,* that in a series of Phase I clinical trials coordinated by the National Cancer Institute, "the complete plus partial response rate (a 50% or greater decrease in the product of the perpendicular diameters of measurable tumor masses) was only two percent. Only two patients (0.16 percent) achieved a complete remission. . . ."

The once sacred patient-physician relationship is now compromised by a host of overseers, including well-meaning hospital tumor boards, fat and frightened pharmaceutical companies, a thoroughly confused Food & Drug Administration, greedy, withholding insurance companies, and arbitrary Medicare and health maintenance organization (HMO) regulations.

Many cancer patients never discover a real doctor along the treatment trail. They are visited by a plethora of people in white coats, all of whom have the meter running during their brief, mute visits. If a crisis arises late at night or on a Friday or over the weekend, it is often impossible to locate any physician at all. It is well and good for the state to insist that decisions regarding patient care should reside with those who are licensed to practice medicine, but too frequently the licensed practitioners are simply not there. When they are, they have been instructed to ignore their intuition and their knowledge and their skills, and conform to unbending conventional practices.

In theory, new cancer therapies are withheld from the public until proof of efficacy and safety is firmly established. Ironically, almost all of those treatments which have passed muster are so toxic that they poison and kill thousands of patients every year.

The other side of the coin is a failure by the National Cancer Institute to provide funds to test the several low-toxicity therapies that have achieved dramatic remissions among many of the most refractory cancers. Good therapies abound here and abroad, but without powerful government or pharmaceutical company sponsorship they remain underused, underexposed, unexplored, unrefined, and primitive. The home-grown treatments are pompously condemned out-of-hand as "unproven methods" or "quackery," while those from abroad are either similarly suppressed or, more often than not, just ignored. In neither case are they given a fair trial.

The pressures against fair clinical testing are substantial. In June of 1986 Congressman Guy Molinari (R-NY) (and eventually 37 other congressmen and senators) petitioned the Congressional Office of Technology Assessment, to perform a dual task. First, it was to test one of the most popular "alternative" cancer therapies, Lawrence Burton's Immune Augmentive Therapy. Second, it was asked to set forth evaluative procedures for other unorthodox cancer treatments. It took the OTA a full three years to recommend, not surprisingly, an old-fashioned (and unnecessarily cumbersome) randomized controlled trial—which effectively put aside all evidence of Burton's successes. After bitter infighting among its consultants, the OTA panel has still been unable to produce a consensus on how to evaluate alternative therapies.

Some guidelines have been relaxed. Some patients may now import unapproved prescribed medications for personal use from abroad and the government has initiated a timid "parallel track" program whereby some patients are allowed experimental treatments "off-study." Still, unconscionable delays in getting new therapies to cancer patients are the rule, not the exception.

A Canadian physician's effective total androgen blockage therapy for prostate cancer was detailed in a plethora of papers appearing in peer-review medical journals beginning in 1985. They demonstrated the clear superiority of Dr. Fernand Labrie's results in advanced cases over the traditional and relatively ineffectual castration, female hormones and radiation treatments. Dr. Labrie was finally invited to present his findings to an American Cancer Society Science Writers Seminar that same year.

Finally, four years later the *Oncologist's Clinical Update* newsletter described it in its December 1989 issue as a "newer" treatment and "the best currently available palliative therapy for men with advanced prostate cancer and can reasonably be regarded as state-of-the-art therapy." Meanwhile, advanced prostate cancer patients have been subjected to and, for the most part, are still subjected to the old inferior treatments of radical surgery, crippling radiation, and feminizing hormones.

For nearly two decades, European medical journals have described the unique remissions obtained in some of the most difficult-to-treat tumors by an extraordinarily versatile alkylating agent called ifosfamide. Finally, its pioneer developer, Dr. med. Wolfgang Scheef of Bonn, West Germany, showed in the March 1979 *Cancer Treatment Reports,* the National Cancer Institute's most prestigious journal, that the major toxicities associated with this drug could be completely alleviated with Mesna, a rescue agent. *Yet it was not till 10 years later that the Food & Drug Administration finally approved this lifesaving agent for use in the United States.* Two precious years were lost as unsophisticated (to put it kindly) FDA officials tested it for tumor-killing power and then concluded it was worthless. National Cancer Institute experts, aghast at this blunder, informed the agency that Mesna's only claimed purpose was protection of the urinary tract against the ifosfamide's side effects—which function it performed superbly.

There are literally dozens of other examples of proven valuable therapies which today are being withheld from cancer patients, either by suppression, condemnation, ignorance or neglect.

The inability of the FDA and the NCI to make available promptly useful new therapies has hurt cancer patients in many ways. The Federal government's enforcement of medical conformity has encouraged state and local bodies to follow suit and persecute medical dissidents on their own.

Many cancer patients must rely upon what a chauvinist Medicare (Medicare refuses to reimburse Americans for treatments they may only find abroad) or their HMO can provide or their insurance company will allow.

Today, the insurers increasingly are declining to reimburse patients not only for unorthodox remedies, but for the various government-sponsored experimental chemotherapy combinations. None of the commonly used polychemotherapy schemes, by the way, has ever been approved by the FDA.

National Cancer Institute data purport to show that approximately one half of cancer's victims live at least five years after diagnosis. Many experts, including the country's most respected epidemiologists, challenge this figure as grossly exaggerated. Indeed, the United States General Accounting Office in March of 1987 accused the National Cancer Institute of presenting statistics with "biases [that] can artificially inflate the actual improvement in patient survival."

The health care system itself has ridden roughshod over such basic human rights as the right to choose one's own medicine. Patients who insist on other than the orthodox recipes are compelled to serve as guinea pigs in order to obtain a last ditch chance at survival.

Randomized, double-blinded, controlled clinical trials are not necessary to identify "breakthrough" treatments. As proof of efficacy, they are entirely superfluous. Treatments which bring about statistically significant improved remissions in normally refractory, resistant tumors in small populations, deserve the most serious attention and prompt assay in larger trials. Randomized, blind trials have an important role to play in determining fine points of protocol definition later on. But should a qualified doctor ever be told that he must turn his patient population into guinea pigs if he wishes to try a new treatment method?

Promising new agents should not be used as bait to enroll desperate human beings into researchers' numbers games.

The hostage of this system is none other than the desperate, pitiful cancer patient, in whose name all the funds were voted, the wallets fattened, and the bureaucrats hired and empowered. The war against cancer failed as pathetically as our Viet Nam war failed. The dollars were channeled into fabulous profits and perquisites for the providers, but they never seemed to buy cures. The condition of the cancer patient can be improved only by substantial and drastic changes at every level of the system.

Doctors and patients need to be liberated from the medical bureaucracy's politics. When there is no curative conventional treatment, doctors should be free to try the unconventional. Innovative therapies do not always succeed on patients with advanced disease, but even when they fail, patient and physician may enjoy the soul-felt satisfaction of having given their best to the battle for life.

As a start toward improving the patient's welfare, CANHELP, Inc., a medical information and referral service, herewith proposes adoption of the following basic rights for the cancer patient.

A Bill of Rights for the Cancer Patient

1. The Right to Choose One's Own Medical Therapy

Every cancer patient shall have an inalienable right to choose any therapy, regardless of provenance, regardless of experimental status, and regardless of approval or lack of approval by any third party. The physician's principal role is that of expert medical surrogate and counselor for the patient. With informed patient consent, the physician thus should be able to prescribe any diagnostic test or treatment, which, in the physician's judgment, may prove beneficial. This should not relieve the physician of the obligation to treat the patient with competence, caution and compassion, or to provide upon request a documented therapeutic rationale. But no longer should a physician be required to restrict his or her practice to locally popular or "approved" treatments and protocols.

2. The Right to Information About One's Disease

Patients shall have the right to know as much as they care to know about their condition. Physicians shall stay in touch with their patients and inform them of their progress and answer their reasonable questions; failure to so inform them should constitute grounds for disciplinary action or for charges of fraud and malpractice. At all times, the patients' medical records shall be available to patients upon their request. Physicians shall scrupulously inform their patients about:

a. The reasons for selecting a particular treatment plan.
b. The reasons for rejecting alternatives.
c. The risks and benefits of relevant therapies.
d. The survival possibilities and probabilities with the therapy selected for them, and whether the treatment is designed as potentially curative or merely palliative.
e. Their condition at all times, and particularly whether they appear to be improving or deteriorating.
f. In the event the treatment appears ineffective, what other options may be considered.

3. The Right to Fair Treatment Evaluations

Since the cancer patient has the sole right to decide how he or she shall be treated, the Kefauver-Harris amendments to the Federal Food, Drug & Cosmetics Act of 1938 should be repealed. This ambiguous legislation has encouraged a stifling conformity and discouraged innovation. Toxic and ineffectual treatments from powerful pharmaceutical companies have been approved, while nontoxic, effective treatments from independent investigators have been spurned. Time-wasting, inefficient, and extravagant testing procedures do not protect the public; they hurt the public by keeping possibly helpful therapies from them and needlessly increasing morbidity and mortality rates. The current drug testing program should be scrapped and replaced by one more consonant with real patient needs. Powers usurped by the Food & Drug Administration's should be returned to the physician and the patient, whence they were expropriated. This agency's proper function in oncology and hematology should be to collect and disseminate accurate information about all cancer treatments. It should, further, actively assist scientists and physicians of modest means to assess and develop their therapies. Although the FDA denies that it dictates to physicians what they may and may not do for their patients, its well-documented history of oppressing innovative researcher-physicians belies its piety. This oppression should cease in all of its subtle and nonsubtle forms.

4. The Right to Humane and Efficient Medical Care

Patients shall have the right not to be forced to enroll in randomized experimental trials in order to obtain new therapeutic agents. This would prevent scarce new treatments from being abused as a means of blackmailing patients. Any physician using such experimental options, however, shall be obliged to report results promptly and comprehensively. While government agencies may recommend protocols, any physician will have the right to modify those protocols for the patient's benefit. The present clinical therapy testing system has turned out to be a nightmare of pseudoscientific arrogance. It is impossible to pinpoint a single treatment breakthrough issuing from this system which could not have been produced from a more humane and efficient testing procedure. Current procedures are predicated on a mistake and a sin. The mistake lies in the false assumption that the randomized, blind-control design alone produces significant scientific results. The sin lies in treating human beings as laboratory animals. In addition to informing their patients of probable results and side effects from such experiments, participating physicians should disclose any conceivable conflict-of-interest, including and particularly, any compensation they or their sponsors or institutions may receive for enrolling patients in these trials. Far too many patients have been induced to participate in questionable clinical experiments wherein the sole goal has been to evaluate drug activity without any compensatory benefit for the patient. Actual patient benefits stemming from such participation have been practically nil. It is high time to expose the sham of the experimental trial game.

5. The Right to Comprehensive Insurance Coverage

Third party insurance carriers, including Medicare and HMO plans, shall reimburse cancer patients for any reasonably priced cancer therapies— be they conventional, experimental, alternative or complementary therapies—

when prescribed by licensed treating physicians. Criteria of treatment propriety shall be the province exclusively of patient and physician, not the insurer or any government agency or any advocacy group. The decision to choose a cancer therapy is one no patient can afford to take lightly or capriciously. Cancer patients pay with their lives for an erroneous selection, and thus they take most solemnly their decision. The right of the patient to choose his or her own treatment is the cornerstone of civilized cancer care.

6. The Right to Have One's Physician Held Free From Inappropriate Civil Lawsuits

The patient's right to humane treatment depends upon the physician's right to be free to treat the patient conscientiously, without harassment, without relentless second-guessing by third parties, and without the burden of having to parry malicious and nuisance lawsuits. Litigation is a poor way to solve patient care-related problems, albeit occasionally the only way. Unfortunately, the resort to litigation has not succeeded in eliminating the impaired or venal physician, but it has increased health care costs unconscionably, shrunk the supply of capable practitioners in high-risk categories, and encouraged cynicism and mistrust between patient and physician. Legislation should be enacted to protect the physician and hospitals from frivolous legal action. Greedy attorneys, thoughtless and ungrateful patients, sentimental juries and reckless judges have contributed to the destruction of the intimate bond between physician and patient. Mischance and accidents must not be interpreted as malice, nor so punished. This chilling, addictive American litigiousness effectively discourages physicians from treating patients by their best lights. It creates an irresistible temptation to work instead from a fatuous cookbook and overlook possibilities for innovative, and successful healing.

7. The Right of the Public to an Open, Universal Tumor Registry

Cancer should be a legally reportable disease. Physicians should be obliged to monitor the progress of their cancer patients as long as possible and shall submit regular reports to a universal tumor registry. This will provide a deeper, more accurate view of cancer epidemiology and clarify which treatments work or do not work. Without such a universal registry, treatment validity will remain as it is now: a matter of guesswork, distortion, propaganda, and notoriously subject to political manipulation. The public's access to these data should be unrestricted, save for narrow safeguards protecting the personal identities of individual persons.

8. The Right to Strict Observance by the United States Government of the 1964 Declaration of Helsinki Recommendations Guiding Doctors in Clinical Research

Patients participating in clinical research have the right to know that they alone must be the primary benefactors of trials, and not serve merely as guinea pigs. The Helsinki Declaration to which this country is signatory stipulates that, among other things "the doctor must be free to use a new therapeutic measure, if in his judgment it offers hope of saving life, reestablishing health or alleviating suffering" and "The doctor can combine clinical research with professional care . . . only to the extent that clinical research is justified by its therapeutic value for the patient." Violations of the Helsinki Declaration's protections against patient abuse shall constitute grounds for the imposition of disciplinary sanctions and provide a cause of action for civil lawsuits.

Appendix C

THE HEALTHCARE RIGHTS AMENDMENT

The proposed Healthcare Rights Amendment to the United States Constitution gathered nearly 100,000 signatures before its originator, the Coalition for Alternatives in Nutrition and Healthcare (CANAH), ceased to exist. Benjamin Rush, M.D., a signer of the Declaration of Independence and famous Revolutionary War physician, insisted that the Constitution should make special provisions for medical freedom of choice—otherwise, he predicted, an "undercover dictatorship" would dictate medical practices and procedures in this country. Medical freedom of choice lost out and was not enumerated in the Bill of Rights.

The modern Healthcare Rights Amendment will be revived as soon as a member of Congress has the integrity to sponsor it. People who support this concept should write to their local representatives in Congress (House of Representatives, Washington, DC 20515, and Senate Office Building, Washington, DC 20510) expressing their desire for freedom of choice in health care and nutrition. Ask your congressperson to introduce and work for a health-care rights amendment that would spell out the constitutional right to freedom of choice in medicine.

Catherine J. Frompovich, former president of CANAH, writes:

> Vested interest groups, certain individuals and trade associations, the American Medical Association in particular, have launched legal procedures against medical doctors who employ in their practice such modalities as natural nutrition, chelation therapy, vitamin/mineral supplementation and other means commonly referred to as alternate healthcare modalities which may not be in agreement with orthodox medicine. Practitioner and patient alike, have been brought

up before the bars of justice and peer review with heretofore unknown medical inquisition-like techniques. WE THE PEOPLE believe this is unconstitutional, and therefore propose this amendment.

WE THE PEOPLE want to bring to the attention of the Congress of the United States, the serious problems which we feel exist in our country with regard to the right to and freedom of choice in self-determination and healthcare.

WE THE PEOPLE believe the time has come for everyone to act responsibly with regard to the right to self-determination in healthcare. We believe no one, and in particular the government itself, should deny and/or abrogate one's personal and God-given right to self-determination in healthcare.

WE THE PEOPLE want the right to legally be treated and seek the professional counsel of any and all alternate healthcare professionals at any time for ourselves, our children and our posterity.

WE THE PEOPLE believe there is no other way to guarantee this unalienable right and dignity of self-determination in healthcare than by establishing it within the framework of the Constitution of the United States of America.

WE THE PEOPLE request that all members of Congress introduce legislation to effectuate the passing of Amendment XXVII the Healthcare Rights Amendment.

The Healthcare Rights Amendment

Photocopy, sign, and send to:

Senator _____
U.S. Senate
Washington, DC 20510

Dear Senator _____ :

Please introduce legislation to effectuate the following amendment to the U.S. Constitution: *Amendment XXVII, the Healthcare Rights Amendment.*

Section 1. The Congress shall make no law which restricts any individual's right to choose and to practice the type of healthcare they shall elect for themselves or their children for the prevention or treatment of any disease, injury, illness or ailment of the body or the mind.

Section 2. The Congress shall have the power to enforce, by appropriate legislation, the provisions of this article.

Section 3. This amendment shall take effect immediately after the date of ratification.

Thank you for working to guarantee my constitutional rights to freedom of choice in healthcare and the right to self-determination in healthcare.

Name _____

Address_____

_____

Interested organizations or persons can contact Catherine J. Frompovich, Ph.D., Government Relations Specialist, P.O. Box 399, Richlandtown, PA 18955; 215-346-8461.

Appendix D

IMPORTATION OF UNAPPROVED DRUGS FOR PERSONAL USE

For many years, the FDA has had guidelines that allow district offices to exercise discretion when determining whether or not to allow entry, for personal use only, of drugs sold abroad but not approved in the United States. When permission is granted, the petitioner may import just enough of the drug for up to three months' personal use. Several unapproved drugs that some consider of therapeutic benefit for AIDS and AIDS-related conditions have thus been allowed entry into the country.

People usually bring such products into the country in their baggage when they return from abroad. These drugs may also be imported by mail. The FDA's policy on mail importation as of December 11, 1989, is that if there is no evidence of unreasonable risk, fraud, or promotion, permissive discretion may be applied and the product mailed providing:

- The product was purchased for personal use.
- The product is not for commercial distribution, and the amount of the product is not excessive (that is, there is just enough for up to three months' use).
- The intended use of the product is appropriately identified.
- The patient seeking to import the product affirms in writing that it is for his or her own use and provides the name and address of the licensed physician in the United States who is responsible for directing the treatment with the product.

If the imported product is considered fraudulent or dangerous, or if it is promoted for use in the United States despite a lack of approval, the FDA issues "import alerts." Up to July 27, 1988, there were forty import alerts restricting entry of medical products considered fraudulent or unsafe. These restricted products included laetrile, Immuno-Augmentative Therapy agents, and products promoted by Dr. Hans Nieper of West Germany. On January 27, 1992, the FDA issued Import Alert Number 66-57: "Automatic Detention of Foreign Manufactured Unapproved Prescription Drugs Promoted to Individuals in the U.S." This alert lists some firms that have products on automatic detention because of promotional activities.

The latest information on the FDA's policy on importing drugs can be obtained from local FDA offices or by writing to:

United States Department of Health and Human Services
Public Health Service
Food and Drug Administration (HFI-35)
5600 Fishers Lane
Rockville, MD 20857

INDEX